Bernhard Hadolt, Andrea Stöckl (eds.)
Hope and Uncertainty in Health and Medicine



**Health, Communication and Society** | Volume 5

**Bernhard Hadolt** (PhD) is a social anthropologist with a specialisation in medical anthropology. He is a senior lecturer and director of studies at the Department of Social and Cultural Anthropology at the University of Vienna.
**Andrea Stöckl** (PhD) is a medical anthropologist and practising psychotherapist, working in Innsbruck, Austria. She has been a lecturer at the School of Medicine, Health Policy, and Practices at the University of East Anglia, UK, until 2021.

Bernhard Hadolt, Andrea Stöckl (eds.)

# Hope and Uncertainty in Health and Medicine

## Imagining the Pragmatics of Medical Potential

[transcript]

**Bibliographic information published by the Deutsche Nationalbibliothek**
The Deutsche Nationalbibliothek lists this publication in the Deutsche Nationalbibliografie; detailed bibliographic data are available in the Internet at https://dnb.dnb.de/



**First published in 2024 by transcript Verlag, Bielefeld**


Cover layout: Maria Arndt, Bielefeld
Cover illustration: Bernhard Hadolt
Printed by: Majuskel Medienproduktion GmbH, Wetzlar
https://doi.org/10.14361/9783839467626
Print-ISBN: 978-3-8376-6762-2
PDF-ISBN: 978-3-8394-6762-6
ISSN of series: 2940-1828
eISSN of series: 2940-1836

Printed on permanent acid-free text paper.

# Contents

# Introduction
## Hope and Uncertainty in Health and Medicine

*Bernhard Hadolt and Andrea Stöckl*

This edited volume originates from the *XI Medical Anthropology at Home (MAAH) Conference* "Transfigurations of Uncertainty in Health and Medicine," held at the University of Vienna and the Schüttkasten Geras, Austria, in October 2021.[1] Most chapters assembled here have been discussed in a draft version at this four-day working conference. True to the tradition of MAAH conferences, the conference was held at a pleasant and somewhat remote venue, providing an ideal setting for intense scholarly work and collaboration. This event marked a significant moment, as it was the first in-person international academic gathering for most participants after the disruptions caused by the COVID-19 pandemic, due to which it had to be postponed twice. The palpable joy and relief of being able to meet and collaborate face-to-face set the tone for the conference. Initially centred around the theme of transfigurations of uncertainty, the communal rejuvenation and scholarly exchange inspired the idea for this volume, bringing the theme of hope into a more prominent position.

In our interconnected and polycentric world, certainty and uncertainty of knowledge are central to how health and medicine are organised, experienced, and practised. Despite the rapidly growing extension of evidence-based knowledge, this very knowledge, its reliability, validity, and relevance, has become contested. Sometimes populism, scepticism, or plain hostility towards science, and "alternative facts" and "fake news" replace informed debates. This crisis of knowledge-informed practices becomes particularly relevant in contexts of suffering, illness, and dying when the viability and well-being of oneself and those close to us are at stake. In these moments, traditional ways of coping are called into question. As medical

1 We, the conference organisers, would like to thank the University of Vienna for its financial and organisational support for both the conference and this publication, and Clemens Schmid for his valuable assistance in organising the conference and providing technical support. We would also like to express our gratitude to the staff at transcript, especially Dagmar Buchwald and Katharina Kotschurin, for their dedicated and patient support with this publication.

anthropologists have already long ago emphasised, the pursuit of certainty, but also the value of uncertainty has been a defining feature in most medical practices, as Van der Geest demonstrates in his contribution to this volume. This is the case especially for diagnosis and subsequent treatment options (e.g., Jenkins et al. 2005; Lupton 1995; Nissen and Risør 2018; Street 2014; Van Dongen 1998; Whyte 1997). In this modality, this quest and the uncertainty that arises are inherent in medical practice per se but also result from the interconnectedness of diverse heterogeneous social domains and processes. These are linked to factors such as neoliberalism, the leaping pace of technological innovation, and shifting political alliances, to count a few (Andersen, this volume).

As an analytical tool, uncertainty can be conceptualised as a genuine epistemological crisis in current medical practice and an ontological state for patients and practitioners immersed in the above-described nexus. What are the key modes of current uncertainties in health and medicine, and how do they emerge? How do they shape and yield medical practices, discourses, and environments? How can we make sense of the dynamic interconnectivity that links medicine with many other societal domains, such as policymaking, public administration, scientific research, the private profit-making sector, humanitarian work, the media, religion, or law? In which ways are they generating forms of uncertainty? How can we comprehend health-related phenomena and the implicated uncertainties as they manifest and change over time—sometimes incrementally, sometimes abruptly—in different practices, configurations, and atmospheres? Finally, how can we make sense of the apprehensions, concerns, hopes, imagined futures, and feelings of the people who affect and are affected by such processes as they constitute themselves in their specific life-world? These questions informed our conference in essential ways.

In health and medicine, imagining what the future holds is essential in propelling people into action. This is true not only at the level of individuals who envision and carry out everyday activities and long-term plans but also for institutional practices framed by and unfolding within socio-political ecologies and transfigurations (Adams et al. 2009; Kehr et al. 2019; Mattes et al. 2020; Taussig et al. 2013). Hope and uncertainty, as key affective and knowledge-related modalities of such imaginations, assume meanings in policing and managing health, illness, and wellbeing (Novas 2006; Chattoo, this volume). Alongside "risk talk," medical practice has always been underpinned by a discourse on hope and the potentiality for a better future (Fainzang 2017; Good et al. 1990; Konrad 2005; Mattingly 2010). The proclaimed medical revolutions, such as the definite cancer cure, have characterised medical popular discourse and imagination ever since the significant technological revolutions of the 19th and 20th centuries. Contemporary versions of such discourses focus on the usages of synthetic biology, gene editing, and Big Data and artificial intelligence (Kirksey 2021). The digitalisation of medicine and patients' health care data has informed public debates for the last twenty years. They gained new momentum with the hype around powerful artificial intelligence tools like ChatGPT in 2023 (Ruckenstein and Schüll 2017; see also Heitger, this volume). Public health officials often employ a discourse of the "technical fix" of medical problems (Layne 2000) and of prevention and risk to tame uncertainty by framing questions of factuality and potentiality in terms of probability (Stöckl 2010; Taussig et al. 2013; Modelhart, this volume). In doing so, they contribute to a general climate of uncertainty, for example, in debates about controlling epidemics and pandemics. This approach is increasingly politicised, particularly concerning the future impact of climate change on health and illness and what is referred to as planetary health (Singer et al. 2022; Baer and Singer 2023).

When examining medical technologies, infrastructures, and materialities, the technological advances of diagnostic and therapeutic medical procedures and the—expected and unexpected—field of action that they afford have both facilitated and impeded innovation (Hogle 2005; Lock 2013; Mattes 2019; Reinsch, this volume). This is partly due to the pace at which bureaucracy and the specific governance of its application often lag. In the UK, for instance, policymakers allow for the innovative use of ultrasound in the private sector for keepsake purposes but prohibit its portable use for diagnostics in general practitioner surgeries (Smajdor and Stöckl 2018). The increasing need for individual data protection has significantly augmented bureaucratic burdens on researchers and medical practitioners, leading to new professional roles such as data managers and artificial intelligence specialists. These emerging professions deal with the spaces of uncertainty that Big Data and its sophisticated processing produce (Hunt et al. 2017). Technologically intensive medical procedures, such as remote surgery, alter the dynamics between medical practitioners and patients as well as between different generations of practitioners. Body parts and substances are being further decontextualized from real humans and re-contextualised in new ways than ever in medical history (Landecker 2000; Waldby and Mitchell 2006; Hadolt, this volume). Tablet computers, mobile phones, and various software applications are increasingly used in settings such as psychotherapy (Stöckl, this volume). In rural areas of the Global South, medical information, such as ultrasound images, is transmitted to specialised medical centres for diagnostic purposes, creating an impression of diagnostic certainty (Hunt et al. 2017; Lupton 2018; Oudshoorn 2011). While these technologies offer an opportunity for improved diagnosis, they also contribute to the lack of funding for rural areas. The relationship between the Global South and the Global North affects how medical products and services are produced and distributed and how ideas, materials, and people travel. This relationship also shapes research practices, including clinical trials, stem cell research, and their associated ethical dilemmas (Abdalla 2018; Cohen 2005; Müller-Rockstroh 2012; Sunder Rajan 2007).

The dual nature of uncertainty and hope is also evident in moral quandaries and health policing. Ethical and moral dilemmas in medicine and medical research practice have contributed to the development of new legal practices in some countries but not in others, e.g., fostering medical tourism within and beyond the EU due to these disparities (e.g., De Looze 2016; Inhorn 2003; Petryna et al. 2006; Wailoo et al. 2010). The commodification of health, particularly in the case of personalized medical devices such as self-tracking wearables and ultrasound keepsakes, has furthered this trend. They introduce new means of quantifying and economizing health and healthcare, including changes in health insurance regimes (Farrington and Lynch 2018; Heitger, this volume). The advent of gene editing raises moral questions about accessibility and equity in its benefits (Kirksey 2021). Biorepositories, while helping to identify trends in population health, often oversimplify individuals into mere data points removed from their diverse life contexts. At the public health level, various modes of moralities and new alliances, such as those between NGOs and large corporations, e.g., in vaccination policies funded by big businesses, are observed (Graham 2016). Unregulated technologies generate vast amounts of data, which could potentially be used to shape public health policies in ways that might favour stakeholders' interests over the public good. There is a widespread demand for certainty from the public, medical practitioners, researchers, and companies, a demand that policymakers, legal courts, and public health, with their discourse on probability, often struggle to fulfill.

The role of affectivities and social atmospheres must also be addressed when examining hope and uncertainty in health and medicine. Emotions, affects, and feelings not only play a part in how individuals make decisions about their care for themselves and others (Hadolt 2018; Démolis, Buclin and Foley, this volume; Hsu, this volume) but also significantly impact organisational practices and policy making in public health (Martin 2007; Novas 2006; Fortin and Lessard, this volume; Risør and Nissen, this volume). As uncertainties proliferate, so do anxieties. Policymakers often rely on psychological concepts such as resilience and coping strategies rather than addressing anxieties. This fosters a trend toward expecting populations to be more resilient, particularly in facing health challenges related to aging, lifestyle choices, and climate change. The emphasis on self-optimization and individual responsibility in policymaking contributes to new subjectivities of health and illness, often creating a misleading sense of certainty based on quantifiable data (Rose 2007). At the individual level, people frequently cope with these uncertainties and responsibilities by turning to conspiracy theories and misinformation, such as the unfounded belief about vaccinations and refugees being responsible for spreading diseases (Drążkiewicz 2023).

This volume is organised into four parts: (1) *Pragmatics of hope and uncertainty* explores the broader conceptual and moral aspects of uncertainty and hope in healthcare, challenging traditional medical reasoning and underscoring the value of embracing ambiguity in medical ethics and decision-making. (2) *The techno-sphere* investigates the role of emerging technologies in medical and health-related practices and identities, examining the intertwining of medical uncertainty and potential implicated in medical advancements in self-knowing, therapeutic, and diagnostic decision-making, and novel understandings of bodily processes. (3) *Health management* analyses the adaptation of health policies and practices in response to technological and socio-material shifts, addressing issues like antimicrobial resistance, polypharmacy, and the development of tele-mental health. (4) Finally, the part on *Individual and socially distributed emotions* focuses on the affective and social dimensions within health contexts, discussing the interplay of affectivity and sociality in negotiations about medical diagnosis, the experience of (non)recovery in chronic conditions, and socio-material practices surrounding fermented foods and their health benefits.

## Pragmatics of hope and uncertainty

We enter the discourse with a section on pragmatics of hope and uncertainty. This section explores the broader conceptual and moral implications of uncertainty in meaning-making in health and medicine, opening the space for a nuanced balance between embracing uncertainty and navigating ethical responsibilities in complex medical scenarios.

Sjaak van der Geest invites us to ponder whether uncertainty might also be a good thing and whether we should embrace it rather than try to eliminate it. He takes us on a journey through debates from philosophy to moral and spiritual guidance to art and psychology, showing that the importance of accepting uncertainty is increasingly debated as a standpoint. There is even "wisdom" and "courage"' to be found in not knowing, and "agnosticism" is gaining acknowledgment as the only "rational" position, not just in religious contexts. He reflects upon debates in anthropology, and here especially in medical anthropology, with the unease to conceptualize the human person as a rational being or as a machine and argues that rationality became rationalization in that we do things and produce a reason afterwards. In his deliberation on the embrace of uncertainty, Van der Geest also reminds us that being able to do so might be a privilege that not all social actors can embrace, e.g., doctors who must decide to treat someone regardless of whether the intervention might work or not. Yet, he concludes, there is growing recognition that uncertainty could be seen as a superior way of knowing and, contrary to what we might believe, is not a "destroyer of hope."

Sylvie Fortin and Sabrina Lessard follow this introduction to the theme by analysing fieldwork carried out in Paris and Montreal in paediatric intensive care and haematology-oncology units as well as in geriatric hospital wards and long-term care facilities. They explore how the evolving landscape of medical and pharmaceutical advancements blurs the lines between disease-directed and palliative care, especially as formerly fatal illnesses become chronic. This transformation alters the therapeutic project in cases of life-limiting illnesses or critical conditions. Physicians are sometimes inclined towards a palliative approach, providing active treatments that prolong life, whether briefly or for an extended period, while prioritizing patient comfort. Alternatively, the promise of scientific research and innovation can inspire a more proactive medical approach, fuelling a cycle of hope and trust. Fortin and Lessard draw our attention to issues of timeliness: when biomedicine is seen as supporting life, a trade-off between enduring never-ending treatments now for potentially better times ahead becomes apparent. They show how doctors and other healthcare providers grapple with this balance between immediate quality of life and life extension, challenging traditional notions of care and ethical responsibilities. In settings characterised by uncertainty, hope, and trust, the moral roles of doctors and other healthcare providers as caregivers are complex, sustaining action, even in the face of the likelihood of death.

## The techno-sphere

The second part of the collection deals with the increasing impact of the techno-sphere on our understanding of what it means to be human or, indeed, to become a human being. It investigates how emerging (and old) health practices and technologies, including self-tracking and novel medical treatments, are reshaping medical and health-related practices both inside and outside hospital settings, presenting both challenges and opportunities for shifting policies, comprehension, and ways of dealing with health problems.

Anna Heitger starts the discussion with a chapter that focuses on the practice of self-tracking in health and fitness. Drawing on ethnographic research conducted between 2017 and 2019 with users of self-tracking technologies and self-tracking start-ups in Vienna and Berlin, she explores how self-tracking as a practice and entrepreneurship intersects with the broader themes of health management, the role of technology in personal wellbeing, and the quest for deeper self-knowledge through data. Heitger argues that self-tracking practices, which lie at the fringes of medical expertise, challenge the traditional boundaries between medical and non-medical practices. They foster a new way of "doing health" by quantifying activities, bodily states, and processes, making health a continuous individual responsibility. It transforms health from being a state to an ongoing practice in which users navigate their lives and well-being as informed, responsible citizen and consumers. The self-tracked body, constantly objectified in its quantifiable aspects e.g., water intake, heart rate, and sleep pattern, becomes the site of both concern and doing health, where users attempt to take charge of their health-related behaviour. While the past appears as fixed, represented by the recorded data that can be accessed at any time, the potential for change lies in the openness of the very present and the ontological uncertainty of the body's future state, opening possible pathways to better future wellbeing and thus creating a sense of hope in a broad, more general way. Heitger concludes that self-tracking technologies and their mobilisation in "doing health" can be interpreted as part of an increasing individualization, responsibilisation, and economization of health in general.

In her ethnography, based on fieldwork carried out between 2017 and 2019, Sangeeta Chattoo takes us to another continent, namely India. She delves into the experiences of patients and their carers dealing with thalassemia, a severe, potentially life-threatening blood disorder, and their decision-making regarding the use of thalidomide, a controversial treatment within clinical literature and practice. Her chapter highlights the complexities and uncertainties inherent in choosing this novel therapy within the broader context of a "political economy of hope and caring," challenging conventional understandings of medical evidence. The ongoing debate about thalidomide's safety and effectiveness in treating thalassemia highlights the intricate hierarchy in clinical practice that determines how evidence is used to justify medical improvisation and change. Chattoo aims to understand the motivations and therapeutic paths of those seeking new treatments amidst uncertainty and financial burden. The analysis is framed theoretically around the concepts of potentiality and precarity. It sheds light on the importance of the context in which the material reality of the disease and the risks, uncertainties, and hopes associated with new treatments unfold over time. This exploration into uncharted therapeutic terrain blurs the lines between treatment and cure, shifting the focus to the everyday, often mundane aspects of ongoing care. This perspective challenges us to consider the "ordinary, chronic and cruddy" nature of care in the face of chronic illness. With her contribution, Chattoo also contributes to an understanding of how novel therapies create new perspectives on timeliness.

Stefan Reinsch's chapter further explores how novel technologies are changing the perception and implementation of medical interventions in clinical practice. Based on his ethnographic studies with German women, Reinsch describes how since 2012 pregnant women in Germany have been able to opt for non-invasive prenatal testing (NIPT) for inherited genetic conditions. This test, which only requires a blood sample from the mother, presents a safer alternative to amniocentesis, which carries a risk of inducing miscarriage. He argues that in societies driven by neoliberal and techno-scientific values, the "elimination of risk" and the "promise of knowledge" are powerful cultural narratives. Using two detailed case studies of women's involvement in NIPT, Reinsch examines how the introduction of NIPT affects the way prenatal genetic diagnostics are perceived and utilized. He notes that while NIPT aids in normalizing prenatal genetic testing, it also brings with it new uncertainties, particularly regarding potential disability and its impact on family dynamics. He argues that women are not only succumbing to technology; rather, some use NIPT pragmatically as a means of gaining knowledge, viewing it as a tool in the logic of testing and preventing disability. Conversely, other women decide against NIPT, wary of its implicit demands and obligations. Instead, in an alternative but complementary logic of caring, they prioritize the embodied and experiential knowledge they gain from the natural course of pregnancy and their developing bond with their unborn child. Reinsch's work thus illuminates the nuanced ways women navigate the evolving landscape of prenatal technology, balancing the promises of scientific advancement with personal beliefs and values.

Bernhard Hadolt's contribution, the last in this part of the book, also deals with reproduction. Drawing on ethnographic fieldwork in Austrian fertility clinics, Hadolt explores the complex interplay of hope, uncertainty, and temporality that defines In-vitro fertilization (IVF) as social practice in important ways. In following IVF users through the dramatic ups and downs of their quest for a baby, he highlights the situated and intentional nature of IVF users' experiences, underscoring their essentially pragmatic stance and the pivotal role of hope as a driving force in navigating the uncertainties and challenges of the treatment process. This hope, however, is not unbridled but is carefully modulated to balance the desire for a successful outcome with the risk of potential failure. The author argues that hope, in its relationally distributed form, is an integral part of the social practice of IVF, organizing the actions and decisions of those involved and sustaining IVF treatment. In this regard, Hadolt points to the unique temporal dynamics of IVF, where the journey towards pregnancy is marked by distinct phases, each with its own emotional and practical challenges. The cumulative nature of IVF, where each step must be successfully mastered to maintain the possibility of pregnancy, creates a temporal structure characterized by immediate, short-term goals juxtaposed with the overarching goal of achieving pregnancy and parenthood. Hope resides in uncertainty about *what is*, *what will happen*, and *how best to deal with it*. Using knowledge as a tool to manage uncertainty can paradoxically increase it, as is evident in the final phase of IVF treatment, embryo transfer, and implantation. Detailed medical knowledge about what can "go wrong," inconclusive pregnancy test results and certain bodily feelings may lead to situations where being pregnant is not simply binary but can be understood in gradations as being "a little bit pregnant" that requires work to make the pregnancy "real."

## Health management

In the third part of the book, we look at how health management and governance deal with the challenges brought about by the developments in the technosphere. This section delves into how these developments, along with broader socio-material issues related to ways of living and the pandemic crisis, reshape practices, policies, and perceptions within the health sector.

We first follow Rikke Sand Andersen's analysis of the rise in solo living as a global trend and its repercussions on the politics of care. Andersen explains that in Denmark, where she conducted extensive ethnographic fieldwork on the topic from 2020 to 2021, solo living is supported by an egalitarian approach to caregiving and is considered a conventional lifestyle choice. However, in many societies, solo living intersects with the ongoing normalization of family and private homes as primary settings for caregiving. Drawing on critical feminist care theory and discussions of vulnerability to understand human subjectivity, Andersen embarks on a journey to uncover the evolving landscape of the social organization of care work in Denmark. Furthermore, she explores the vulnerabilities and social dynamics that become apparent within these emerging contexts. Through a careful examination of two cases of two cancer patients living alone, Andersen investigates how individuals living alone navigate their daily lives within the realm of cancer care. Reminding us that vulnerability is not an inherently personal trait but is instead shaped by structures of power, privilege, and oppression, she identifies two key types of what she considers emerging vulnerabilities: relational vulnerabilities, which refer to the growing social and moral tensions that surface when seeking access to care, and vulnerabilities to the self, which Andersen defines as "the loss of abilities to engage in world-making activities." She argues that care politics itself is the "architect" of human vulnerabilities, producing both relational vulnerabilities and vulnerabilities to the self. The current interplay between caregiving and embodied existence in Denmark makes solo living in severe disease possible yet extraordinarily challenging.

Antonia Modelhart's chapter looks at antimicrobial resistance (AMR) in German hospitals and the threat that AMR poses to both global health and the individual health of patients and those working there. Based on interviews Modelhart conducted with hospital hygiene specialists who work in and outside of hospitals in Hamburg, Germany (mainly nurses and physicians, but also researchers in academia and patients), she describes how these professionals understand and deal with the increasing challenge of bacterial resistance and the decreasing effectiveness of antibiotics. Using the analytical lens of microbiopolitics and the intricate dynamics and negotiations involved in managing microbial life, she examines the vibrant interactions between humans and microbes as they manifest in hospital hygiene policies and practices employed by hospital hygiene management teams. Given the fundamental uncertainty concerning bacterial composition, patient resilience, the case-specific effectiveness of antimicrobial therapy, and the uncertain future of antibiotics in general, these practices, among which risk-adapted screening of patients is critical, are characterised by a careful case-by-case and day-to-day assessment and governance of microbe-human interactions that consider the specific "microbiologies" at a place as they evolve. Modelhart argues that this approach to dealing with the risk of antimicrobial resistance echoes post-Pasteurian biopolitical thinking. This promotes a more nuanced understanding of microbial life that acknowledges the ubiquitous and often beneficial presence of microbes and their complex relationships with human health. It promotes hygiene strategies that aim at managing bacterial compositions and preventing infection rather than eliminating colonization.

In the next chapter in this section, Rachel Démolis, Thierry Buclin, and Rose-Anna Foley discuss the complex and often overlooked issue of polypharmacy among older people in Switzerland. The authors shed light on the paradoxical reality faced by these polymedicated elderly patients, who find themselves in a dilemma between the need to take multiple drugs for chronic conditions and the awareness of potential adverse effects and insufficient research on drug interactions. The authors explore the subjective experiences of these elderly patients and how they give meaning to these experiences. They describe how they find strategies in dealing with iatrogenic risk and related uncertainty and perceive and interpret their illnesses and healthcare practices. This exploration is framed within a larger socio-cultural context, considering the impact of economic, institutional, cultural, and political factors on the patients' narratives and healthcare experiences. Démolis, Buclin, and Foley argue for an approach to understanding such health dynamics that moves beyond the conventional analysis of macro-social dimensions that determine health behaviour. Instead, they emphasise a more fluid and interactive process in which the roles of health professionals, health insurance policies, and patients are not static; they evolve concerning patients' "lay vigilance" over their polypharmacy, highlighting the importance of considering patient agency. Patients' control over the temporality in which they live, whether in terms of linear "chronos time" or "kairotic moments" (as in medication accidents), is crucial here.

In the last chapter in the third section, Andrea Stöckl, a social-cultural anthropologist and a psychotherapist by training, reflects on her experiences as a newly qualified psychotherapist practicing in pandemic times in Austria. Using an auto-ethnographic perspective and focussing on somatic attention, she analyses the impact of delivering online therapy and the challenges of bringing together ethical and legal regulations, technical knowledge, and the need for clients to remain in contact when everything else seemed to fall apart. She sets her own experiences in the context of the rapidly changing field of telemedicine and mental health. Clients have actively driven this change because of the ever-growing demand for psychological help in uncertain times. While the professional body of psychotherapists in Austria has viewed the delivery of mental health care via technology with scepticism due to their stance that it is the direct interpersonal relationship between therapist and client that drives the healing process, clients have welcomed the integration of tools such as Skype, Zoom and WhatsApp because it allowed them to engage in the therapy process from the comfort and safe space of their own home. Legal considerations propose that therapists had no special training in online training, were not aware of the pitfalls of data protection issues, and thus would find it difficult to guarantee the privacy of the treatment. Continuous professional training has caught up with these issues in the meantime. Privacy is one of the cornerstones of successful therapy. Thus, the notion of trust would have to be renegotiated to make an already impossible professional relationship more certain and trustworthy. Stöckl looks at some areas of the relationship between clients and therapists that might have to be rewritten while using online therapy, one of them being the corporeal part of the encounter.

## Individual and socially distributed emotions

We have arrived at the book's last section, which looks at individual and socially distributed emotions. In this section, we take a journey from Norway to Spain and France, and finally to Switzerland, exploring the affective and social dynamics of health and illness related to diagnosis-making, fighting for recovery, and the culinary art of producing and consuming fermented foods.

Mette Bech Risør and Nina Nissen examine the diagnostic processes surrounding chronic fatigue syndrome (CFS) as they take shape in Norway. They argue that despite the perception of biomedical knowledge as indisputable, there is often a significant level of epistemic uncertainty associated with these processes. This uncertainty is particularly pronounced when symptoms do not conform to established disease models. Drawing from their ethnographic fieldwork conducted at a Norwegian university hospital, they show that this discrepancy frequently arises in cases of chronic fatigue, leading to complex processes of diagnostic negotiations in which, against the backdrop of various factors such as health agendas, bodily experiences, and relational competences, the mutual and situational involvement of the actors (doctors, psychologists, occupational therapists, patients) is central. The authors emphasize that the affective aspects of the clinical encounter play a pivotal role in comprehending the diagnostic journey, showing that these encounters are influenced by biomedical expertise, institutional routines, and the neoliberal approach to healthcare, all of which contribute to a multifaceted web of concerns and interests involving all participants. By drawing on the notions of affective atmosphere and affective attunement, Risør and Nissen show how patients and health professionals, and health professionals with each other, become affectively aligned or synchronised in an intersubjective process of diagnostic assessment, contributing to the potential for change, understanding, and movement in the diagnostic and treatment processes. Highlighting the affinity between affect, hope, and potential, the authors suggest that hope anticipates what has not yet materialized, and the disposition of hopefulness can have a transformative effect on suffering individuals; hope is an "ability to affect and be affected by the world".

The second chapter in this section by Lina Masana takes us not only to Spain and France but also on a journey through the lives of people who live with locked-in syndrome (LIS). LIS, which in most cases results from a stroke in the brainstem or in connection with neurodegenerative disease, is characterised by the fact that those affected are, to varying degrees, unable to move (quadriplegic) or speak (anarthric), while remaining conscious, mentally alert, and able to see, hear, and feel, and most importantly by its poor and highly uncertain prognosis. In her chapter, Masana explores LIS with a focus on the challenge of this rare medical condition to the notion of recovery among healthcare professionals, patients, and their families. Based on ethnographic research about people living with LIS carried out in France and Spain from 2019 to 2021, she looks at the lived experience of LIS from the perspective of those suffering from it as they "fight" for recovery. The author argues that living with LIS and the prospects of recovery are marked by what she calls the "certain uncertainty of LIS": very few may fully recover from LIS, some may not recover at all, and many will experience varying degrees of partial recovery. Mapping the high variability of LIS in the illness trajectories of those affected, Masana shows that fighting for recovery comes with significant financial, emotional, and moral burdens. It requires access to technical aids and continuous, specialized professional care over the years, coupled with the persistence and personal commitment of those affected. Nevertheless, some individuals dedicate themselves tirelessly to this process, while others do not. The reasons include various factors such as personal health situation, professional support, family backing, living conditions, and financial resources. Essentially, the pursuit of recovery with LIS is an endeavour against uncertainty and odds and a challenge to medical prognosis. It is, Masana says, about regaining control over their changed lives and bodies. She concludes by pointing out that "fighting" for recovery in LIS is controversial because the notion assumes a medically created certainty based on inherent uncertainties.

In the final chapter of this volume, Elisabeth Hsu takes us on a very real journey through mountainous and rural parts of Switzerland. Her inquiry focuses on the distinctive aspects of various culinary techniques that facilitate fermentation and how these methods and the connected social practices foster socialities that have potential health benefits. Drawing on various chance encounters that Hsu made over the years during her visits to Switzerland, the empirical basis for her analysis is detailed ethnographic snapshots rather than the outcome of a systematic research project. She presents four vignettes that relate to the lived experience of people involved in the various processes around the production and consumption of fermented food: wine and cheese-making in the Italian-speaking canton Ticino, government-supported community events involving the consumption of alcoholic beverages during the *Adventszeit* (the period before Christmas) in villages at the French-speaking border in the region of the Jura and the Romansch-speaking part of the Engadin respectively, and a baked cake in the German-speaking canton of Appenzell.

Based on her delicately written descriptions of her encounters with the socialities that form around fermentation, Hsu argues that they best be understood as "figurations of fermentation", emphasising affective processes and atmospheric changes that also include alterations in the "body ecologic". Despite the many uncertainties inherent to processes of fermentation, fermentation as a socio-ecological figuration is a way of place-making, "empotment" in Hsu's terms. By forming and cultivating connections and interspecies dependences with the local environment and its specific materiality, fermentation as a "culinary art" both contributes to the specific materiality of a particular place and fosters a sense of connectedness and belonging for those humans "enskilled" in producing and consuming fermented foods.

In sum, this volume presents a rich tapestry of perspectives on hope and uncertainty in health and medicine. It offers insights into how these phenomena are experienced, navigated, and managed across various cultural, social, and institutional contexts and how they are entangled with the infrastructure and material culture within and beyond medicine. The volume aims to deepen our understanding of the complexities and dynamics at the intersection of health, hope, and uncertainty through its diversity of contributions.

## References

Abdalla, Mustafa. 2018. Transfigurative Experiences of Sickness: Medical Regimes, Disease Commodification, and Professional Patients in Egypt. Zeitschrift für Ethnologie 143(1): 21–39.

Adams, Vincanne, M. Michelle Murphy, and Adele E. Clarke. 2009. Anticipation: Technoscience, Life, Affect, Temporality. Subjectivity 28: 246–265.

Baer, Hans, and Merrill Singer. 2023. Planetary Health: Capitalism, Ecology and Eco-Socialism. Capitalism Nature Socialism 34(4): 20–38.

Cohen, Lawrence. 2005. Operability, Bioavailability, and Exception. *In* Global Assemblages: Technology, Politics, and Ethics as Anthropological Problems. Aihwa Ong and Stephen J. Collier, eds. Pp. 79–90. Malden: Blackwell Publishing.

Drążkiewicz, Elżbieta. 2023. Are You With Us or Against Us?: Studying Conflicts Over Conspiracy Theories and Overcoming the Great Conspiratorial Divide. Anthropology in Action 30(1): 12–23.

De Looze, Karen. 2016. India's Kidney Belt and Medical Tourism: A Double-Edged Sword. *In* Organ Transplantation in Times of Donor Shortage. Ralf J. Jox, Galia Assadi, and Georg Marckmann, eds. Pp. 271–284. Heidelberg: Springer.

Fainzang, Sylvie. 2017. Self-Medication and Society: Mirages of Autonomy. London: Routledge.

Farrington, Conor, and Rebecca Lynch. 2018. Personal Medical Devices: People and Technology in the Context of Health, *In* Quantified Lives and Vital Data: Exploring Health and Technology through Personal Medical Devices. Rebecca Lynch and Conor Farrington, eds. Pp. 3–16. London: Palgrave Macmillan.

Good, Mary-Jo DelVeechio, Byron J. Good, Cynthia Schaffer, and Stuart E. Lind. 1990. American Oncology and the Discourse of Hope. Culture, Medicine and Psychiatry 14(1): 59–79.

Graham, Janice. 2016. Ambiguous Capture: Collaborative Capitalism and the Meningitis Vaccine Project. Medical Anthropology 35(5): 419–432.

Hadolt, Bernhard. 2018. A Desire for Knowing: Ontological Uncertainty, Diagnostic Evidence and Generative Affectivity in Pre-symptomatic Genetic Counselling. *In* Diagnostic Fluidity: Working with Uncertainty and Mutability. Nina Nissen and Mette Bech Risør, eds. Pp. 129–147. Tarragona: Publicacions URV.

Hogle, Linda F. 2005. Enhancement Technologies and the Body. Annual Review of Anthropology 34(1): 695–716.

Hunt, Linda M., Hannah S. Bell, Allison M. Baker, and Heather A. Howard. 2017. Electronic Health Records and the Disappearing Patient. Medical Anthropology Quarterly 31(3): 403–421.

Jenkins, Richard, Hanne Jessen, and Vibeke Steffen, eds. 2005. Managing Uncertainty: Ethnographic Studies of Illness, Risk and the Struggle for Control. Copenhagen: Museum Tusculanum Press.

Inhorn, Marcia Claire. 2003. Local Babies, Global Science: Gender, Religion, and In Vitro Fertilization in Egypt. London: Routledge.

Kehr, Janina, Hansjörg Dilger, and Peter van Eeuwijk. 2019. Transfigurations of Health and the Moral Economy of Medicine: Subjectivities, Materialities, Values. Zeitschrift Für Ethnologie 143(1): 1–20.

Kirksey, Eben. 2021. The Mutant Project: Inside the Global Race to Genetically Modify Humans. Bristol: Bristol University Press.

Konrad, Monica. 2005. Narrating the New Predictive Genetics: Ethics, Ethnography, and Science. Cambridge: Cambridge University Press.

Landecker, Hannah. 2000. Immortality, In Vitro: A History of the HeLa Cell Line. *In* Biotechnology and Culture: Bodies, Anxieties, Ethics. Paul E. Brodwin, ed. Pp. 53–72. Bloomington: Indiana University Press.

Landecker, Hannah. 2007. Culturing Life: How Cells Became Technologies. Cambridge, MA: Harvard University Press.

Layne, Linda L. 2000. The Cultural Fix: An Anthropological Contribution to Science and Technology Studies. Science, Technology & Human Values 25(4): 492–519.

Lock, Margaret. 2013. The Epigenome and Nature/Nurture Reunification: A Challenge for Anthropology. Medical Anthropology 32(4): 291–308.

Lupton, Deborah. 1995. The Imperative of Health: Public Health and the Regulated Body. London: Sage.

Lupton, Deborah 2018. Digital Health: Critical and Cross-Disciplinary Perspectives. New York: Routledge.

Martin, Emily. 2007. Bipolar Expeditions: Mania and Depression in American Culture. Princeton: Princeton University Press.

Mattes, Dominik. 2019. Fierce Medicines, Fragile Socialities: Grounding Global HIV Treatment in Tanzania. Oxford: Berghahn.

Mattes, Dominik, Bernhard Hadolt, and Brigit Obrist. 2020. Introduction: Rethinking Sociality and Health through Transfiguration. MAT-Medical Anthropology Theory 7(1): 66–86.

Mattingly, Cheryl F. 2010. The Paradox of Hope: Journeys through a Clinical Borderland. Berkeley, CA: University of California Press

Müller-Rockstroh, Babette. 2012. Appropriate and Appropriated Technology: Lessons Learned from Ultrasound in Tanzania. Medical Anthropology 31(3): 196–212.

Nissen, Nina, and Mette Bech Risør, eds. 2018. Diagnostic Fluidity: Working with Uncertainty and Mutability. Tarragona: URV Publicacions.

Novas, Carlos. 2006. The Political Economy of Hope: Patients' Organizations, Science and Biovalue. BioSocieties 1(3): 289–305.

Oudshoorn, Nelly. 2011. Telecare: Technologies and the Transformation of Healthcare. New York: Palgrave Macmillan.

Petryna, Adriana, Andrew Lakoff, and Arthur Kleinman, eds. 2006. Global Pharmaceuticals: Ethics, Markets, Practices. Durham: Duke University Press.

Rose, Nikolas. 2007. Politics of Life Itself: Biomedicine, Power and Subjectivity in the Twenty-First Century. Princeton, N.J.; Oxford: Princeton Univ. Press.

Ruckenstein, Minna, and Natasha Dow Schüll. 2017. The Datafication of Health. Annual Review of Anthropology 46(1): 261–278.

Singer, Merrill, Eleanor Shoreman-Ouimet, and Ashley Graham. 2022. Climate Change and Health. *In* A Companion to Medical Anthropology, Second Edition. Second edition. Merrill Singer, Pamela I. Erickson, and César Abadía-Barrero, eds. Pp. 429–441. Hoboken, NJ: Wiley Blackwell.

Smajdor, Anna, and Andrea Stöckl. 2018. PMDs and the Moral Specialness of Medicine: An Analysis of the "Keepsake Ultrasound". *In* Quantified Lives and Vital Data. Rebecca Lynch and Conor Farrington, eds. Pp. 155–178. London: Palgrave Macmillan.

Stöckl, Andrea. 2010. Public Discourses and Policymaking: The HPV Vaccination from the European Perspective. *In* Three Shots at Prevention: The HPV Vaccine and the Politics of Medicine's Simple Solutions. Keith Wailoo, Julie Livingston, Steven Epstein, and Robert Aronowitz, eds. Pp. 254–269. Baltimore: Johns Hopkins University Press.

Street, Alice. 2014. Biomedicine in an Unstable Place: Infrastructure and Personhood in a Papua New Guinean Hospital. Durham: Duke University Press.

Sunder Rajan, Kaushik. 2006. Biocapital: The Constitution of Postgenomic Life. Durham: Duke University Press.

2007. Experimental Values: Indian Clinical Trials and Surplus Health. New Left Review 45(2007): 67–88.

Taussig, Karen-Sue, Klaus Hoeyer, and Stefan Helmreich. 2013. The Anthropology of Potentiality in Biomedicine: An Introduction to Supplement 7. Current Anthropology 54(S7): S3–S14.

Van Dongen, Els. 1998. 'I Wish a Happy End': Hope in the Lives of Chronic Schizophrenic Patients. Anthropology & Medicine 5(2): 169–192.

Wailoo, Keith, Julie Livingston, Steven Epstein, and Robert Aronowitz, eds. 2010. Three Shots at Prevention: The HPV Vaccine and the Politics of Medicine's Simple Solutions. Baltimore: Johns Hopkins University Press.

Waldby, Catherine, and Robert Mitchell. 2006. Tissue Economies: Blood, Organs, and Cell Lines in Late Capitalism. Durham: Duke University Press.

Whyte, Susan Reynolds. 1997. Questioning Misfortune: The Pragmatics of Uncertainty in Eastern Uganda. Cambridge: Cambridge University Press.

# Part I: Pragmatics of Hope and Uncertainty

# 1 Embracing Uncertainty

*Sjaak van der Geest*

Uncertainty has been an all-pervasive part of my biography. Needless to explain that being brought up in a devout Christian tradition that teaches absolute truth (in spite of a famous biblical passage in which the protagonist rhetorically asks, "What is truth?"), one is constantly in doubt about these unproven truths. Interestingly, that very same epistemological not-knowing has been made the cornerstone of believing. Faith based on knowledge would not be faith but simply knowledge. Faith is defined as a leap into the unknown, as trust in what cannot be perceived by any of our (only) five senses or concluded by logical deduction. "Credo quia absurdum" (I believe because it is absurd) became a favourite response by theologians (from Tertullian to Kierkegaard) to sceptics of religion. I hope that this autobiographical starting point makes my paper a suitable contribution to this collection of articles about hope and uncertainty at home, in the sense that it reflects on my most intimate "home", myself.

This somewhat chaotic assembly of ruminations is similar to the fieldnotes that anthropologists collect and organise as a first step to writing an article or book. In this case[1], the "field" is the desk where I conduct my "interviews" with colleagues and authors from other disciplines and write down quotes from their work that may serve my envisaged article. I have made an attempt to organise the thoughts and quotations that I have collected so far into four categories or sections: (1) philosophical debates; (2) uncertainty in search of certainty (knowledge); (3) certainty as a tool to cover up uncertainty in human encounters; and (4) embracing uncertainty/agnosticism. Throughout these four steps run the continuously shifting appreciations of certainty and uncertainty. The context in which these changing appreciations occur is the domain of medical anthropology and the wider field of human experience in general.

The original idea of the first *Medical Anthropology at Home* conference in 1998 (and thereafter) was to discuss and tinker with draft papers in order to make them bet-

1 This chapter is based on a paper presented at the *XI Medical Anthropology at Home (MAAH)* Conference "Transfigurations of Uncertainty in Health and Medicine" (2021, Schüttkasten Geras, Austria). I am grateful to the participants for their comments on the draft paper and to the editors of this volume for their finishing touches.

ter. "Perfect" papers were not welcome because they offered nothing to tinker with. Because of this tradition, I decided to submit this text about uncertainty in an uncertain state, which reflects my own state of mind. Both content and form reveal my doubts about claims of certainty in all walks of life and my growing acceptance of unavoidable and honest uncertainty. Ironically, it forces me to ignore Max Weber's admonition that complexity requires precise and unambiguous language. I have often cited him to convince colleagues or students to be more precise and clearer when the subject matter of a text is imprecise and unclear: "Scharfe Scheidung ist in der Realität oft nicht möglich, klare Begriffe sind aber dann deshalb um so nötiger" (Weber 1976: 123).

But before presenting my thoughts about uncertainty, I want to commemorate the seminal article by Murray Last (1981), who in his eloquent way drew our attention to the importance of "knowing about not knowing". Anthropologists have gone out of their way to "tap" people's knowledge about anything one can imagine, but never took an interest in what people did *not* know and what that ignorance meant in their daily life. Murray Last put not-knowing on the anthropological agenda and has been a great inspiration for me at several junctions of my anthropological work, including this one.

## Debates in philosophy

Obviously, delving into philosophical treatises on epistemology and human anxiety when facing the unknown is a "mer à boire". For this occasion, I limit myself—arbitrarily—to two themes. The first theme relates to Pyrrhonism. Pyrrho was a Greek philosopher about whom little is known, but his ideas about scepticism regarding knowledge have survived thanks to the writings of Sextus Empiricus, who lived in the 3rd or 2nd century BC.

> The main principle of Pyrrho's thought is expressed by the word *acatalepsia*, which connotes the ability to withhold assent from doctrines regarding the truth of things in their own nature; against every statement its contradiction may be advanced with equal justification.
> Pyrrhonists withhold assent about non-evident propositions, that is, dogma. They disputed that the dogmatists had found truth regarding non-evident matters. For any non-evident matter, a Pyrrhonist tries to make the arguments for and against such that the matter cannot be concluded, thus suspending belief. According to Pyrrhonism, even the statement that nothing can be known is dogmatic. They thus attempted to make their scepticism universal, and to escape the reproach of basing it upon a fresh dogmatism. Mental imperturbability (*ataraxia*) was the result to be attained by cultivating such a frame of mind. (Wikipedia, accessed 10–03–2020)

This early epistemological scepticism, combined with the calm acceptance of its ensuing uncertainty, strikes me as surprisingly modern (reflected in, for example, Spinoza, Bayle, Hume, Wittgenstein) and has pushed me to investigate my own scepticism, as I try to do in this essay. I soon realised that the philosophical discussions and debates were overwhelming: I would be doomed to achieve at most some simple reinventions of the wheel. Nevertheless, I thought it useful to take the philosophical theme of scepticism and suspending (or giving up) knowing into anthropological reasoning, and medical anthropology in particular.

The Dutch sociologist Johan Goudsblom preceded me in this endeavour. He describes in his published doctoral thesis (1960) the unintended consequences of long-term developments in European philosophy and—more generally—culture. Starting with Socrates, he followed "[...] the development of the 'truth commandment' which pushed great thinkers ever further, undermining each other's and finally their own certainties". The following quote from his impressive study (also translated into English in 1980) refers to Pyrrhonism.

> Pyrrho casts doubt even on the authority of reason, for if reason is completely dissociated from the sensory world, what does it have to offer when it comes to understanding the world we live in? Is not this knowledge a delusion, too? The one is as fraudulent as the other:
>
> "Neither our perceptions nor our judgments teach us to know truth or untruth. Therefore we must not trust either our senses or our reason, but must remain without opinion, unmoved, inclining neither to one side nor to the other. Whatever the matter in question may be, we shall say that one can neither deny nor confirm it, or that one must simultaneously confirm and deny it" (Aristocles on Pyrrho, quoted by Brochard 1932: 54).
>
> Pyrrho could be called a silenced Socrates—someone who knows that the truth is inaccessible and has rejected all striving, even the search for truth, is vain. [...] he makes a virtue of necessity and adopts the stance of *the wise man's superior detachment* [...] [F]or Pyrrho the philosopher is an impartial and serene observer, who knows that the distinction between truth and falsehood, between good and evil, is too obscure for human beings, and who has only one moral lesson to teach: be brave and leave one another in peace. (Goudsblom 1980: 114; my italics)

Clearly, Goudsblom does not follow the radical viewpoint of Pyrrhonism; to "be brave and leave one another in peace" does not really make sense for an author who intends to share his ideas about human thought and cultural development. His stand is similar to the comments by Jerry Green, who also points at the internal contradiction in Pyrrho's agnostic scepticism. How can one "who refused to make assertions about the world outside of perceptual or intellectual appearances" make such a statement? (Green 2017: 335). Knowing or not-knowing, we are all caught by contradictions as soon as we start speaking about knowledge.

The second theme in my philosophical quandary presented itself almost sixty years ago, when I studied philosophy. Maurice Merleau-Ponty was my teacher's favourite philosopher at that time. One of the concepts of the French philosopher that grabbed me then and has remained with me ever since was "maudite lucidité".

> *Abstract* concepts are too easily assumed to represent the reality from where they have been taken. Merleau-Ponty used the indication *précoce lucidité* (precocious lucidity) to reject this assumption (Merleau-Ponty 1960: 32). He emphasised the obscure and bodily existence of human beings which is overlooked by a too rational approach. In more general terms, he emphasised the unreal character of philosophical theories about human beings that exclusively on the basis of reasoning formulate an explanation. A related term by Merleau-Ponty was *maudite lucidité* (accursed lucidity). (ibid.: 33) (Unknown source, my translation from Dutch)

Human reality is complex, dynamic and subjective and cannot be reduced to a simple statistical quantity. Because of its concrete yet ephemeral nature, reality can never be completely and "lucidly" known according to Merleau-Ponty. Should I therefore refrain from speaking clearly about uncertainty and its social and psychological implications?

## Uncertainty in the search for certainty

Focusing on medical anthropology, uncertainty is overwhelmingly regarded as a problem or obstacle in the quest for certain knowledge, by physicians and caregivers as well as by patients and their relatives. Medicine was once described in a Dutch medical PhD dissertation as a "factory of reassurance", providing patients with certain knowledge about the state of their condition. Equally, physicians reassure themselves by being able to reassure their patients.

In probably the first extensive hospital ethnography, *Experiment Perilous*, Renée Fox (1987 [1959]) sketches the ambiguity of progressing biomedical science in a metabolic research group in a US hospital. All physicians are confronted with problems of uncertainty. Some of these result from their own incomplete or imperfect mastery of the available medical knowledge and skills; others derive from limitations in current medical knowledge; and still others grow out of difficulties in distinguishing between personal ignorance or ineptitude and the limitations of medical science.

> In a sense, the physicians of the Metabolic Group can be thought of as specialists in problems of uncertainty—particularly those uncertainties related to limits of present medical knowledge. As clinical investigators, it was their special role to work on the periphery of what is medically known [...]. (Fox 1987[1959]: 28)

The above quote points at the uncertainty that disturbs the research team looking for effective solutions for their patients and struggling with ill-understood mechanisms of the human body. In the next quote, Fox cites a doctor who explains that every step forward in mastering knowledge produces new uncertainties. In addition, discoveries that lead to improved knowledge are often not the outcome of rigid testing and scientific reasoning but of coincidence, serendipity.

> The advances in knowledge and skill which their work effected helped to clarify and occasionally even dispel some of these uncertainties. But at the same time, as in all research, these gains in knowledge frequently uncovered new problems of uncertainties to be explored. "Things multiply. You solve one problem, and you're faced with two others. Things you didn't know once become obvious. But then other things you didn't even know existed arise [...]." (Fox 1987 [1959]: 29)

Patients too are worried by the uncertainties that doctors encounter and by the unpredictability of their condition and the experimental treatments they undergo. Their uncertainty is complicated by the ambiguities of their incomprehensible disease. As one patient expressed:

> This is a very peculiar disease I've got. It's got all kind of phases, and God only knows what phase you're in at what point. The doctors can't tell you exactly [...]. After you've had this for a while, you either go in one direction or another. You reach a point where you either get better, or you get worse. And there's no foolproof way of telling in advance which way you are going to go [...]. (Fox 1987 [1959]: 127)

Patients' anxieties are tempered by instilling hope and encouragement, which is not so much based on knowledge but on empathy and is at the same time an attempt to keep the atmosphere on the ward positive. These encouragements are given by the medical staff as well as by fellow patients. Abraham de Swaan (1983: 161–219) described such a "regime of hope" in a Dutch cancer hospital, much to the chagrin of the hospital authorities, who regarded the observation as belittling their medical competence and being harmful to their patients (Van der Geest 1989).

Managing uncertainty is also a theme in Susan Whyte's (1997) *Questioning Misfortune*, an ethnography about HIV/AIDS in Eastern Uganda. Whyte's central intuition focuses on the pragmatism of the Bunyole people in their confrontation with misfortune and uncertainty. They are unable to create safety in their existence, despite the diagnostic techniques and explanations available to them. Their solution is a *modus vivendi* with uncertainty that Susan Whyte interprets through the "pragmatism" of the US philosopher John Dewey. According to Dewey, people try to defuse their conditions of constant uncertainty not with ideas but with actions. Thoughts are not so much the drivers of our actions, but rather the result. Acting goes before thinking. If people are rational, it is mainly because they are rationalising.

The many suspicions and accusations, rituals and medical acts that Bunyole people attempt are mostly psychologically effective. They give those involved the feeling that they are doing something and not watching helplessly. Not optimism, but—in William James' terminology—meleorism: maybe it gets a little better, a little hope in a mass of uncertainty. It is a life in the "subjunctive mode" (subjunctive "wishful thinking"). Whyte quotes Byron Good, who talks of "[...] trafficking in human possibilities rather than in settled certainties" (Whyte 1997: 24).

Twenty-five years after Fox's provocative hospital ethnography, Paul Atkinson (1984) published a rebuttal of her view on medical uncertainty in the training of medical students, which in Fox's terms was or should be a "training for uncertainty" (see also Fox 1957). Atkinson argued that Fox had seduced her readers with "the elegance of her presentation and the sheer fascination of her subject matter", but that in reality, uncertainty is a normal part of medical (and any other) research. In everyday language: Fox exaggerated the anxiety and stress that students and teachers suffer as a result of not-knowing:

> [...] issues of 'certainty' and 'uncertainty' are not mutually exclusive. They are not all-or-nothing orientations to work and knowledge on the part of 'scientists', 'professional practitioners' or 'lay' members. (Atkinson 1984: 954)

I do not think that Fox was unaware of this and I am not surprised that she declined the editor's invitation to respond. Arguing the obvious produces only embarrassment. Her 1959 study did in fact argue what was less obvious at the time: that the alleged solid body of medical science was in fact strewn with uncertainties that remained largely unspoken of, certainly in front of patients.

Nearly fifty years after Fox's publication, Hillen and co-authors (2017) raised the question of if and how uncertainty tolerance (UT) can be measured in medical settings. The implication of the term UT is clear: uncertainty is an unwelcome but unavoidable phenomenon in health care (and other domains of life), so there is no choice but to tolerate it. But how far should our tolerance go? An analysis of 18 existing measures of uncertainty and tolerance teaches the authors that the concept of uncertainty is a muddled mix of a wide variety of human experiences and opinions. Definitions of uncertainty may range, for example:

> [...] from the possibility that a negative or potentially harmful event may occur to the period of anticipation prior to such an event, to the notion that negative events may occur and there is no definitive way of predicting such events. (Hillen et al. 2017: 65)

As long as this muddle exists, the objective of "calculating" how much uncertainty people can bear (if that would be possible at all) remains unreachable. "Researchers use [...] the same terms to signify different things, and different terms to signify the same thing" (Hillen et al. 2017: 67). To overcome this obstacle, the authors set out to propose an all-encompassing definition that would allow for intelligent measuring and comparing a tolerance of uncertainty.

The authors offer the following working definition of uncertainty tolerance: "The set of negative and positive psychological response (cognitive, emotional, and behavioural) provoked by the conscious awareness of ignorance about particular aspects of the world" (ibid.: 71). The implied definition of uncertainty in this working definition is a "conscious awareness of ignorance about particular aspects of the world" (ibid.: 64). I wonder if this working definition will lead to more clarity and practical usability for future research on coping with or rather embracing uncertainty. I agree that it is desirable that research in medical settings provides suggestions for solving existing problems, but how likely is this to succeed if the problem at hand is transformed and reduced to the (quantifiable) lucidity that Merleau-Ponty criticised and rejected?

I was more intrigued by the experience-nearness and diversity of the quoted reactions to (un)certainty that the authors collected from the 28 sources they examined. They gave me a sense of the lived reality of uncertainty that would be hard to catch in a clever definition. My perception of these quotes resembles Schutz's notion of "natural attitude", common sense or everyday practical reasoning and practical activity. "Such thinking as usual is characteristic of the person 'in the street', who is content to rely unquestioningly on such common sense" (quoted from Atkinson 1984: 954). Let me, as a "person in the street", present some of these quotes from Hillen et al.'s collection.

> Embracing *uncertainty*:
> There is something exciting about being kept in suspense.
> I like the mystery that there are some things in medicine we'll never know.
>
> *Disliking/fearing uncertainty*:
> When I can't clearly discern situations, I get apprehensive.
> I have a lot of respect for consultants who always come up with a definite answer.
> I am dissatisfied when the specialist does not make a diagnosis.
> I like things to be ordered and in place, both at work and at home.
> I feel anxious when things are changing. (Hillen et al. 2017: 67)

In a table listing reactions to uncertainty, negative ones (aversion, denial, discomfort, anger, stress, worry, anxiety, confusion) greatly outnumber the positive ones (enjoyment, attraction). “Embracing” seems far away, particularly in medical settings.

## "Certainty" as a social strategy

Another title for this section could have been “False claims of certainty” or “The pretence of certainty” or “Certainty to cover up uncertainty”. Claiming to be certain of something or somebody is a powerful tool to position oneself above others, that can be exercised in the most diverse contexts. It therefore deserves anthropological attention. Murray Last's article, mentioned above, describes this social strategy among healers in Northern Nigeria, who practise medicine without much understanding of the illness or of their own treatment. Yet they act and speak as if they know. To quote the author:

> I am suggesting here that the origin of ‘not-knowing’ lies in the break-up of traditional medicine as a system; and from this not-knowing there has developed first, a secrecy which tries to conceal the lack of knowledge and certainty; and second, a scepticism in which people suspect that no one really ‘knows’; that there is no system. But the social conventions of politeness—as well as people's real need to find a cure for their ills—keep the veils of secrecy and scepticism sufficiently in place, for themselves and for others. (Last 1981: 391)

Doubtful claims of knowledge are common in medical settings where physicians or nurses are short-staffed, lack time and have insufficient diagnostic equipment to be certain about their patients' type of disease and appropriate cure. Alice Street (2014) carried out research in a hospital in Papua New Guinea and describes such a situation. Biomedicine, renowned for its enormous evidence-based body of knowledge, is enacted in this overcrowded hospital as a murky and dark field of uncertainty. Doctors are often forced to act without knowing. Reality on the ground contrasts starkly with the book reality they met during their training. They have no choice but to keep up the appearance of knowledge and to “improvise”, an elegant euphemism for a frustrating practice. Admitting their uncertainty would be disastrous for both the medical staff and the patients (see also Street 2011).

But even in well-equipped medical settings, uncertainty dwells, as we have seen in Fox's monograph and the discussion around it, and may, occasionally, force medical professionals to hide their ignorance in order not to upset their patients. “The doctor gives me a medicine to cure his own uncertainty” is the title of a Dutch article I once read (exact reference lost).

A similar observation could be made with regard to religious language that overrules the doubts of the faithful, believers and non-believers. No one has a monopoly on the truth about what exists outside our perception and sensory experience. That unknown world provides, of course, free ground for speculation, belief and hope, but can never be claimed to be known. Sermons during funerals, in which death is denied in metaphoric language that may be taken literally by some attendees, is a case in point. Rituals after death are prominent occasions where the thoughts and convictions of the deceased (and those attending) are hijacked by an "all-knowing" officiant. Doubts are chased away. If that happens, we can rightly speak of oppressive and misplaced certainty. But the converse also applies; the conviction that religious beliefs are false (and therefore must be eradicated) cannot be founded on certain knowledge for the same reason.

Returning to the medical field: Arthur Frank (2001) and Gerhard Nijhof (2000; 2018), two scholars who were themselves patients, both mention the irritating experience of medical staff members who claim to know everything about their condition and suffering. Such an attitude overrules and "steals" the patient's experiential knowledge. "A claim to know the other's suffering takes away part of that other's integrity" (Frank 2001: 359). A similar thing happens in the rules and discussions around euthanasia in my country, the Netherlands: doctors—not patients—decide whether the patient's suffering is truly "unbearable".

Personally, I find the common saying in ordinary conversation— "I know exactly what you mean" or "I fully understand you"—irritating and arrogant. The words could be uttered in a comforting context to support the other, in which case the text does not need to be taken literally (yet, I would still not appreciate such condescending empathy). I also do not intend to deny our capability of intuitively sensing what the other person is saying or thinking (otherwise any type of conversation would be impossible, cf. Fonagy and Allisson 2014). I rather refer to the common use of these terms in debates when one person tries to defeat the other by discrediting him/her based on what the other may think, in an attempt to interpret or rather misinterpret his/her spoken words. In other words: by stealing and turning around what the other meant to say. Claiming to know what other people think is not only annoying and arrogant, as I just mentioned, but also naïve and silly.

Joel Robbins (2008), who did fieldwork in a small community of Urapmin people in Papua New Guinea, encountered what he called a language ideology of opacity. When people speak, they do not express their real thoughts and intentions. What they have in mind and plan to do, for example, remains unsaid, opaque. Those listening to the speaker know this and will not pursue with questions about what they mean (as anthropologists tend to do), but respect and accept the opacity. Insisting on what is behind the words is regarded as rude and an intrusion of the speaker's privacy.

> I came to think of Urapmin ideas about opacity, and the failure of speech to carry the thoughts of others, as linked to a broad conception of what we might call "psy-

> chic privacy." People's minds are private places, and invading their privacy by finding out what they really think would, were it possible, be a serious personal violation. (Robbins 2008: 426)

Reading his article, I thought: Is it different in my own society? Perhaps to some degree, but also "at home" in our own conversations, we know—or at least should know—that we never know what the other really means when speaking and that insisting on more information may be regarded as bad-mannered. Moreover, it is well-known that words are convenient tools to hide our thoughts.

## Embracing uncertainty

The embrace of uncertainty is likely to be a reaction to the various abuses and unwarranted claims of certain knowledge. I had hoped that a collection of ethnographic studies of doubt, edited by Mathijs Pelkmans (2013a), would enlighten me on how people manage to live peacefully with uncertainty. It did to some extent. In his introduction, Pelkmans points out that doubt and uncertainty are two different things. Doubt is a temporary and changing condition; it facilitates action to reach a conclusion that provides clarity. Doubting between two (or more) possible actions pushes for a choice. It is in fact knowledge about two (or more) possible truths that eventually prioritises one. For Descartes, "doubt was his instrument to reach solid foundations of knowledge, after which doubt ceased to be relevant and could be discarded" (Pelkmans 2013b: 8). Indeed, "[...] doubt cannot be at rest, whereas uncertainty cannot be wilfully employed" (ibid.: 4). Thus doubt is "activated uncertainty" (ibid.: 16).

> Doubt and uncertainty are related concepts, but uncertainty lacks the agency that is implicit in doubt. People may live in uncertainty because the times are uncertain, but although it is possible to live in doubt, it would be odd to blame this on doubtful circumstances. While uncertainty rests in the situation, doubt is located in the actor. (ibid.: 17)

Having said this, Pelkmans then turns to the contribution of Maurice Bloch (2013) in his edited volume. Bloch deviates from Pelkmans' conceptual distinctions and describes how people in a small community in Madagascar "remain in doubt" ("and quite comfortably so") about certain issues he discussed with them. In Pelkmans' words:

> These seemingly contradictory positions can be reconciled, though, by pointing out that there are different ways to deal with the restlessness of doubt. Without presuming to give an exhaustive enumeration I suggest that restlessness can be

> halted by: (a) diverting one's attention, so that the object of doubt is no longer in the spotlight; (b) reinterpreting the object of doubt in a way that makes it less 'dubious'; (c) denying that doubt is doubt; or (d) removing the alternative when confronted with two possibilities. (ibid.: 20)

For my paper, I intended (but failed) to explore these four ways of remaining in doubt (*accepting uncertainty*) without becoming crazy or desperate. At the same time, I doubt if these mental manoeuvres will bring me to my initial inspiration, which is not about *accepting* uncertainty but about *embracing* it. My concern is the paradoxical phenomenon that uncertainty—in certain circumstances—is a superior type of knowledge, more reliable and honest than certainty.

## Positioning embrace

The simplest version of the objective of anthropological fieldwork is to get to know other people, to try to find out what they do and think and to make sense of it. But from the beginning, researchers were conscious of the fact that they themselves were part of the discoveries they made. In his description of sexual life among Trobrianders, Malinowski (1932: xxv) admitted that anthropology attracted him mainly as the best way to get to know himself. And Evans-Pritchard is told to have said that the main reason he travelled all the way to the Azande was not that he wanted to describe the life of a remote African tribe but that he was trying to fathom what rationality is: solving a personal question by meeting people who believed in witchcraft (source not found).

This type of reflexivity regarding fieldwork became more common in the 1970s and has lasted until today, as we all know. The most extreme form is the type of autoethnography in which the "others" have become figurants in the author's search for his/her own self. Critics, like Charlotte Davis (2008: 216), have warned that social enquiry about others could thus disappear altogether. Such "getting lost in subjectivity" has received many pejorative labels, such as "navel-gazing", "narcissism", "self-absorption", "exhibitionism" and "self-voyeurism".

The fieldwork for this chapter was carried out at my desk and started off with a personal question: How do I stand in my encounters with uncertainty? Many authors of various disciplines were my interlocutors, some of whom made their entry into this chapter. Of course, I was curious as to what they would tell me about their views, but in secret I had already made up my mind, at least to a large extent. One could almost say that I had my conclusion ready before I started my "interviews". That conclusion was that uncertainty is (or should be) increasingly experienced as something to be welcomed in a world where everything needs to be certain, transparent and proven. Errors, whether in politics, business, science, sport, insurance, transport, the internet, education, sex, gender or medicine, are not tolerated. Ministers who make a mistake have to "crawl through the dust", as the Dutch expression goes, and doctors who misdiagnose may be sued. Accepting, even embracing, a bit of uncertainty offers a relief in the midst of this tyranny of strictness and "true" knowledge.

The recognition of uncertainty or not-knowing, I believed, is making remarkable advances in the most diverse fields of academic as well as popular writing, from philosophy to moral and spiritual guidance, from art to psychology. Internet discussions emphasise the importance of accepting uncertainty and speak of the "wisdom" and "courage" of not-knowing. "Agnosticism" is increasingly recognised as a "rational" position, not only in matters of religion. Confessing to not-knowing is regarded as honesty, in contrast to false claims of knowledge, as I pointed out earlier.

Talking of confession, I admit that I was selective in my choice of interlocutors; I chose those who I thought were on my side or those who defended the need for certainty in a way that I believed could serve my purpose. But what came out of this self-exploration through communication with my interlocutors? Did my pre-conceived "conclusion" change during my roaming through the views and arguments of others? Yes, it did, in particular with regard to uncertainty in medical settings. Medical work is probably the least likely place where not-knowing on the part of professionals is tolerated and where uncertainty among patients and relatives can lead to grave anxiety. But to be honest, I knew this. Expecting that, for example, uncertainty about the duration or end of medical treatment would be calmly accepted was a bit of wishful thinking since some cases that I personally witnessed and admired. It is doubtful, however, that such mental imperturbability (*ataraxia*) in medical settings will become more common in the near future.

In wider contexts, I do, however, discern a growing appreciation of uncertainty, as I mentioned before: the appearance of a paradoxical phenomenon that uncertainty—in certain circumstances—is regarded as a superior type of knowledge, more reliable and honest than certainty, and not a destroyer of hope. Or, as someone suggested in Hillen et al. (2017: 67), life will be more exciting and intense if it keeps some mysteries that we may never scientifically uncover. The greatest mystery, which haunts and excites me at the same time, is Leibnitz's famous—simple and baffling—question: "Warum gibt es überhaupt etwas und nicht vielmehr nichts?" ("Why is there something at all and not rather nothing?").

Having arrived at the end of my desk-centred "soul-searching", a last thought presents itself and adds to the doubts that I have shared throughout this chapter: Is enjoying uncertainty not a luxury that only a few can afford? This view was eloquently phrased in a column in a Dutch newspaper:

> [...] I often see doubt and nuance as something gratuitous. That endless on the one hand-on the other hand is a luxury for the living room, for thinkers, poets,

> writers who can continue to philosophise and do not have to decide anything. Judges cannot afford that. Surgeons can't. Drivers can't. In the end, in every organisation (country, school, family) doubts have to give way to making decisions. (Hertzberger 2020; my translation)

The outcome of my "fieldwork" may be disappointing and my title should perhaps have been more modest, for example "accepting uncertainty". But even if the end of my journey is unsatisfactory, the journey itself was instructive and rewarding.

## References

Atkinson, Paul. 1984. Training for Certainty. Social Science & Medicine 19(9): 949–956.

Bloch, Maurice. 2013. Types of Shared Doubt in the Flow of a Discussion. *In* Ethnographies of Doubt: Faith and Uncertainty in Contemporary Societies. Mathijs Pelkmans, ed. Pp. 43–58. London and New York: I.B. Tauris.

Brochard, Victor.1932. Les sceptiques Grecs. Paris: Imprimerie nationale.

Davis, Charlotte A. 2008. Reflexive Ethnography: A Guide to Researching Selves and Others (second edition). London and New York: Routledge.

De Swaan, Abraham.1983. De mens is de mens een zorg: Opstellen 1971–1981 [Untranslatable: Essays 1971–1981]. Amsterdam: Meulenhof.

Fonagy, Peter, and Elizabeth Allison. 2014. The Role of Mentalizing and Epistemic Trust in the Therapeutic Relationship. Psychotherapy 51: 372–380.

Fox, Renée. 1957. Training for Uncertainty. *In* The Student Physician. R.K. Merton, G. Reader and P.L. Kendall, eds. Pp. 207–241. Cambridge, MA: Harvard University.

Fox, Renée 1987 [1959]. Experiment Perilous: Physicians and Patients Facing the Unknown. Glencoe: Free Press.

Frank, Arthur. 2001. Can We Research Suffering? Qualitative Health Research 11(3): 353–362.

Goudsblom, Johan. 1980 [first Dutch publication 1960]. Nihilism and Culture. Oxford: Basil Blackwell.

Green, Jerry. 2017. Was Pyrrho an Pyrrhonian? Peiron 50(3): 335–365.

Hertzberger, Rosanne. 2020. Minister is nu juist geloofwaardiger. NRC 4 Sept. 2020.

Hillen, Marij A., Caitlin M. Gutheil, Tania D. Strout, Ellen M.A. Smets, Paul K.J. Han. 2017. Tolerance of Uncertainty: Conceptual Analysis, Integrative Model, and Implications for Healthcare. Social Science & Medicine 180: 62–75.

Last, Murray. 1981. The Importance of Knowing about Not-Knowing. Social Science & Medicine. Part B: Medical Anthropology 15(3): 387–392.

Malinowski, Bronislaw. 1932. The Sexual Life of Savages in North-West Melanesia. London: Routledge & Kegan Paul.

Merleau-Ponty, Maurice. 1960. Signes. Paris: Morrison, JR & MA.

Nijhof, Gerhard. 2018. Sickness Work: Personal Reflections of a Sociologist. Singapore: Palgrave/Macmillan.

Nijhof, Gerhard. 2000. 'Openheid' in kwalitatieve interviews ter discussie ['Openness' in qualitative interviews discussed]. KWALON 5(1): 4–10.

Pelkmans, Mathijs. 2013a. (ed.) Ethnographies of Doubt: Faith and Uncertainty in Contemporary Societies. London and New York: I.B. Tauris.

Nijhof, Gerhard. 2013b. Outline for an Ethnography of Doubt. *In*: Ethnographies of Doubt: Faith and Uncertainty in Contemporary Societies, Mathijs Pelkmans, ed. Pp. 1–42. London and New York: I.B. Tauris.

Robbins, Joel. 2008. On Not Knowing Other Minds: Confession, Intention and Linguistic Exchange in a Papuan New Guinea Community. Anthropological Quarterly 81(2): 421–430.

Street, Alice. 2011. Artefacts of Not-Knowing: The Medical Record, the Diagnosis and the Production of Uncertainty in Papua New Guinean Biomedicine. Social Studies of Science 41(6): 815–834.

Street, Alice. 2014. Biomedicine in an Unstable Place: Infrastructure and Personhood in a Papua New Guinean Hospital. Durham and London: Duke University Press.

Van der Geest, Sjaak. 1989. Censorship and Medical Sociology in the Netherlands. Social Science & Medicine 28(12): 1339–1341.

Weber, Max. 1976 [1922]. Wirtschaft und Gesellschaft: Grundriß der Verstehenden Soziologie. Tübingen: Mohr.

Whyte, Susan Reynolds. 1997. Questioning Misfortune: The Pragmatics of Uncertainty in Eastern Uganda. Cambridge, UK: Cambridge University Press.

Wikipedia. (2020). Pyrrhonism (https://en.wikipedia.org/wiki/Pyrrhonism, accessed 10–03–2020).

# 2 Hope, Trust, Medical Action, and Care

## The Moral Challenges of Practising Medicine Today

*Sylvie Fortin and Sabrina Lessard*

> Being mortal is about the struggle to cope with the constraints of our biology, with the limits set by genes and cells and flesh and bone. Medical science has given us remarkable power to push against these limits, and the potential value of this power was a central reason I became a doctor. But again and again, I have seen the damage we in medicine do when we fail to acknowledge that such power is finite and always will be.
> *(Gawande 2014: 259)*

> More than ever, contemporary medicine has the potential for relief and torture, and this torture is, of course, always carried out in the name of possible relief.
> *(Our translation, Sicard 2012: 500)*

Isha, a 12-year-old boy, was a patient on the hematology-oncology ward in a leading pediatric hospital in Canada. He fell ill shortly after his ninth birthday and was diagnosed with leukemia. Chemotherapy and radiation proved insufficient, so Isha underwent a bone marrow transplant. Following a relapse, Isha's mother, Aanandhi[1], pleaded with the oncology team for a second bone marrow transplant although the protocol for second transplants did not favor a new graft. Aanandhi was very proactive in searching for alternate medical strategies and hoped that

1 Aanandhi, her husband (Isha's stepfather), and Isha immigrated from South America to Canada a few years ago. Aanandhi's family (her mother and brothers) also immigrated, some to Canada, others to the United States. Aanandhi, her husband, and Isha are fluent English speakers.

> Isha would eventually overcome his invasive and life-threatening illness. Her relationship with the healthcare team was somewhat tense; she did not think they were doing their best. As Isha's medical dossier (2007–2009) affirmed, "there are no curative therapies available for this unfortunate child. I (the treating doctor) hope the family will come around to our suggestion of palliative therapy." Yet support care was rejected by the family and experimental treatments resumed. The healthcare team experienced conflicting interests: those of the mother versus those of the young patient. (Field notes, Toronto, November 2009)

Isha's story and many others, as well as several encounters with healthcare providers (HCPs), gave way to the question at the core of this paper: How do HCPs portray their moral role with young and old patients where uncertainty and great illness are part of everyday life? This question is raised in a context of medical and pharmaceutical progress where the boundaries between disease-directed care and palliative care are porous. The chronicity of once lethal illnesses transforms the therapeutic project, where prolonging life is often the consensus and where death is largely concentrated in old age, although not exclusively. Questioning this moral role is also part of a societal context where "dying with dignity"[2] and autonomy are strongly valued. Beyond the promotion of a contemporary ideal, "strong democratic" values support this "dying with dignity" in the intimacy of care, as "a conception of human dignity that makes possible a journey to the edge of death" (Our translation, Hirsch 2012: 16).

When faced with bleak prognoses, doctors may resort to a palliative approach by offering active treatments that prolong life for a (short or long) time while ensuring the most comfort for their patients. They may also choose medical action as research and scientific innovation foster hope, which in turn feeds trust (leading to a bond between the family and the doctor), which feeds hope. This spiral causes HCPs to want to honor this trust and hope by outplaying the prognosis, if at all possible.

Taking care in these uncertain paths is also a challenge. In an attempt to reconfigure the patient-family-doctor relationship into one of partnership where decisions evolve horizontally, poor prognosis, technology, and trust may become allies in distancing all parties from what Gawande (2014) calls "what matters in the end". The HCPs we met with were engaged in supporting families who had to negotiate these uncertain paths and in doing so sometimes abandoned their patients. Hirsch's (2004) call for non-abandonment[3] is not an easy one. And perhaps, room must be

2 Commission spéciale sur la question de mourir dans la dignité, Assemblée nationale du Québec (assnat.qc.ca). Rapport *Mourir dans la dignité*, 2012: 11. https://numerique.banq.qc.ca/patrimoine/details/52327/2103522

3 Hirsch, French professor of medicine and medical ethics, refers to this duty of non-abandonment as a core ethical stance. It is a moral (and political) commitment required by the medical profession, if "we" are to live in an environment (such as the hospital) of solidarity, humanity, solicitude.

made for another perspective in this partnership, one that acknowledges from the onset the legitimacy of supportive care alongside disease-directed care in the area of life-threatening and life-limiting diseases. Yet, families tend to reject palliative care because it is strongly associated with end-of-life care and death. Paradoxically, if it were implicit to all who enter the realm of such illnesses that death is a possibility, life would perhaps find itself enhanced.

The overarching weight of biomedicine, the promises of research, and how this impacts the standard of care give way to a whirling spiral of healthcare drivers (Kaufman 2015)[4]. Both medical staff and families are entwined, bringing them forward into action as the only path even when (near) death is the probable outcome. Again, Gawande (2014) reminds us of our mortal condition: thinking of medicine as a support to life is perhaps a preferable ethos to that of sacrificing time now (with never-ending treatments) for time tomorrow.

The *colloque singulier* (doctor-patient bond) that frames the care provider-patient relationship is a core feature of the medical code of ethics (Hardi 2013). This bond may be challenged by emerging and ordinary therapeutic possibilities. These possibilities may also challenge the meaning of care that refers both to taking care (of someone), in relation to the other, and a therapeutic action aimed at a specific disease or bodily function (Worms 2010). Beyond medical progress, when the ultimate goal of medicine is to maintain life or not to let die, where and when can life coming to an end be acknowledged? These possibilities and in some ways the moral goals of medicine are entwined as strengths and weaknesses of this same medicine. They provide hope while distancing recognition of our common finitude. Can it be otherwise?

Much can be said regarding the moral role of HCPs. If we accept that morality refers to conceptions of right and wrong, just and unjust, acceptable and reprehensible, these conceptions are in turn based on values considered fundamental in a given environment. From these conceptions derive norms that define acceptable practices and, in so doing, we say that morals guide individual and collective practices (Massé 2015). This reminds us of the always situated character of morality (Ricoeur 2001a) or to put it differently, the local anchorage of morality and by extension the plurality of local moral worlds (Kleinman 1999). Now, if the encounter between HCPs and patients is to be a *colloque singulier* as understood by Canguilhem (2011[1966]), a perspective that is far from unanimous (Foucault 1966), this encounter is nonetheless al-

4 We are referring to Kaufman's (2015: 6–7) Chain of Health Care Drivers: (1) Biomedical research industry, (2) U.S. federal health insurance program and private medical insurance, (3) Reimbursable therapy by insurance as standard of care, (4) Standard therapies become ethically necessary and difficult to refuse. Although our local medical system (in Quebec) is public, medical insurance companies may offer better hospital facilities and give access to private ones, but they take no part in therapy management.

ways situated with a diversity of HCPs and patients at its heart. Koksvik (et al. 2022) nonetheless refer to the prominent place of action in medicine, an "action ethos" that promotes active treatment over therapeutic abstention. They also mention the sharing of information with the patient and the search for a certain horizontality in the contemporary care provider-patient relationship as an integral part of their moral role as HCPs and "taking care". When serious illness occurs, can death be part of this "taking care"?

Regarding the particular settings explored in this paper, where young and older patients as well as their caregivers are challenged by poor prognosis and end-of-life issues, how do physicians and other HCPs perceive and negotiate the tension between life now and prolonged life? How do they perceive their moral role? What is right? When is it enough? Can a "good life" embrace letting go and allowing a person to die?

In this chapter, we seek to understand the moral role of HCPs in the context of serious illness and poor prognosis. We explore the imminent moral issues of end-of-life decision-making and question whether there is a threshold at which it becomes legitimate to consider death and how this threshold defines what is "acceptable" at the end of life. These questions are supported by various ethnographic studies conducted in pediatric (Fortin) and geriatric (Lessard) settings. They allow us to consider the instability of notions of "good" or "right" in the practice (or in the moral role?) of HCPs when a patient is going through a major illness with a poor prognosis.

Thus, we invite the reader to delve into the realms of children and older adults. With children, we examine the moral role of HCPs and how this role is transcribed into practice. We then explore with the older adults how decisions about therapeutic orientation are constructed around a moral evaluation of what is considered right and enough. Finally, we offer a discussion of what we call "the moral threshold of acceptability".

## The setting

The data and thoughts shared in this paper stem from ethnographically informed studies carried out in both pediatric and geriatric settings. Fortin's work in pediatric settings across Canada (Montreal, Toronto, and Vancouver) and in France (Paris) between 2004 and 2020 focused on the many challenges of high-tech medicine, particularly in hematology-oncology and intensive care units but also in general pediatrics and palliative care. Lessard's work focused (and continues to focus) on practices surrounding older adults who were dying in a geriatric hospital ward and a long-term care (LTC) facility in Montreal (2017–2018). She is specifically interested in the moral aspects that promote or hinder end-of-life care for older adults living with multiple chronic and degenerative diseases. In contrast to the pediatric environment, where there seems to be few (or no) limits to therapeutic action, both the geriatric unit and the LTC home favor a medical posture of humility "with regard to power over life" (Collège des médecins du Québec 2008: 22) that embraces the limits of medicine, although everything seems possible in our medicalized world.

For these studies, long-term observations and (many) one-to-one interviews with HCPs and families formed the basic data. In addition, taking part in many informal discussions, various team meetings, ethics consultations, and an array of teaching activities made the hospital environment somewhat a home milieu over time. While Fortin's research topics favored collecting data over time and included diversity issues (Can the clinic be a space of plural values and norms?), both authors focused on the decision-making process when facing poor prognosis, mostly in relapse episodes among the youngest children and older adults.

In both settings, young and older patients as well as families and doctors bond in decision-making processes: in both cases, the therapeutic possibilities seem never-ending, once again illustrating that how and when to stop or when to embrace a palliative approach is a complex issue. How doctors and other HCPs perceive and negotiate this tension between life now and prolonged life may, in turn, challenge the notion of care and its ethical stance.

## Realms of the young

Advances in pediatric haemato-oncology allow glimpses of cancer as a controllable chronic illness rather than a lethal disease (Fortin and Le Gall 2022). One treatment follows another without necessarily seeking to "defeat cancer". Are we perhaps at the point where we want to defeat the finitude of life at all costs?

Even if therapies are announced as experimental, the hope they sustain seems to underscore the fact that they are ... experimental. Can a mother or father say "no" to these therapies? Is it too much to ask of them? Hope is inspired by medical quests (DelVecchio Good 2001). It is at once needed when facing poor prognosis and detrimental to generating alternate care paths from active treatment to life enhancing treatment. Hope is also nurtured by the trusting relationship, so dear to HCPs and families alike and central to the patient-family-HCP partnership, that guides the decision-making process. This trust nurtures hope: for a life to come, whatever that may be (Mattingly 2010). So, in a way, a strong family-HCP relationship as well as medical progress team up in sustaining hope that may, at some point, inhibit therapeutic options aimed at improving the patient's quality of life rather than a disease-directed approach (Sercu et al. 2018). Yet, as Fortin's fieldwork has revealed, we have both hope and sustained aggressive action, although some of this action is intended to improve life (palliative intent through active care).[5] How do HCPs perceive their moral role in such settings where disease-directed action prevails even when (near) death is the probable outcome?

## Clinicians' moral worlds

Some believe that the doctor's moral role is to dialogue with the patient, convey information, and explain possible treatment options, all the while putting the patient first.

> In my opinion, the doctor's moral role is to engage in a dialogue with the patient in which they provide [...] all the objective data available [...] not just objective elements, but elements of professional experience. And then, their moral role, in my opinion, is to ensure that the discussion with the patient includes the patient's values and experience and that in the end, a decision is more or less made and that the modalities are also more or less defined as to how this decision will be challenged if new elements appear or if people are tired with the decisions that have been made. (Dr D., senior physician, Montreal, May 2017)

It is important to listen to one's patients because the therapeutic trajectory can move depending on their understanding of the situation and their changing needs. This attention is not given once and for all, it must be situated and resituated as the clinical context changes.

We are referring to the patient, but our fieldwork indicates that it is usually the parents who want to try everything. Where is the patient's voice in such situations? Should we abandon the patient to support their parents?

Yet, according to Dr D. until recently, with the explosion of treatment options in oncology[6], doctors didn't "decide" anything. If there was a treatment protocol with proven efficacy to treat the disease, the protocol had to be applied. So the clinician's moral duty here consisted of being well versed in the medical-scientific literature. Otherwise, there was the possibility of a clinical trial. Parents, who "share a culture of innovation with us", generally tended to favor this option, he says. Thus, when faced with these two options, "we go ahead with the treatments". When there is no known treatment, a decision must be made, and "the vast majority of parents and patients choose what is possible". In doing so, "we are not abandoning the patient", we are

5 Hope as a key issue in the practice of medicine is further discussed in Fortin et al. 2021.

6 Advances that have given rise to treatments that are generally less toxic, unlike those of the past, which were usually much more toxic and deleterious for patients.

giving them a chance, however slim, to overcome the disease (for a time), especially in a new context where the toxicity of these possibilities is reduced.[7]

The moral role of the clinician is also interpreted by some as the cornerstone of any therapeutic relationship. The physician is a guide who bears a responsibility:

> It's a huge role—you can't make mistakes. Thank God, the weight and responsibility are collective—I'm not alone as a doctor [we are a team[8]], but [the fact remains that] when you're in a relationship with a patient, as soon as you're in a therapeutic relationship, you're a doctor. We're rarely 15 doctors. [...] And so, your role is a major one. You absolutely have to be aware of that. That we have a moral role. [...] We will influence. And influence in a major way. You have to be aware of that [...]. (Dr H., senior physician, Montreal, June 2017)

Similarly, a colleague stated that "this power should not be abused" while also saying that it is his duty "to honor the trust" that parents demonstrate (Dr O., senior physician, Paris, November 2019).

This responsibility extends to "bringing about acceptance", that is, communicating the possibilities:

> In fact, your major role as a doctor in this triangle, this partnership [with the family] is to get the patient (which is often easier) and the parents to accept the situation. [...] From the very beginning, you open up the possibilities [...], you inform them about everything. You want the child to get out of the situation—that's not the problem—but you inform them of the possibilities. One of the possibilities is healing. It's a possibility, okay? There is also the possibility of not being cured, the possibility of chronic illness, the possibility of death. And the more things progress, the more they evolve, the more things move towards these different possibilities. But it is absolutely necessary to make them visible, to make them meaningful. People must make these possibilities their own and they must not fight against them. (Dr H., senior physician, Montreal, June 2017)

---

7 And we remain in a curative perspective, or at the very least, in an impression of a curative trajectory.

8 (Medical) team decision-making is not discussed in this chapter. Again, in Fortin et al. 2021, we discuss this issue and affirm that voices that call for action in team meetings seem to carry more weight than others. Actually, silences in meetings generally foreshadow some kind of disagreement but it is rarely voiced as such. This is particularly so in field work that took place in Québec. In the French context, although meetings remain top down (like in Quebec), disagreements amongst physicians are generally voiced (in a lively manner) but it is unclear how treatments are furthered after these discussions take place. Our data is limited in this regard (field work having been interrupted by COVID pandemic). In light of what was collected, we could state that although alternate treatment perspectives may be voiced in team meetings, the vivid hierarchy within medicine leaves the decision to the "top" physicians.

Paradoxically, this same physician said, "if there is a one percent chance of beating the disease, we should go for it". In doing so, the recognition of death goes hand in hand with therapeutic activities that are oriented towards healing, even when this is not an illusion but a very distant possibility. Note that the cases reported here are generally not situations of first diagnosis of a disease, but rather situations of relapse (first, second, third ... after a period of remission of highly variable duration).

(Biomedical) research and clinical trials are no strangers to these postures. Subscribing to them gives rise to choices about how the patient and their family want to experience what happens next. These choices create a duty for the doctor:

> Often, of course, families are not sure how to judge the value of a certain research protocol from a scientific point of view. So, they ask me, "What would you do if it were your child?" That's the basic question, always ... and I have to answer, "It can vary depending on the disease [the doctor then hits the table], depending on research projects as well [idem]." [...] My goal is to get all three messages across palliative care, standard care, and research. And then, depending on what the family wants, I will expand on one of these aspects. [...] It's a dynamic thing, that is to say, it can vary depending on the person in the family with whom I'm talking. Also, the mum and dad, they don't necessarily have the same point of view. The child, when they're small, they're often taken out of the discussion by the parents, as they prefer to keep things between them and the doctors. But when children are older [over 14 years old in Quebec], like Arthur[9], they are able to make their own decisions, and we really take into account what they are asking for and what the parents want. (Dr T., senior physician, Montreal, April 2017)

## A few blind spots

For some, information sharing and support are the driving forces. For others, the driving force is based on the "best interests of the child" even if that means, paradoxically, going a bit against the parents' opinion (Dr D.). This best interest does not mean neglecting the duty of an alliance with the family, an alliance that is "built and rebuilt" throughout the therapeutic trajectory. To quote a nurse in a hematology-oncology care unit in Paris:

> The challenge of advanced medicine is not [only] to see the research but to see the best interest of the child first and foremost [...] and to always keep that in mind. What is in the best interest of the child? Is it that their parents be there during care or is it in the best interest of the child to tell the mother, "Well, if you

9 For an in-depth account of Arthur's story, see Fortin and Le Gall 2022.

> don't mind, please leave because things go better when you're not here". (Our translation, Angela, nurse, Paris, December 2019)

At the same time, a doctor will say without question that the pediatrician must look after the child, ensure their care, and that the parents are partners here. But if the parents are opposed to a therapeutic directive which will have an impact on the quality of care and the child's future, "the parents must be disregarded" (Dr B., senior physician, Toronto, October 2009). A colleague agrees, "I have a responsibility in society to defend the child." (Dr G., senior physician, Toronto, September 2009). However, this emphasis on the child's "protection" is not given outright, as Isha's story suggests:

> Joan [nurse] informed me that the parents, especially the mother, were always pushing for treatment. They applied for a drug in the U.S. The [medical] team had been reluctant to give active treatment for a while now and actually considered Isha [a 12-year-old boy] a palliative patient. Regarding this specific drug from the U.S., the team was against giving it because they knew it could have a severe impact on the boy (and thereby reduce his quality of life). His mum, however, insisted upon it. The nurse actually said that "she [the mother] had to do it," meaning that it was her role to fight for her child.
>
> Interestingly, Joan mentioned a few times that the boy expressed "tiredness" and "wanting to go home" to the medical team. He, however, did not express this when his mother was around, and she either did not know, or did not take it into consideration.
>
> Ultimately, Isha was given the new drug and, sadly, went into multiple organ failure, which was one of the known risks of the treatment. Joan said that he died quite quickly. (Observation notes, oncology unit, Toronto, November 2009)

In an interview, Joan stated:

> I struggle with the fact that [quantity of time prevails over quality of time]. Sometimes we are really pushing that research and pushing these medical innovations but not necessarily able to explain to families what this might look like. And that yes, there's this that might be able to give you more time, but what kind of time? I feel like that's one of our weaknesses, it's really explaining what kind of quality that child is going to have.

And regarding Isha:

> We had a patient where we all struggled with the way we had moved forward with the treatment. We knew there was no chance to cure, and we felt that the

> primary doctor was offering too many options for the family and that Isha wasn't receiving any quality of life. And the nurses struggled with that because he often voiced to us that he didn't want any more, but of course, when the physician would ask, Mum would be there, and he wanted to please Mum and he knew she wanted everything. So, we had an internal struggle. [...] I would try to share some of the comments that her child had made with her, trying to do it with as little judgement as possible, because it was very difficult, but she was ... it was ... [a difficult relationship], it wasn't the best example of a really good therapeutic relationship ... so it made it really, really challenging to have those open discussions with her. She really could not see our nursing perspective. (Joan, senior nurse, Toronto, October 2009)

When asked about the ethical challenges of contemporary hematology-oncology practice (it was 2009 at the time), a young doctor in the same unit spoke of Isha:

> I mean it's oncology, so there's ethics every day and every minute. Probably the big issues I've come across just over the last year or two are usually around either patient or family autonomy or around end-of-life care. So, you know, from an autonomy point of view, a family who doesn't want their child to know that they have cancer or who doesn't want the child to know that they're dying or etc., etc., etc., and all the sort of issues that arise from an end-of-life care point of view, when there is a disconnect between ... in a situation when a cure is no longer a feasible option for a particular child. What then is in the child's best interest when the treating team has a different idea of what that may be for the child or the family? So you know, when a cure is not an option, is giving toxic medication to give [sustain] hope appropriate? And if a family desperately wants this experimental very toxic chemotherapy to be given, even though you really don't think there is any realistic cure and you think it will just bring side effects, what do you do? (Dr G., junior physician, Toronto, October 2009)

## Realms of the older adults: Are they so different?

In the geriatric context, the incurability of disorders affecting older people who are admitted to geriatric units or LTC homes is common. While we can hope for a relative recovery, especially for people suffering from acute illnesses, or to slow down the decline of chronic illnesses, people living in these settings will not be cured of their conditions. It is around quality of life that efforts will primarily be concentrated.

Although most patients were frail older adults, palliative and end-of-life care was usually only initiated hours or days before death, when offered. According to one long-term care doctor, this "end of life" is usually more of a decision than an unequivocal state of affairs. Like him, many HCPs question what the end of life is, or at least observe the absence of clear markers that delineate it. This doctor then evoked two types of life endings: the unavoidable and the avoidable. The first results in an inevitable death, despite the care provided. The second is a death that could have been avoided if the therapeutic intensity had been different. In this second case, it is a matter of choosing not to carry out certain interventions that could have prolonged life. We may therefore consider the acute care episode as a window of opportunity as Kitzinger and Kitzinger (2013) would say, where the withdrawal or abstention from treatment leaves room for the possibility of dying.

In short, according to doctors, recognition of the end of life is a matter of clearly having no more possible therapeutic options or, alternatively, not wanting to consider possible options for prolonging life. It is the critical point where one is faced with two options and must choose between prolonging life or considering death.

Circumscribing the end of life implies distinguishing the sick from the dying, the curable from the incurable (Rossi 2010). These boundaries are shifting and porous. The passage from one category to another gives rise to a change in the person's status (and level of care) and, in so doing, affects the ways of doing and saying of the actors involved. Beyond an operational definition of the sick and the dying person, the challenge is to recognize the transition from one category to the other at the "right" moment. Thus, according to the perspective of HCPs, relatives, and sometimes, older adults, there is a critical point of what is considered right and enough where the recognition of dying becomes a moral issue. How can we recognize that life is ending beyond the clinical notion of end of life?

## Ms Moretti's story

Ms Moretti, a 90-year-old woman and with an advanced major neurocognitive disorder, refused to eat and drink. These refusals had been occurring quite frequently for a year and were usually accompanied by an infection. Her family, who was very present, demanded active care (antibiotics and artificial hydration) during each acute care episode. At a certain point, the family was considering the use of a gastric tube to allow Ms Moretti to be fed. These situations raised questions among many HCPs about the appropriateness of the interventions, especially with respect to Ms Moretti's quality of life. As a nurse stated:

> She (Ms Moretti) was a resident […] I could see that she was not able to express herself, but her family, I thought that they were very hard on her. She was given invasive treatments. You could see in her eyes, in her look, that she was tired. I found that terrible. But we can't judge, they are human after all. The doctor managed to convince the family to let her go a little bit. But it was really difficult. It was spread out over several months; there were IVs, a lot of treatments. I found it invasive to keep her alive. She had no quality of life. She stayed in bed, we got her

> up, she was entirely dependent. (Our translation, Mel, senior nurse, LTC home in Montreal, August 2017)

According to several HCPs, Ms Moretti was kept alive for a long time because her family wanted her to receive active treatment. The head of the unit and the doctor believed that it was essential to "put their foot down if her health condition deteriorated again" and speak out in favor of comfort care over active care. They had to support the family on their journey towards accepting Ms Moretti's impending death.

One doctor felt that it can be difficult to decide what to do when you don't know the wishes of the sick person.

> So, at that point, I think that we can't go completely against what the whole family wants when the person can no longer respond, especially if we don't know what that person would have wanted in that situation. [...] For example, if a family asks us to place an IV on a patient who is at the end of their life, is it inevitable that they will die? Well, obviously, if we put in an IV, we delay that deadline because we are hydrating artificially. (Dr Damato, LTC home in Montreal, September 2017)

A few days after Ms Moretti's nth refusal to eat and drink, the doctor met with the family and explained that Ms Moretti's decline was part of the normal course of the disease and that no active treatment would benefit her. End-of-life care was offered. Ms Moretti benefitted from this care for a few days before taking her last breath surrounded by her loved ones.

Although many doctors and nurses have testified to the family's central role in decision-making, the final decision remains a medical prerogative, at least for seniors. The concept of shared decision-making and partnership is ambiguous. The information shared with the family by HCPs is weighted according to what the team believes the family is able to accept.

The healthcare team's decision[10] to stop or refrain from treatment can thus give the impression that it is part of the natural course of a terminal illness. One doctor's words speak for themselves:

> It takes the guilt out of it if you tell them that this is what you think, this is where you are, this is what you should do. It's often a relief for them not to have to make that decision themselves. It's not that we decide 100 percent. Those who object will object. [...] But for others, it takes the weight off their shoulders when we decide for them. (Dr Damato, LTC home in Montreal, September 2017)

10 Decisions among members of the health care team regarding end-of-life care are generally made by consensus. However, some differences may emerge when physicians follow the wishes of families (to continue care) while nurses may not believe this is in the best interest of the patient.

In this type of situation, debate is avoided, and the decision does not have to be justified. The family defers to the recommendations of the HCPs as to the steps to be taken, and thus does not have to take part in the final decision, that is, the decision that would mean the end of their loved one's life. This mode of action, while it may be described as "paternalistic", relieves the family of the tragedy of the undecidable.

HCPs see their moral role as one of protecting the ill person who can no longer express themselves, or even of advocating for the respect of their wishes, when known or still perceived (then described as a fatigue of living). They also see it as "doing good", with respect and without judgement.

What does it mean, especially when the approaching death is not recognized by all? How does the moral role of HCPs translate into practice? What legitimizes, from a moral perspective, the option of considering death? What is the threshold that defines what is "acceptable" at the end of life?

## The moral threshold of acceptability

Isha's and Ms Moretti's stories illustrate the discomfort that some HCPs experience when active treatment continues while death looms. Isha's HCPs, however, did not challenge Isha's mother's request for the drug, nor did they warn her about the fatal consequences it could, and did, have on her son. On the other hand, in Ms Moretti's case, after several episodes of active care, the caregivers decided, by mutual agreement, to bypass the therapeutic possibilities by proposing that there was nothing more to be done. Ms Moretti was then able to live her last moments with her family while benefitting from comfort care. Does this mean that, unlike children whose lives are considered precious, the lives of older people are expendable? Isn't this sacredness, or lack of sacredness, of life, so typical of the global North and its perspective inherited from Enlightenment ideas prevalent and formed in the 18th century in the West? It is rooted in the positive connotations attributed to childhood as opposed to the negative connotations attributed to old age, which is associated with dependence, senescence, and frailty (Baker and McCullough 2009)?

According to Biehl (2013), there are categories of people who are allowed to die because of their perceived lower social status. Glaser and Strauss (1964) referred to the different social value of the dying regarding ethnic affiliation in particular, but also according to age group. More recently, Králová (2021) reiterated the inequalities in status and the impact of these inequalities on the experience of care, despite the dynamism and agency of the people concerned. Kaufman (2006: 23) also proposed that neurocognitive disorders (dementia) act "as a rationale for facilitating death."

If there is (cultural) ambivalence about whether (an older adult's) life no longer having meaning is reason enough to consider death, it is sometimes the very status of "living" that becomes difficult to pin down, define, or even justify (Soulières 2019).

And from the perspective of Lessard's field, this is not only relevant in the context of people who suffer from neurocognitive disorders, but also in the context of older people whose physical decline is very advanced.

It is this moral threshold, where it becomes more acceptable, legitimate, even desirable, for a person to die, that we wish to focus on. In our work, some people are looking for a threshold at which it would be right to stop curative treatments. Others question the very idea of having to stop, as the possibilities are now minimally toxic, or minimally invasive, reducing the notion of therapeutic overkill to nothing, or almost nothing. It is also around this threshold that "regimes of living" (Lakoff and Collier 2009), or perhaps here we could say "regimes of dying", seems to be operating to give substance to an action guide of negotiation of what is considered right and enough. Moreover, according to Broom et al. (2014), negotiation becomes more important when the lines of action are uncertain, which is particularly the case when it comes to pursuing futile treatments and redirecting care. Care, especially that which is played out at the very end of a senior's life (particularly in the case of Ms Moretti), often seems to be family-oriented to some degree. The subjectivity of the (sick) elder is relayed to the representations that the HCPs or relatives have of what is acceptable for the older person.

If this threshold is difficult to define for older adults, how can we consider this same threshold for children? How can we explain the silence of the HCPs around Isha? When does it become acceptable to tend towards a comfort perspective rather than a curative approach? Is their silence intertwined with the tension between a horizontal vision of the HCP-patient relationship rather than a vertical, top-down approach? Does this partnership with the family become deleterious to the patient at a certain point? Is it similar to the hope of a miracle treatment, however improbable? Although Du Pont-Thibodeau (2017) has demonstrated that end-of-life care is more easily proposed and implemented for babies in neonatology than for older children, Fortin's results show that action is often required for children of all ages, at least in oncology. Don't some pediatric oncologists say, "if there is a one percent chance of beating the disease, we should go for it"? Among the older adults in our study, the end-of-life stories where negotiation took place were those where the integrity of the body seemed particularly compromised and where consensus on the course of action to be taken was not a given at the outset. In all the stories documented by Lessard (2021), the legitimacy of dying was built around the threshold at which action was no longer justified, when the integrity of the body was compromised, and quality of life was absent (from the point of view of the physicians and sometimes also of the relatives).

According to Rose (2001), human existence, whether individual or collective, is based on bodily existence. This would explain why the immobile, suffering body, in great decline becomes from then on the place where the moral threshold of what is considered right and enough is manifested, at least among older adults. Among children, another dynamic seems to be at work, one in which youth and its importance in our societies prevails over everything, as in Isha's case. In this way, if the inert, lifeless body of an older person seems to flout human dignity and therefore makes death morally acceptable, it seems that this morality is less well defined among children. And even among older adults, acceptance of an impending death is often delayed and delays the care that could alleviate the suffering, if not of the family members, at least of the patient.

Suffering of the dying older person cannot be legitimized and accepted as it is no longer an obligatory passage towards a better life. Unlike with children, for whom any hope of recovery, however slight, can lead to a denial, by both physicians and parents, that the child's suffering will be endless. Hence their rejection of a perspective of care aiming at comfort and life now rather than the hope of a life after. Suffering becomes from then on either "tolerable" or "intolerable" and, thereby, a denied or legitimately accepted death (Bueno-Gómez 2017). This makes it an object that is subject to moral judgement.

The attainment of the moral threshold of what is considered right and enough is subjective; it depends on who makes the evaluation and that person's judgement. Not all HCPs have the same perspective on this moment. It is a work of interpretation that takes place over time, based on evaluation criteria that are objective and biomedical as well as subjective, such as quality of life and the patient's perceived or expressed desire to die. This evaluation is also experiential, i.e., it is part of the biographical history of the people making the judgement. This moral evaluation is also inscribed in power relationships between the different actors, care services, and types of curative or palliative medicine.

In the end, we come back to a tension that has been discussed many times in our fields of knowledge, that is, the attention paid to life in itself or to living (Fassin 2000). Despite the sustained work of HCPs with both children and older adults, this tension between life and living remains despite the progress of various policies affirming the fundamental right of people of all ages and all backgrounds to "die with dignity". The fact remains that the moral role of the various protagonists is inscribed in a plurality of worlds: at its center, there is an inalienable reminder of the unique, asymmetrical character of the clinical encounter, between the person who is suffering and the one whose knowledge and know-how are aimed at alleviating the suffering (Ricoeur 2001b). Perhaps we could simply write that "taking care" is a common value in life and death and that this taking care takes precedence in the moral field of HCPs. This care is a key notion both before and after life and dying; it is at the heart of the tension between life now and prolonged life.

## Concluding remarks

This incursion into the realms of pediatrics and geriatrics where terminal illness, life, and death are juxtaposed, reminds us of the extent to which therapeutic orientations are mixed with possibilities. In a therapeutic context that values a multiplicity of voices, we have questioned the moral role of the caregivers and, even more so, the moral roles of HCPs.

Regarding the pediatric settings, it seems that the French team, while listening to the families, remains "top down" in its intervention, taking "the best interests of the patient" to heart. The Quebec and Toronto teams, on the other hand, are more oriented towards a horizontal relationship with the family, in keeping with the "patient as partner" approach that the Quebec healthcare system holds dear. Of course, the patient is at the heart of everyone's concern, but unlike the French team, the families' choices seem to take precedence over those of the pediatric patients. Nevertheless, as Clemente (2015) observed, when faced with a poor prognosis, optimism prevails, and death is overlooked.

In both Montreal and Paris, the therapeutic orientation is still compartmentalized within the curative; there is a lack of input from those who could advocate for patients or alternative therapeutic strategies, particularly a palliative orientation. Yet, the duty of non-abandonment is an inclusive duty, attentive to a plurality of voices, capable of opening up a discussion on possibilities—not only in the field of curative care but also in that of support (Jouannet 1999). It is taking care (in all its complexities) that is at stake, care as a moral commitment, as a duty of non-abandonment.

As for the realms of the older adults, as in Ms Moretti's story, the doctors' decision to limit the curative approach spared the family the impression of giving in to death rather than doing everything possible to maintain life. If the "top down" decision-making mode used by the attending doctor can be described as paternalistic, it nonetheless provided support for the family and a way to better cope with the impending death of their loved one. "Doing good" does not necessarily mean providing active care or comfort care, but rather following an approach that must be constantly validated depending on the history of the patient and their loved ones.

However, the fact remains that both Isha's and Ms Moretti's stories give us glimpses of the encounter between young and old age in that the prolongation of life seems to be a central value that guides action when doubt hovers. This doubt may or may not be shared by all HCPs, by HCPs and the family, or by HCPs, the patient, and the family. How then can we move forward if not by recognizing a potentially dominant posture, that of taking care as a primary value? Can we think of the encounter between patient and caregiver in this light?

The discomfort of death is certain—clinicians approach it with difficulty, as do families. Could we consider death (even faintly) as a possibility alongside serious illness? And would a collaborative approach guided by horizontal relationships among HCPs be a way to do this?

In short, beyond these issues or perhaps through them, our "multi-faced relationships" to the numerous complexities of medicine further (or contribute to) our understanding of a world constantly in the making. As Kehr et al. (2018: 2) and many others have asked: "How do moral, medical, political, and economic values and norms shape health-related subjectivities and processes of subjectivation, and how do understandings and definitions of being human change accordingly?" In this way, the many challenges of medical decision-making are a window into how medical progress shapes our views on life, death, and dying. They also provide insight on medicine as a political site as well as a moral one.

## References


Baker, B. Robert, and Laurence B. McCullough. 2009. Medical Ethics through the Life Cycle in Europe and the Americas. *In* The Cambridge World History of Medical Ethics. Robert B. Baker and Laurence B. McCullough, eds. Pp. 137–162. Cambridge: Cambridge University Press.

Biehl, João. 2013. Vita: Life in a Zone of Social Abandonment. Berkeley: University of California Press.

Broom, Alex, Emma Kirby, Phillip Good, Julia Wootton, Patsy Yates, and Janet Hardy. 2014. Negotiating Futility, Managing Emotions: Nursing the Transition to Palliative Care. Qualitative Health Research 25(3): 299–309.

Bueno-Gómez, Noelia. 2017. Conceptualizing Suffering and Pain. Philosophy, Ethics, and Humanities in Medicine 12(1): 7.

Canguilhem, George. 2011 [1966]. Le normal et le pathologique. Paris: Presses Universitaires de France.

Clemente, Ignasi. 2015. Uncertain Futures: Communication and Culture in Childhood Cancer Treatment. Oxford (UK): Wiley Blackwell.

Collègue des médecins du Québec. 2008. Pour des soins appropriés au début, tout au long et en fin de vie. Montréal: Rapport du groupe de travail en éthique clinique. Collègue des médecins du Québec.

DelVecchio Good, Mary-Jo. 2001. The Biotechnical Embrace. Culture, Medicine and Psychiatry 25: 395–410.

Du Pont-Thibodeau, Amélie. 2017. Les nouveau-nés: des personnes pas comme les autres. Ph.D. dissertation, Sciences biomédicales. Montréal: Université de Montréal.

Fassin, Didier. 2000. Entre politiques du vivant et politiques de la vie: Pour une anthropologie de la santé. Anthropologie et sociétés 24(1): 95–116.

Fortin, Sylvie, Josiane Le Gall, Michel Duval, and Antoine Payot. 2021. Decision-making and Poor Prognosis: When Death is Silenced by Action. Medical Anthropology 41(2): 183–196.

Fortin, Sylvie, and Josiane Le Gall. 2022. Prolonging Life or Envisioning Death. *In* Subjectivities and Afflictions in Medical Anthropology. Angel Martinez-Hernáez and Lina Masana, eds. Pp. 81–100. Newcastel upon Tyne: Cambridge Scholars Publishing.

Foucault, Michel. 1966. Messages et bruits. Le Concours médical 43: 6285–6286.

Gawande, Atul. 2014. Being Mortal: Medicine and What Matters in the End. New York: Metropolitan Books.

Glaser, Barney, and Anselm Strauss. 1964. Social Loss of Dying Patients. The American Journal of Nursing 64(6): 119–121.

Hardi, Anne-Chantal. 2013. Du colloque singulier à l'éthique médicale. *In* Travailler à guérir. Anne-Chantal Hardi, ed. Pp. 23–24. Rennes: Presses de l'EHESP.

Hirsch, Emmanuel. 2004. Le devoir de non-abandon: Pour une éthique hospitalière et du soin. Paris: Éditions du Cerf.

Hirsch, Emmanuel. 2012. Fragilité et vulnérabilité de nos positions face à la mort. *In* Fins de vie, éthique et société. Emmanuel Hirsch, ed. Pp. 13–17. Toulouse: Éditions Érès.

Jouannet, Pierre. 1999. Principes éthiques, pouvoir médical et responsabilités du praticien. Theme issue, "Le pouvoir médical," Pouvoirs 89. Paris: Éditions du Seuil.

Kaufman, Sharon. 2006. Dementia-Near-Death and Life Itself. *In* Thinking About Dementia. Annette Leibing and Lawrence Cohen, ed. Pp. 23–42. New Brunswick: Rutgers University Press.

Kaufman, Sharon. 2015. Ordinary Medicine: Extraordinary Treatments, Longer Lives, and Where to Draw the Line. Durham & London: Duke University Press

Kleinman, Arthur. 1999. Moral Experience and Ethical Reflection: Can Ethnography Reconcile Them? A Quandary for 'The New Bioethics'. Daedalus 128(4): 69–97.

Kehr, Janina, Hansjorg Dilger, and Peter Van Eeuwijk. 2018. Transfigurations of Health and the Moral Economy of Medicine: Subjectivities, Materialities, Values. Zeitschrift für Ethnologie 143: 1–20.

Kitzinger, Jenny, and Celia Kitzinger. 2013. The 'Window of Opportunity' for Death after Severe Brain Injury: Family Experiences. Sociology of Health and Illness 35(7): 1095–112.

Královà, Jana. 2021. Social Death in 2020: Covid-19, Which Lives Matter and Which Deaths Count? *In* Death, Grief and Loss in the Context of COVID-19. Panagiotis Pentaris, ed. Pp. 77–89. London: Routledge.

Koksvik, Gitte Hanssen, Naomi Richards, Sheri Mila Gerson, Lars Johan Materstvedt, and David Clark. 2022. Medicalization, Suffering and Control at the End of Life: The Interplay of Deep Continuous Palliative Sedation and Assisted Dying. Health 26(4): 512–531.

Lakoff, Andrew, and Stephen Collier. 2009 Ethics and the Anthropology of Modern Reason. Anthropological Theory 4(4): 419–434.

Lessard, Sabrina. 2021. Pratiques (sociales) entourant le mourir des personnes du grand âge dans deux institutions publiques montréalaises. Thèse de doctorat en anthropologie. Montréal: Université de Montréal

Massé, Raymond. 2015. Anthropologie de la morale et de l'éthique. Québec: Presses de l'Université Laval.

Mattingly, Cheryl. F. 2010. The Paradox of Hope: Journeys through a Clinical Borderland. Berkeley, CA: University of California Press.

Ricoeur, Paul. 2001a. De la morale à l'éthique et aux éthiques. *In* Le Juste 2. Paul Ricoeur, ed. Pp. 55–68. Paris: Éditions Esprit

Ricoeur, Paul. 2001b. Les trois niveaux du jugement médical. *In* Le Juste 2. Paul Ricoeur, ed. Pp. 227–243. Paris: Éditions Esprit.

Rose, Nikolas. 2001. The Politics of Life Itself. Theory, Culture & Society 18(6): 1–30.

Rossi, Illario. 2010. Culture palliative: pour anticiper et accueillir la mort. Revue international des soins palliatifs 24(1): 37–43.

Sercu, Marie, Ilse Beyens, Marc Cosyns, Fien Mertns, Myriam Deveugle, and Peter Pype. 2018. Rethinking End-of-Life Care and Palliative Care: Learning from the Illness Trajectories and Lives Experiences of Terminally Ill Patients and their Family Carers. Qualitative Health Research 28(14): 2220–2238.

Sicard, Didier. 2012. Le coup de grâce. *In* Fins de vie, éthique et société. Emmanuel Hirsch, ed. Pp. 499–501. Toulouse: Éditions Érès.

Soulières, Maryse. 2019. Des personnes à part entière? Ethnographie auprès de résidents atteints de troubles neuro-cognitifs majeurs au stade avancé en centre d'hébergement. Thèse de doctorat en anthropologie. Montréal: Université de Montréal.

Worms, Frédéric. 2010. Le moment du soin. Paris: Presses Universitaires de France.

# Part II: The Techno-Sphere

# 3 Self-Tracking Practices of "Doing Health"

## Mobilizations of Data and Technological Inscriptions of (Un)Certainty

*Anna Heitger*

### Introduction

"Look", Tom says, showing me the screen of his smartphone. We are in a tiny smoothie and snacks bar in Vienna. He works here a few days a week in the late mornings. Later in the day, he will run to the fitness center where to exercise and work as a fitness coach. "Here you can see my performance on the app. And here", he scrolls down a bit, "I can see how I did yesterday... Or here, for example, I get a summary of last week. It's all in there." On the display, I see data organized into various sections with different categories such as running, walking, heart rate, calorie consumption, and so on. He scrolls so fast through the app I cannot make out many details, but at this point in my ethnographic research I am already familiar enough with the way these self-tracking apps operate: The app receives data from a wearable tracking device. In Tom's case, this is a so-called "smartwatch" he wears around the wrist. The device's built-in sensor technologies enable the recording of different kinds of bodily information, and this data is then visualized on the screen of the user's smartphone app. How does Tom engage with this data, though, what does it tell him and how does it become meaningful in practice?

Self-tracking technologies such as Tom's smartwatch give rise to quite different kinds of practices—not only because of the variety of software and hardware, or the specific bodily activity tracked and translated into data, but also because of the ways they can become meaningful as well as useful for different actors on different scales. For Tom, but also for Tessa and Sarah, who became the main participants in my research, self-tracking is first and foremost a tool for understanding one's body. More precisely, it is about understanding it *better*—as in getting closer to particular kinds of information of the body, an underlying truth that can be uncovered, accessed, and known with the help of technological mediation. To engage in self-tracking not only provides them a novel kind of knowledge about their body and its doings, but the recorded data is supposed to be used to adapt these doings, adjusting them accordingly. Self-tracking is about managing the body, taking (good) care of it.

## "Doing health"

My notion of "doing health" refers precisely to the increasing reach of the particular logic of self-tracking into the field of medicine and health: Through the systematic and purposeful quantification enabled by these technologies, the body and specific activities, states and processes become knowable in new ways which open up new possibilities for management and control of bodies. In the field of self-tracking, health becomes something that is *done* in an ongoing way. It is about *becoming* healthy, as in an ontological sense (Deleuze and Guattari 1987). Rather than a bodily property in opposition to a lack of health in a dichotomous sense, health is enacted as a project that requires specific and active doings of care.

My concern, then, is for anthropology, and for medical anthropology specifically, to take notice of the diverse current endeavors of implementing self-tracking into health care systems, to engage with the logic of managing bodies that self-tracking practices emerge from, and to take seriously actual as well as potential effects of these shifts of doing health. I contend that this shifting notion of health is becoming increasingly pervasive and normative: By developing and applying measures and measurements, doings are captured into a feedback loop; signals are recorded, quantified, and fed back to the individual to trigger a process of ongoing adjustment. The current advancements in the tech development sector result in more precise and thus more "objective" technological measurements and an increased accessibility as well as affordability of these features. But more than that, the scope of self-tracking itself is continuously expanding in critical ways through explorations of new possibilities for measurement and recording of more and more aspects of human being-in-the-world. It is thus crucial to consider the ways in which these measurements become potentially powerful and to ask what is at stake when German health insurance companies, for example, aim at implementing self-tracking technologies into their programs and policies. I argue that this altered understanding of "health-as-doing" that requires particular attention, as well as the integration of technological tools to generate knowledge and instructions on how to "do" health, emerges with/in new uncertainties about the body and its being-in-the-world. I will further explore the affectivities that emerge with self-tracking and how, in the different modes of doing health encountered in my field(s), uncertainties become mobilized and distributed across different sites.

## Methods, field sites and theoretical approach

My research on self-tracking technologies took place from 2017 to 2019 across different field sites in Vienna and Berlin. After an autoethnographic self-experiment as a first exploratory approach to self-tracking, I focused on individual practices of moving-through-the-world with self-tracking technologies. I conducted ethnographic research in Vienna over a period of three months, employing participant observation, informal conversations, and semi-structured interviews in research with several individuals who regularly engage in self-tracking. The core of my analysis of user practices builds on data from research with Tessa, Tom and Sarah who allowed me to accompany them during their tracking routines. Although they are situated in different settings and engage in different kinds of self-tracking, they are in the same age group (25 to 35 years), the three of them are able-bodied, part of the dominant white mainstream society in Austria, speak fluent German, and working as employees. Their technological knowledge and skills differ to some extent, but they must be considered as technologically savvy. All in all, they fit the ideal of the user that is configured into the technological design, which enables rather smooth interactions with their respective self-tracking technology.

In a second step, and to get a better understanding of these technologies not as given but as emerging from situated practices of technological design, I approached diverse start-ups with a focus on self-tracking technologies. I conducted semi-structured interviews and had several informal conversations with different people in three tech start-ups in 2019 in Berlin to gather insights into perspectives and practices of design. If gaining access to self-tracking start-ups within the highly competitive field of technological innovation already posed a considerable challenge, I hit an invisible wall in my attempts of "studying up" when trying to get access to stakeholders of health insurance companies, with all my interview requests to gain information on their efforts of integrating self-tracking technologies into their programs being denied. Therefore, I needed to resort to publicly accessible information, but also obtained further insights in interviews with tech designers who would discuss the issue with me.

In my analysis, I aim at bringing together different methods, field sites and more-than-human agency constitutive of the phenomenon of self-tracking. To analytically consider self-tracking in terms of practice theory proves useful insofar as it grasps different actors as parts of practices instead of assuming human-technology relationality either in terms of individual autonomy or technological determinism. Instead, a practice theoretical lens allows for considering the ways in which different kinds of technologies, subjectivities, and bodies come into being with/in practices. To conceptualize the human-technology interface, I furthermore found the notion of the "script" particularly helpful. Madeleine Akrich (1992) proposed to think of technological design as script: Technologies are scripted with implicit assumptions, values, understandings, but most importantly with instructions for doings, for how to engage with the technology in question. The script-approach has been further developed by various scholars concerned with the ways in which technologies through their design delegate competencies, actions and responsibilities, and the ways these scripts are potentially challenged and re-scripted (see for example Oudshoorn et al. 2004). Suchman (2007), in turn, describes what she calls the *strategic vagueness* of the technological script, in contrast to a more *pre*scriptive-like understanding of the concept. In my analysis, I mobilize this approach to consider the ways in which self-tracking technologies become scripted with/in design, and to consider the affordances of these technological scripts in emerging practices of usage and the multiple kinds of doings they evoke.

## Self-tracking in practice: Data discussion

Drawing on ethnographic material on self-tracking in both user and designer practices, I focus specifically on doing health as a meaningful mode of engagement with/in self-tracking practices. After a short discussion of the term self-tracking (2.1), I will discuss emerging self-tracking practices as they mobilize self-tracked data (2.2), particular doings of health and the ways these are scripted into technological design (2.3), and finally provide insights into ongoing projects of implementing self-tracked data into health care and health insurance in the German context (2.4). In the last part (2.5), I interrogate my material specifically in terms of the affectivities and multiple kinds of uncertainties that emerge with/in self-tracking technologies.

### Introducing the phenomenon of self-tracking

What exactly *are* self-tracking technologies and what kind of self-tracking practices am I discussing in this paper?

To describe self-tracking as a set of dispersed yet interrelated technologies, practices, and increasingly also policies, has proven a peculiar task since the very beginning of my research. When I started looking into the field of self-tracking in 2017, I had only a vague idea of something of the kind of a smartphone app you use to track how many steps you walk a day. The phenomenon I will call self-tracking here is discussed under varying terms—such as "quantification of the self" or "lifelogging", with of course diverse German translations of these terms. This was certainly a challenge for my research regarding literature and public media discourse as well as setting up the field research, but it also says something important about the heterogeneous and fragmented character of these technologies: They emerge not necessarily as a novel innovation but find their way into standard smartphones, sports gear, and even into items as familiar as a wristwatch. The idea of tracking activities or tasks itself is not radically new, and thus affords for smooth and often almost unnoticeable integration into everyday activities. I found that indeed many people make use of self-tracking functions without identifying or thinking about these practices as self-tracking—the most prominent example being the step tracking function that does not require any additional knowledge or equipment. Tom and other individuals I encountered in my research who engage in self-tracking practices in a purposeful and in an elaborated way just refer to the name of the app, or of the brand of the technology they use. Technology developers, in turn, situate their work within fields such as fitness, lifestyle or the medical sector, for example, but not necessarily in terms of self-tracking in an explicit way.

The lack of an encompassing term points to the fact that these technologies are dispersed across different scales, actors, and practices rather than comprising a coherent field with a specific directionality. Indeed, the scope of self-tracking seems to be expansionary, towards increasingly elaborate tracking of activities, bodily states and processes also with/in practices in the field of medicine and health. The notion of self-tracking as a perspective on the abstract entirety of these phenomena has proven a useful tool for my analysis of the particular logic these emerge with/in. And while some of the readers might have already had an idea of what self-tracking is about, it is crucial to notice the elusive ways in which these technologies operate as they emerge with/in diverse and fragmented practices and policies across different sites.

Thereby, public discussion, evaluation and critique are largely averted, or at least significantly delayed (see also Farrington and Lynch 2018: 5)—while the size of the billion-dollar market of data-generating technologies rapidly increasing (Matthewman 2018: 34). All the more important it is to put a spotlight on self-tracking practices and the notions of health they emerge with/in. The recent years have seen a rise of scholarly engagement with these novel forms of data generation and evoked critical analyses of what has been called "datafication" (e.g., Lupton 2016, Sumartojo et. al. 2016, Schüll and Ruckenstein 2017) of various aspects of life. While Lynch and Farrington (2018) propose a framing of data tracking technologies as "personal medical devices" in their anthology "Quantified Lives and Vital Data" and my analysis tries to center the very practice(s) of self-tracking, in which these technologies emerge—rather than taking these as point of departure. Arguably, the logic of self-tracking largely evades established boundaries of what is considered "medical" and instead alters practices of doing health across diverse contexts and fields.

## Mobilizations of data at the human-technology interface

Self-tracking technologies measure, record, and capture signals from the body and turn them into data points that become accessible on different types of screens, e.g., smartphones or smartwatches. From the ongoing flow of being-in-the-world, individual units of an embodied being-in-the-world emerge as data points in this kind of measurement. This has an intriguing effect on the temporality of being-in-the-world: These units of being-in-the-world emerge as data points allocated within seconds, minutes, days, weeks, and years and effectively establish being within a linear temporality. As these recordings happen ongoingly, single data points within time accumulate into data sets, retrievable at any given moment—such as the moment described above of Tom showing me the data in his self-tracking app. Different kinds of statistics and other visual analyses organize information into data in meaningful ways. Specifically, these accumulations of data over time are rendered meaningful through generating notions vital to self-tracking practices such as "progress" and "improvement". Similar to Tom's description of how he had been able to improve his fitness performance through self-tracking, Tessa explains in one of our interviews how tracking with a wearable chest strap device helped to improve her running routine:

> In the four years I've been using the app, I've already improved my running speed significantly. But I'm also keeping track of my heart rate and other health factors, you know? And I can always monitor my running routine, you see. Because speed is not the only relevant factor, you have to consider the conditions of the running track, too... like, are there changes in altitude, elevation, ground condition, and so on. Therefore, I get a much better picture of what I'm actually doing, how I'm actually improving and how I can really get better.

The particular dynamic that emerges between the individual and the technological measuring can be understood in terms of a cybernetic logic as feedback-controlled systems (Haraway 1991: 164). Having emerged in the cold war era, cybernetics seem to continue shaping contemporary imaginaries of how technological and human entities interact through design. What is more, it continues shaping tech development practices: Data is established as a common language as medium of regulation between the technology and the body. For example, Tessa describes one situation: Running uphill, she *could sense* how she was running at the same speed, but when she took a look at her app, the data showed her she had "actually" become slower. Here, the distinct quality of the data becomes manifest: The measurements generated by the self-tracking technology Tessa makes use of act as "objectifying data" (Mol 2002: 63). The subjective sense of her being-in-the-world is subordinated to technologically-generated measurements of being-in-the-world. Self-tracking data, in this sense, act as "facts" about the body and the embodied being. In the practices I observed in my research, engaging with these technologically generated "facts" *does* something important in user practices—yet the doings evoked might not necessarily follow the script that is envisioned by tech developers and built into the design.

## Self-tracking practices of "doing health" and processes of responsibilization

Sarah uses a smartwatch like Tom and regularly engages with the data generated through the recording of signals emitted by her body. However, the only data she makes meaningful for herself is the number of the steps she takes during a day:

> Technically, the watch tracks a lot more than the step count, there's an app where you can see all this data, your improvement over time and so on. But so far, I've not even opened the app, I turned off all notifications of the app on my phone. I just need to know the numbers of steps... and these I can easily see on the watch.

Sarah's self-tracking practice does not emerge with/in purposeful physical exercise per se, but rather shapes her moving-through-the-world in significant ways: In her day-to-day life, she engages with the step tracking data, as displayed on the smartwatch screen. Although she affirms that she regularly works out two to three times per week, the only technologically mediated measure relevant to her is the amount of physical movement in her everyday urban life:

> It is a fact that even the most intense training routines cannot make up for a lack of movement in your everyday life. So for example, if I see that I'm still far from my daily goal, maybe I'd walk home instead of taking the bus, or I'd make an extra detour around the block. But I won't let myself go crazy if I don't achieve my steps, either.

The number of steps she takes during a day becomes meaningful for Sarah's practice of doing health as actions that are understood in terms of "choices" within her everyday life, as deliberate decisions she needs to take anew every day through monitoring her performance on the watch. If self-tracking technologies are understood in terms of a script that provides specific instructions for actions, we can see here how a re-scripting of self-tracking is enabled at the technological interface: Sarah never opens the app, she does not care to *know* the data beyond the daily step count produced by her smartwatch. She also takes off the smartwatch at night, even if it could track her sleep cycles. For Tom, on the other hand, the information his smartwatch produces about the quality of the bodily recovery during sleep is important because of what it means for his performance during the daytime. He tells me he had to stop using the wearable at night at some point, however: Knowing his sleep was being tracked made him anxious about the data he was producing by just lying still and made him wake up all the time to check the app.

In contrast to narratives of technological domination and control, the self-tracking practices that emerge here are situated within particular local and temporal contexts as they all bring about different practices of doing health: Tessa uses self-tracking to monitor her running routines as doing health but does not use self-tracking devices throughout the day. Tom engages with the data from his smartwatch in multiple doings, from sleep to lifestyle to physical exercise. Sarah, in turn, uses only one specific aspect of self-tracking that becomes meaningful to her doing health. In my research, it has furthermore become apparent that self-tracking practices are not stable but shifting over time, and are not absolute either. Rather, they are caught up in ongoing processes of negotiation as individuals navigate self-tracking as what could in a Foucauldian sense be understood as "technologies of the self" (see for example Foucault 1997) that link "practices of political government to forms of self-government" (Lemke 2021: 105).

Turning now to practices of design, it is precisely the fragility and indeed the ephemerality of self-tracking in practice(s) that I found tech developers to rather lack a sense of. As already indicated above, self-tracking technology designers configure the user as dutifully engaging with the tracked data and adjusting behavior accordingly in an ongoing way. For them, the objective is both clear and implicit in its normativity: It is about navigating choices and actions in such a way that it fosters the imperative of becoming healthy and to engage in doings I describe as doing health.

Alberto, CEO of a start-up that develops a medical self-tracking technology for the management of body fluids, and in particular of water intake, explains to me:

> There are several reasons why some of our patients need to monitor their water supply—they either drink not enough or too much. Now, we wanted to invent a technology that allows them to do that outside the hospital, to continue to check their water intake, so that they do not have to be hospitalized once again. This way, serious complications and emergencies can be avoided, and, you know, the patients wouldn't have to come back to the hospital all the time to get their water levels back on track.

In this logic, relationalities between different entities emerge as continuous feedback loops (Orr 2006: 107–110) in which signals emitted by one entity are captured by the other and translated into data points, that are transmitted as feedback to the first entity, back again, and so on. Central to this notion is an assumed mechanism of automatic regulation that leads to increased stability of the system: Alberto implicitly expects the future patients of this body fluid management app to use the information to adjust their water intake accordingly in an ongoing way. Thus, the information provided by self-tracking technologies and the novel kind of knowledge that is produced is not neutral and *is* not per se. Rather, it mobilizes with/in a feedback system of constant adjustment of activities and behavior that is already scripted into the design. Alberto's imaginary patient is in a constant process of adjusting water intake as it is recorded by the technology to the desired percentage deemed "healthy" by fine-tuning her doings, i.e., her drinking habits.

In my research, I paid particular attention on how these objectives become scripted into the technological design as imperatives that in user practices will not control but nevertheless significantly shape the emergent doings of health. There is much to say about "the user" that becomes "inscripted" into technological design and its politics—about the implicit gendering, classing, racialization, but also about simple access to the necessary infrastructures (see for example Matthewman 2018: 34). Beyond that, Suchman (2007: 188) has criticized the ways in which individuals are identified exclusively within the relationality to the technology in question, which results in a singularization of the multiplicity of user identities. And indeed, the logic employed by the start-ups I conducted research with, follows such an understanding of the user identified through a problem that needs to be solved and can be managed by being captured within the feedback loop of self-tracking technology. In my conversations with the founder and CEO of a start-up that operates a lifestyle app, the ways in which the technological design implicitly configures not only "the user" but "health" as well became apparent. In the first interview with Norbert, he describes the app's approach as "gamification of health". On a white board, he starts by drawing a horizontal line and explains:

> Here on both ends, you see the extremes, so to say. Here are the unhealthiest, and on the other side the healthiest. These two groups on the outer sides have to be understood as separate groups—they need programs that are specialized for them. But those from the middle, you see, where we would locate actually the majority of people, they can still change their habits and become healthier, do *more* for their health.

What Norbert describes here is an important development in the way the notion of "health" shifts: Within processes of increasing commodification of health, subjects are configured as individuals in terms of consumers that need to navigate not only uncertain futures in terms of the individual at risk, but also the ontological uncertainty of its being in the present. Hence, individuals that previously would have been deemed "healthy" are now being recruited into practices of doing health via different tools of responsibilization, such as the self-tracking technology in question. The implicit imperative is to care for new kinds of knowledge, to engage with bodily data and to adapt and adjust doings to actively counteract the onset of disease and deterioration of the body—which reminds of Rose's (2007) notion of the "vital politics" of our time that are "concerned with our growing capacities to control, manage, engineer, reshape, and modulate the very vital capacities of human beings as living creatures" (2007: 3).

Yet, the imagined automatized regulatory mechanism at the interface of human and technology is not self-evident, but the product of both technological design as well as affective work done by individuals engaging with it: For an individual to look at self-tracked data certainly does not automatically result in an adaptation of doings. The ability to read and understand statistics and visualizations, to relate these to activities and sensed embodied doings, and to modify ongoing doings accordingly must be understood as a task that is indeed demanding and preconditional and in which affectivities and particular kinds of knowledge are mobilized into particular directions—that may or may not match with the configured use. However, self-tracking technologies need to be taken seriously as tools of responsibilization of the individual, and as producing particular practices of doing health—especially in view of current efforts to materialize an integration of self-tracking into health care policies.

## Emerging regimes of "doing health" in insurance policy

The current efforts of health insurance companies in Germany to implement self-tracking technologies reflect an increasing inclination of policymakers to employ technological solutions, and most prominently, wearable devices, for healthcare challenges (Farrington and Lynch (2018: 4). These efforts must be interpreted within ongoing processes of commodification of health and responsibilization of the individual subject as means of biopolitical control: Self-tracking emerges as technological "fix" to "problems" that are presumedly linked to particular kinds of "lifestyle" in urban environments and increasingly sedentary routines, and that can be prevented by doing health in an ongoing way—thus building on a rather mechanical model of social life in a rather patronizing manner (Layne 2000: 493).

While in Austria the attempts to implement self-tracking data into health care seems to be in its early days at the most, developments are more advanced in the German context. Here, almost every health insurance provider is already running different kinds of so-called "bonus programs", which serve as feature of distinction and competition between health insurers on the market. These developments, however, seem to happen outside of political influence of the state as well as far from public discussion about how these processes might put into question the principle of solidarity and equal access to health insurance. With these programs, the insurant can receive a reward or compensation in turn for engaging in different activities, such as attending preventive check-ups. This approach to health care recruits individuals into doings of health that supposedly benefit the individual's quality of life—and at the same time and perhaps more importantly, it is discursively represented as a cost-saving measure from the point of view of health insurance companies.

Whereas the bonus programs were previously conducted through paper booklets, the implementation of self-tracking data is part of a shift towards digitalization of these programs and health care in general. Nowadays, companies increasingly encourage the use of self-tracking, for example by offering to subsidize the acquisition of a self-tracking device. One of the start-ups I had contacted was developing a so-called "white label app" to be integrated into such bonus programs—referring to an app they develop and sell to health insurance companies so that these can brand and provide the app as their own. Back in 2019, Norbert not only told me they were in negotiation with diverse health insurance companies, and that just a few days before our interview, they had been able to finalize negotiations for one specific bonus program. He tells me:

> Ultimately, the goal for health insurance companies is to achieve the shift from a cost reimbursement provider to a health service provider. Not to just pay when the insurant gets sick. But as for today, there's a considerable lack of touchpoints between insurers and insurants—and especially between insurers and their healthy insurants. This is why we need to create what we call touchpoints between the insurer and the insurant. If not, we run the risk of losing the insurants, because nowadays, who hold these digital touchpoints already are Apple and Google Health and the like.

He argues that the growing reach of self-tracking technologies of both Apple and Google Health—both platforms that enable the collection of self-tracked data from different devices into one site—hold a monopole on health data of individuals on a global scale. This, according to Norbert, poses a significant risk and debilitates the position of health insurance companies even more. In order to "keep up" with these developments, he continues, German health insurance providers need to generate their own "touchpoints" to their insurants. Within this ongoing shift of the configuration of the individual—from citizen to consumer—health emerges as a product, and indeed, as *producible.* It would seem as if the notion of "health" that is mobilized here would become broader and more encompassing. However, self-tracking technologies through their design pre-scribe doings of health in very particular ways, so that it seems as if the actual modes of being healthy, and what being healthy means, are in fact narrowed down.

A crucial insight from my research on user and designer practices is that the discrepancy between user configurations produced by tech developers and actual doings of self-tracking in user practices does not come to matter: Take for example Sarah, who might not engage with the tracked data beyond her step count. The tracked data produced by her doings will be fed back into the tracking technology nonetheless, and will become interpreted as if she *was* following the script, so to say. As the data generated in self-tracking practices of users is fed back into the technological design, practices of design are caught up in their own preconfigured feedback loops. The information recorded in user practices cannot be analyzed outside of the technological script, but instead always further reproduces the user configurations it entails; no matter how they are done and possibly re-scripted in practice. As these technological scripts enact a cybernetic logic, even "disobedient" doings, e.g., ignoring instructions, doing activities in the wrong way, or even "lying" by feeding the app with inaccurate data, are simply rendered data points fed back into the system. The "terms and conditions" of self-tracking, so to say, are already established by design and closed to any kind of critique or resistance from within, while the heterogeneous and fragmented nature of these technologies also avert public discussion and debate from the outside, as described before. However empowering they might be as individual strategies for navigating the increasing imperative of doing health, power is distributed rather unequally. That is not to position tech developers as "data-rich" actors holding power as opposed to users as "data-poor" actors in a homogenizing way, as Schüll and Ruckenstein (2007) have warned against. Indeed, designers themselves have to be understood as situated in a highly competitive and fragmented field of tech development, in which they navigate complex affordances in their respective niches. If power becomes bundled, however, into platforms on a larger scale, the risk is that engaging with self-tracking technologies becomes less a possibility for individuals to navigate their being-in-the-world, but an imperative with potentially (socio)material consequences.

## Affectivities and uncertainties of self-tracking practices

In this final part, I will describe more in detail the affectivities mobilized in self-tracking practices as well as the uncertainties they emerge with, and ask how these become distributed across diverse practices, actors and bodies.

I have before shown the ways in which self-tracking technologies become powerful as they produce being with/in a linear temporality and notions of being-in-the-world as a task of ongoing development which becomes normatively charged in terms of "improvement". The doings of user practices produce a subject that is temporally tethered between the past that becomes enacted through data of past doings, and between the future that becomes discernible through the visualizations and statistics. The future is in constant doing, so to say—*becoming* with every new data point that is generated. This is a kind of future directionality that differs from an anticipatory mode, which in the Anthropocene has become a dominant mode of exerting control (see for example Adams et. al 2009): Here actions in the present are directed at predicted or envisioned problems in the future—not to prevent but to navigate them. In self-tracking doings of health, in contrast, "the future" does not as such emerge as point of reference in. The meaning of doing health is produced by actions carried out in the past that are recorded, analyzed and directed towards a possible future through adaptation and adjustment of subsequent actions in an ongoing manner.

Self-tracking technologies that provide predictions of specific kinds of risk such as the body fluid management app, evoke the future in terms of a statistical risk that needs to be navigated—and indeed becomes possible to be navigated—within self-tracking. Here, what is at stake is a specific health concern that comes with a measurable risk. Yet, in technologies that are directed more at evoking doing health as a more encompassing practice, there is no one specific health concern and therefore no specific risk that is being mobilized. What is at stake is the individual's health in the sense of a general wellbeing. If the future health of the individual in this logic is understood as the sum of actions and decisions, each moment in time is important as it produces a consolidation of the kind of health that is done. To engage in self-tracking, then, is to gain control over these ongoing doings, and to decide the directionality of the process of doing health such as Tom, Sarah and Tessa do. They engage with their self-tracked information about how to shape their doing health properly. While the past appears as already written—as data that is retrievable at any given moment—and not changeable anymore, the possibility for action is located in the very present. In this way, self-tracking technologies open up possibilities for adjusting these doings in order to produce health. In this way, potentialities that might be interpreted in terms of hope in a nonspecific, general sense emerge.

The body, in these practices, is rendered the site of concern, and simultaneously as site for doing health. The body itself, but more importantly habits and behavior patterns that are understood as inherently embodied are rendered malleable through measurement. The self-tracked body becomes a hybrid of recordings of bodily information and averages: The information captured by tracking technologies is interpreted, related and analyzed against established standard measures and norms, e.g., optimal water intake, normal heart rate, average of the body mass index (BMI). Uncertainties about the body, its processes and states, become possible to navigate with/in the feedback loops provided by self-tracking devices. On one occasion, Tessa describes how she "didn't have a feeling" for her own body before she started engaging in self-tracking practices. To be able to sense the body subjectively is not enough and indeed misleading, in this logic. In self-tracking, ongoing doings thus become "choices" and "decisions" that get recorded by the tracking device and subsequently fed back to the individual to reflect upon, which in a sense render productive this uncertainty.

Self-tracked data as new kind of knowledge about the body, and ontological uncertainty about the sense of the self as result of not-knowing emerge together with an uncertainty about control and determination of ongoing doings. While the technological recording of signals detected from being-in-the-world generates new knowledge as grounds for further doings, they come with new uncertainties that pertain the tracking itself: Tom, for example, explains to me that the tracking achieves only a very close approximation. He tells me the error rates of different self-tracking devices which he apparently knows by heart. When I ask what this uncertainty about the accuracy does to his practices, he shrugs and says it is such a minimal inaccuracy, it does not matter. And indeed, beyond this single instance, I found that this technological uncertainty does not come to matter in self-tracking practices: The data produced by the self-tracking device is taken as "fact" as it mobilizes further doings. When Tessa, as described above, tells me how the data on the app made her "realize" she had become slower even if she felt she was running at the same speed, the data is enacted as "fact". In relation to the data-as-fact, uncertainty, here, is shifted to her embodied measurement, to her subjective sense of self—instead of causing her to question the accuracy of the information her app displays, for example. This observation is reinforced by statements such as "any training session that is not recorded is no training session", as Tessa explained to me. Only what is tracked by the app is certain and can become meaningful as "fact" about being-in-the-world.

Tech developers do not render meaningful the uncertainties of their technologies either but take the data as "facts" as well, even if they know about uncertainties. Not only do they know about the rate of inaccuracy of their technologies. They also know which standards and the norms they script into the design, and about the potentially uncertain nature of these averages that themselves are subject of modification according to new evidence. When I asked Norbert, the CEO of the lifestyle app, about the possibility to "trick" the app by feeding it with inaccurate information, he laughs and says:

> If someone can really be bothered by lying to the app by entering false information, then so be it. But, you know, you would be betraying yourself. So I can hardly imagine anyone doing this.

The uncertainty about the compliance of users is disregarded and explained away by resorting to the commitment-producing technological script—and becomes eliminated insofar as within the feedback loop, the tracked data is taken as "fact" in tech development processes of further refining and personalizing the technological design. Within this kind of previously described inbuilt automatic regulation, uncertainties become distributed in unequal ways and potentially override and overrule divergent ways of being, sensing, and measuring.

Affectivities of hope and normative understandings of health intersecting with new kinds of information provided by self-tracked data can be potentially empowering for the individual. The ongoing shift towards digitalization is also a shift of personalization of medicine and health care, in which self-tracked data as objectifying knowledge about the body, habits and behavior are becoming more important. This potentially renders the individual as their own "expert" vis à vis generalizing medical knowledge. However, not only is this potential expertise intrinsically produced by a technology scripted according to understandings and desires of tech developers that are well beyond control and contestation by the individual user, but also do the current developments of integrating self-tracked data into health insurance policies indicate a shift in authority, expertise and ownership of the tracked information and data away from the individual. From the side of designers and stakeholders, the openness and malleability of the body is produced with a different kind of hope about the technological manageability of bodies and the health care they need. As already described above, this functional understanding of bodies and individuals as citizens, consumer and part of the labor force reinscribes responsibility for doing health into the subject. It is interesting to consider the fact that the particular notion of "health" emerging from the "problems" self-tracking technologies set out to tackle is increasingly narrow. It might seem a shift towards a more encompassing, holistic approach to health, but it appears that instead, more and more aspects of being-in-the-world become integrated, or "medicalized", in a sense, all the while the particular ways of how to be healthy are increasingly deterministic. An increasing integration of self-tracking technologies into health insurance and health care as outlined above, of course, could further this shift considerably and capture actors, bodies and doings within preconfigured and scripted feedback loops.

Yet another aspect of uncertainty pertains to the question of how exactly insurants as well as insurance companies can benefit from the implementation of these "bonus programs" and the integration of self-tracking technologies, insofar as there is no actual evidence for most of the activities that are promoted as doing health within these practices—or at least not yet. For example, a causal relation between the health of an individual and taking 10.000 steps per day could not yet proven (see Reynolds 2021). In practices of design, these objectives are established at some point, but might not actually correspond to medical insights or the most recent evidence. What is achieved through self-tracking technologies as tools of responsibilization, however, is a recruitment of individuals into doing health as something controllable and adjustable into any desired directions.

## Conclusion

In this chapter, I presented ways of doing health in self-tracking practices emerging with/in processes of increasing urbanization and changing lifestyles, shifting landscapes and bodies leading to critical conditions for human being-in-the-world in late capitalism. Self-tracking as "technology of the self" makes productive the feedback loop of recording bodily information rendered into measurable units and reporting it back as "data" to the individual. I have proposed an understanding of self-tracking practices in their ephemerality that resists conceptualizing the identities of individuals identified as users as fixed, and their practices as coherent, cohesive, and stable. My empirical data has shown practices that are more or less established at the moment of my research, yet emphasized the constant work they require—practices that now, five years later, most probably have shifted in some way or another, that might have become refined, suspended, or abandoned.

In reference to the empirical material, I have discussed the ways in which self-tracked data becomes mobilized into particular doings, and specifically into what I identify as ways of doing health that are directed towards navigating ontological uncertainties about the state and the future of the body and embodied being-in-the-world. Self-tracking technologies enable these doings insofar as they generate objectifying data that opens up possible lines for further doings. As they become powerful tools of responsibilization of individual subjects, an interrogation of the technological script is crucial—even more so in view of ongoing processes of integrating self-tracked data into health insurance companies. The understanding of health that becomes mobilized is shifting from a notion of health as property or state of being towards a more encompassing and indeed ongoing notion of health as doings intrinsically contextualized within linear temporalities. Within this shift and the possibilities enabled by self-tracking technologies to navigate doings of health, affectivities of hope emerge in an open-ended, nonspecific mode. Finally, I have argued that ontological uncertainties about the body and the embodied being-in-the-world, novel technologies and new kinds of knowledge emerge together. Through processes of technologization that are critical to contextualize with/in shifting notions of health, they are distributed in unequal ways across sites, actors, and bodies.

In my attempt to contextualize the ongoing developments in self-tracking technologies and the ways in which these emerging imperatives of doing health become mobilized, these processes can be interpreted in continuity with a logic of cybernetics and a functional understanding of bodies and populations, an increasing individualization, responsibilization and economization of health. It is also interesting to read these processes against new kinds of uncertainties that emerge in the Anthropocene—a growing sense of the porosity of bodies within social and ecological environments, and multiple kinds of evidence from microbiome science or epigenetics, for example, leading to a shifting understanding of human-environment relations in which boundaries between the human and the more-than-human are critically blurred (see for example Heitger et al. 2021). If self-tracking technologies and the re-inscription of choice of an assumed individual human subject are understood as project of (re-)establishing control of bodies and their life conditions in an intrinsically anthropogenic world, their future is more than uncertain.

## References

Adams, Vincanne, Michelle Murphy, and Adele E. Clarke. 2009. Anticipation: Technoscience, Life, Affect, Temporality. Subjectivity 28: 246–265.

Akrich, Madeleine. 1992. The De-Scription of Technical Objects, *In* Shaping Technology/Building Society: Studies in Sociotechnical Change. Wiebke E. Bijker and John Law, eds. Pp. 205–224. Cambridge, MIT Press.

Deleuze, Gilles, and Félix Guattari. 1987. A Thousand Plateaus: Capitalism and Schizophrenia. Minneapolis: University of Minnesota Press.

Farrington, Conor, and Rebecca Lynch. 2018. Personal Medical Devices: People and Technology in the Context of Health, *In* Quantified Lives and Vital Data: Exploring Health and Technology through Personal Medical Devices. Rebecca Lynch and Conor Farrington, eds. Pp. 3–16. London: Palgrave Macmillan.

Foucault, Michel. 1997. Technologies of the Self. *In* Michel Foucault: Ethics, Subjectivity and Truth. The Essential Works of Michel Foucault, 1954–1984, Vol. I. Paul Rabinow, ed. Pp. 223–251. New York: The New Press.

Haraway, Donna. 1991. A Cyborg Manifesto: Science, Technology, and Socialist-Feminism in the Late Twentieth Century. New York: Routledge.

Heitger, Anna, Sabine Biedermann, and Jörg Niewöhner. 2021. More-Than-Human Eating: Reconfiguring Environment | Body | Mind Relations in the Anthropocene. Berliner Blätter 84: 35–48.

Layne, Linda. 2000. The Cultural Fix: An Anthropological Contribution to Science and Technology Studies. Science, Technology, & Human Values 25(4): 492–519.

Lemke, Thomas. 2021. The Government of Things: Foucault and the New Materialisms. New York: New York University Press.

Lupton, Deborah. 2016. The Quantified Self: A Sociology of Self-Tracking. Cambridge Malden, MA: Polity.

Matthewman, Steve. 2018. Theorising Personal Medical Devices. *In* Quantified Lives and Vital Data: Exploring Health and Technology through Personal Medical Devices, Rebecca Lynch and Conor Farrington, eds. Pp. 17–43. London: Palgrave Macmillan.

Mol, Annemarie. 2002. The Body Multiple: Ontology in Medical Practice. Durham: Duke University Press.

Orr, Jackie. 2006. Panic Diaries: A Genealogy of Panic Disorder. Durham: Duke University Press.

Oudshoorn, Nelly, Els Rommes, and Marcelle Stienstra. 2004. Configuring the User as Everybody: Gender and Design Cultures in Information and Communication Technologies. Science, Technology, & Human Values 29 (1): 30–63.

Reynolds, Gretchen. 2021. Do We Really Need to Take 10,000 Steps a Day for Our Health? New York Times. https://www.nytimes.com/2021/07/06/well/move/10000-steps-health.html (last accessed: 30.03.2023).

Rose, Nikolas. 2007. The Politics of Life Itself: Biomedicine, Power and Subjectivity in the Twenty-First Century. Princeton: Princeton University Press.

Schüll, Natasha, and Minna Ruckenstein. 2017. The Datafication of Health. Annual Review of Anthropology 46: 261–278.

Suchman, Lucy. 2007. Human-Machine Reconfigurations: Plans and Situated Actions. Cambridge: Cambridge University Press.

Sumartojo, Shanti, Sarah Pink, Deborah Lupton, and Christine Heyes LaBond. 2016. The Affective Intensities of Datafied Space. Emotion, Space and Society 21: 33–40.

# 4 Precarious Lives, Uncertainty and the Politics of Hope

## Engaging With Novel Therapies for Blood Disorders in India

*Sangeeta Chattoo*

## Introduction

This chapter explores the local, experiential context within which those affected by or caring for a child with thalassaemia choose a particular, so called, *novel* therapy, involving the use of thalidomide and hydroxyurea, which remains controversial within clinical literature and practice. Thalassemia is an inherited blood disorder that causes serious chronic anaemia. The novelty of this treatment circulates within a wider political economy of hope (Good et al. 1990; Novas 2006). A lack of consensus in clinical practice on the safety and efficacy of thalidomide in treating thalassaemia brings home the significance of the hierarchy of methods through which evidence is selected to legitimise innovation and change. However, the processes of (re)constitution and regulation of clinical trials is not the focus of discussion here. Instead, the aim is to analyse the motivations and therapeutic journeys of those seeking this novel treatment despite uncertainty of outcomes and significant financial costs. Theoretically, the analysis hinges on the concepts of potentiality and precarity with uncertainty/hope as the mediating term—drawing our attention to the "ordinary, chronic and cruddy" aspects of everyday milieu within which the materiality of the disease, illness and caring are negotiated (Das 2015; Povellini 2011: 13).

Scientific controversies surrounding the legitimisation and routinisation of new technology and medical interventions can be placed within the remit of "an anthropology of potentiality in biomedicine", following Taussig et al. (2013: S3–S12; also see Bharadwaj 2018, among others). In their eloquent Introduction to the special issue of *Current Anthropology* (2013), they trace etymological roots of potentiality in Greek (*potentia*) and early Latin (*potens/ potence*) implying power/ force/ possessor/ possible/ capable and so on. Interestingly, "potentiality of the negro" was a phrase appropriated during the civil rights movement between the 1960s and 1970s. Hence, the very act of framing something as potential (or controversial) is a political act, invoking ethical choices about how we engage with life and death, health and well-being. The historical shifts in our understanding of an embryo as a person is a classic example. Both as a theoretical concept and an object of study, potentiality reminds us that biomedical knowledge and practice is a dynamic space of contestations over truth, safety, risk and efficacy of treatments (Ford 2019).

Precarity, as a concept, is akin to potentiality since it reflects an inherent uncertainty of outcomes of interventions/ treatments that will only be revealed in time. In tracing its genealogy to the Marxist theory of labour, it implies a generic sense of ontological uncertainty. Here, we are using precarity more specifically to the context of (self)care, following Hyde and Willis (2020 ). As observed by Anne Allison (2014) and others, precarity of care invites a focus on the present, short-term goals rather than a distant future. At the same time, uncertainty of outcome leaves a door open for hope and resilience in the face of a serious illness, whilst reinvigorating investment and hope in innovative therapies (Hinton and Kirk 2017; Good 2010: 275; Brown 2003).

This next section, following a note on methods, outlines the clinical controversy surrounding the use of thalidomide in treating thalassaemia within the Indian context. This is followed by a case study outlining the quest of a father from a North Indian village, seeking this novel therapy for his two children popularly known as *Jhanduwalla ilaj*—set against the backdrop of the struggles of rural families seeking routine care in state hospitals. The third section, takes us right into the clinic of the practitioner, tracing the nuances of his motivation for offering what he called a "novel therapy" with a view to filling a therapeutic gap (Simpson 2007). In the concluding section, I pick up the conceptual threads to analyse the place of *jugaad* (disruptive innovation) as a practice that arises from and mediates the therapeutic space carved by the precarity of caring and the potentiality of an "operational cure". Before we move to the controversy surrounding the use of thalidomide in thalassaemia, a brief description of the methods and the field is important in setting the scene.

## A note on methods and the field: Setting the scene

The arguments and analysis presented here draw on a multi-sited ethnography of public health policies and experiences of inherited blood disorders in India, carried out between 2017–2019.[1] The larger sample included 49 households from three ge-

1 This research was funded by the Economic and Social Research Council (ES/ 15665/1, https://www.york.ac.uk/sociology/research/current-research/inherited-blood-disorders/). I am grateful to all the participants who shared their lives and therapeutic journeys with us. My special thanks to Karl Atkin and Maya Unnithan for their contributions to the project; colleagues at the Institute of Socio-economic Research on Development and Democracy (ISERDD) for their invaluable skills and help fieldwork; and Prayas for their support. I owe a deep intellectual debt to Veena Das for decades of inspiring conversations and what I have borrowed from Affliction. This chapter has benefited substantially from the insightful comments and suggestions of the MAAH panel, especially Rikke S. Andersen and the two Editors.

ographical areas, where a child or an adult had the condition. This chapter is based on case-studies of five families (from the same field-site, S3) who pursued the novel therapy, using in-depth interviews with adult patients and family carers. Each family was interviewed at least twice and followed up on phone during the pandemic. The case studies were written specifically to analyse their engagement with risk and the circumstances within which a decision was made to opt for or discontinue the new treatment. It is important to mention that my initial framing of the novel therapy as being *controversial* has been important in shaping a shifting analytical space and my appreciation for the specificity of the innovative spirit, a point to which I shall return.

We cannot understand the parental quest for a cure and engagement with therapeutic uncertainty related to novel treatments without first locating the disease in its social milieu. The materiality of the disease is enmeshed within persistent struggles of families, marked by striking levels of poverty and inequalities in accessing basic healthcare provided free by the state (Chattoo 2018). Despite cheap diagnostic tests and treatment options available across public and private sectors, including bone-marrow and stem cell transplants promising a cure, only between 5–10 percent of children with beta thalassaemia receive optimal care in India (Parmar et al. 2017). Paradoxically, whilst state healthcare is free for everybody, in principle, 70 percent is accessed in the private sector with huge variations in quality across both the sectors (see Das and Mohpal 2016).

Thalassemia it is an inherited blood disorder that results in severe/ chronic haemoglobin deficiency. Standard treatment involves a strict life-long regimen of red cell transfusions every 3–4 weeks, supplemented by injectable or oral chelation drugs to extract excess iron from the body (caused by the transfusions). The relentless chronicity of the transfusion-chelation routine is painful, involving iatrogenic risks of blood borne infections and iron overload potentially affecting vital organs over time. Some of the parents from a small town in our sample travelled between 70–200 miles to a larger treatment centre to avail safer blood for their children, whilst most had tried several folk, ayurvedic and spiritual remedies, hoping for a cure.

News about new treatments such as stem cell transplants, gene therapy and new medicines travels far online, via *WhatsApp* chat groups conversations at treatment centres where parents/carers and adult patients form close "family like" ties (see Unnithan et al. 2023). That is how I first heard about *Jhanduwalla* (place pseudonym) *illaj* (treatment/ cure), involving a prescription of thalidomide, when I started fieldwork at Site 3. I had not heard of such a treatment for thalassemia either in India or the UK. A quick online search lead me to a clinic advertising the use of thalidomide as a "novel therapy" and an alternate to transfusions. Initially, I was suspicious about yet another "quack" taking advantage of carers who were desperate for a cure. The novelty of this treatment was already framed as part of the historic controversy surrounding the scientific credibility of the use of thalidomide reflected in the clinical literature, for reasons explained below.[2]

## Novel treatment: Controversy, efficacy and safety of thalidomide

Thalidomide remains shrouded in the scandal of birth disorders and miscarriages caused in a cohort of pregnant women who were prescribed the medicine for morning sickness between mid 1950–60s. New versions of the drug are in use for treating epilepsy and malignant blood cancers. A review of clinical literature suggests that some clinicians are less ambivalent regarding the use of thalidomide in thalassaemia and dismiss its efficacy as purely anecdotal (see Manglani and Kini 2017). Others recognise its benefits in raising foetal haemoglobin levels, justifying its use with varying degrees of caution in selecting the "ideal candidates", for whom the benefits override the increased risk (see Chandra et al. 2021). Given the genetic variants, baseline patient characteristics, diagnostic histories and socio-economic factors underpinning outcomes, predefining the "ideal patient" or a single treatment protocol sounds unrealistic. It is difficult imagining how boundaries of risk and safety defined in Europe or North America can be applied to under-resourced healthcare settings being described here. This is not to undermine the importance of setting the bar high and the need for oversight of protocols at a local/national level.

Thalassaemia International Federation (TIF), an influential organisation with a strong clinical focus, who work closely with the WHO and have a wide international membership base of patients' and carers' representatives, posted the following statement on their Facebook page on 30th June 2018:

> TIF has increasingly been receiving questions from patients about the use of Thalidomide in the treatment of thalassaemia, based on the information that some clinics have been treating patients with this drug. TIF wants to clarify and insist that there are no controlled clinical studies to support the use of Thalidomide as a standard of care for the treatment of thalassaemia. The potential that Thalidomide may have as a treatment option for thalassaemia is, currently, only based on case studies. This means that Thalidomide has only been tested in a limited number and specific groups of patients across the world, mainly in India and China, and so results on its efficacy and potential side-effects are limited and not representative.[3]

2 I would like to thank my colleague, Vaibhav Saria, for his contribution to the literature search on thalidomide.

3 https://thalassaemia.org.cy/news/tif-on-thalidomide/

The above statement by TIF was followed by a potted history of thalidomide and its teratogenous side effects, without adopting a formal stance against the use of the drug in thalassemia and sickle cell disorders.

In a similar vein, Sankalp Foundation, one of the leading non-governmental organisations (NGOs) providing clinical care and stem cell transplants for thalassemia patients in Karnataka (India), reviewed the current evidence on thalidomide. They agree that while thalidomide has been reported to enhance red cell production, the safety and efficacy of the drug (for thalassemia) is debatable. Rather than outrightly discrediting use of thalidomide, Sankalp strongly recommend seeking informed consent, communicating the risks to the patients and reporting any adverse events and deaths.[4] Interestingly, neither Sankalp nor TIF referred to a large retrospective cohort study describing the outcomes of a specific protocol used in India, perhaps, since it was not part of a clinical trial (Ramanan and Ketki 2017).

To summarise, the use of thalidomide in treating thalassemia as a highly contested site of therapeutic innovation and policy regulation highlights two important issues: Firstly, given the practical limitations of governance of medical practice (due to scale and complexity of the federal healthcare structure), the notion of informed consent is compromised across healthcare settings in India. Second, as suggested earlier, the use of thalidomide as an experimental therapy in thalassaemia has been reported from other countries. Hence, criticisms of its use in India might be attributed to "epistemic prejudice and geographies of innovation", following Centellas et al. (2019: 3). Based on their ethnography of birthing practices in a poor state like Mississippi in the USA, they define epistemic prejudice as:

> [...] an orientation toward globally relevant knowledge production and influence that denies or underplays local complexity, practice, and insight. [...] We find that epistemic prejudice enables certain assumptions to become taken-for-granted truisms about the world; it facilitates the construction of "facts" on shaky, uncontested, or invalid foundations. Simultaneously, it serves to silence local innovation and creativity, making a kind of paradox of the local, a place that is both so unique and so failed based on cosmopolitan standards that it barely deserves to be taken seriously and therefore has no generalizable insights to provide to other locations. (Centellas et al. 2019: 3)

The process of legitimisation and routinisation of new technology/ medical treatment based on trials is beyond the scope of our discussion here. The question I want to pose is: what motivates a clinician to try novel treatments in which the efficacy and safety are (yet) not well established? This is assuming that an established clinician with a thriving business has a lot at stake and will not jeopardise her reputation

4 https://www.sankalpindia.net/news/thalidomide-thalassemia#main-content

(see Bhardwaj 2015). Second, we must also try and understand the circumstances and rationale underpinning the decision of parents and (adult) patients who choose to accept the (risks) unknowns associated with such treatments? Finally, how does my own framing of the history of thalidomide "controversy" shape the arguments I am presenting here? The "evidence" seems to have already shifted since I wrote the first draft of this chapter for the MAAH workshop in Autumn, 2021. Rather than provide a linear summary in the retrospect, I want to stay with the flux and potentiality of the intervention as I navigated my way through the field. Let us now turn to the therapeutic journeys of parents/patients in pursuit of this novel treatment within a wider political economy of hope (Good et al. 1990; Novas 2006).

## Seeking *Jhanduwalla ilaj*: Precarity of care, uncertainty and hope

Around the time I started fieldwork at Site 3, (2017–18), I heard stories about some of the families in our sample following *Jhanduwalla daktar ka ilaj (doctor's treatment identified by place)*.[5] Given the porousness of the complementary medical systems, health beliefs and knowledge practices, it is common for practitioners across health systems to prescribe allopathic medicines (see Das and Mohpal 2016). Interestingly, only five out of our sample of 59 thalassaemia households had chosen *Jhanduwalla ilaj*, through their hospital network rather than being referred by their clinician. Even though their personal circumstances varied, they came from the same state (Site 3). The following case-study provides a synopsis of what I defined earlier as precarity of caring, especially in rural areas, in securing regular transfusions they considered to be safe, in the first instance.

In April 2018, Rajan Singh (ISERDD colleague) and I went to meet Prakash and Rani, Papu and Hansa (their children who were under18 and had thalassaemia). They lived in a village about nine miles away from the District hospital in town (Site 3), tucked away from the bus route along the highway. Whilst we were finding our way across unmarked village streets and houses without numbers, Papu met us half- way and recognised Rajan from his previous visit. The family lived in a relatively large, *pucca* (concrete) house (a sign of being relatively better off), with a mud *chullah* (oven) used for heating water in the courtyard. His paternal grandmother, in her long customary *ghoonghat* (veil) covering her face, welcomed and invited us to sit on a *manji* (jute-string-bed), as we waited for Prakash. It was coming to the end of the Winter-harvest season and most of the men and women were busy in the fields, we were told. Rani only made a brief appearance to serve us water and refreshments, assisted by Papu, but did not join in the conversation, given the local custom of deference

5 The names of places and participants have been anonymised throughout the chapter.

women must show to generation and gender. Her mother-in-law, however, was listening carefully and occasionally interjected. We were soon joined by Prakash, one of his brothers, nephew and a neighbour who sat in listening but did not contribute to the discussion.

Clearly, Prakash was the main carer who navigated the medical system, accompanied his children for their hospital appointments and looked after their medications. His nephew helped him financially and whenever they needed help in taking the children to the hospital. There was a sense of desperation in Prakash's voice as he described the routine of taking time off farming to take Papu and Hansa, on public transport (subsidised for patients), for their monthly transfusions to the state hospital about 80 miles away. At times they stayed overnight, involving further expenses. This is a journey they had to undertake every 2–4 weeks since, at the time, the district hospital closer home did not have a blood separation machine. He preferred the long journey to the city hospital, to access separated blood for the children, knowing the harmful impact of whole blood transfusions. Co-ordinating their treatment schedule with the demands of farming, however, was not easy despite the practical support from his nephew. Prakash recollected the time when Hans's transfusion was delayed due to the pressures of harvest taking priority over her routine care.

Prakash was moved to tears when he echoed what I had heard from other parents. He did not know how long his children would live, perhaps 20–25 years, he ruminated. It was quite sad to hear him say, "[...] sewa karunga, dil se, jab tak hen"! (literally, "I will serve them with my heart and soul, until they live"). This expression of *sewa* (care) is a reversal of what parents expect from their children as they get older. He had tried spiritual remedies, votive offerings and other treatments to no avail. At times, he was upset at his *kismet* (poor luck) at having two children who had a difficult, painful condition for which they would need transfusions all their lives.

Unfortunately, such a prognostic vision of a brief life, reinforced by the knowledge of other families losing a child in their 20s, affected the life choices for children with thalassaemia. Papu said that he had not been able to continue school beyond the 8th standard since he found cycling both ways quite tiring. Instead, he now helped his mother with the household chores and went to the fields with his father. In contrast, Prakash said proudly, "Our daughter is really clever and very good at her studies. She needs our support and we are focusing on her education now. We don't expect her to do any housework. You will meet her. She will be back soon".

So, how did he first hear about the *Jhandhuwalla ilaj*, I asked. Prakash responded:

> All the friends at the hospital and the [...] group (naming the city) talked about it. Then we were invited to the camp (educational meeting) on 7th May [world thalassemia day] by the Society [the main patient support group based in another city] and parents were talking about it. Then four of us [parents] from the hospital

> decided to travel to jhandhuwalla (a distance of 580 miles, a journey over 24 hours by bus and train).

Prakash and the children had met the doctor three times, in person. The first time, they travelled as a group of four (affected) families. The consultation fee was 3.000 rupees (for both) and the doctor was nice and patient. He explained everything in detail using a graph, showing how the hb (haemoglobin) would behave, coming down before registering a steady rise. Several tests including a DNA analysis were ordered to confirm the type of thalassemia the children had, each costing 7500 rupees. They were (re)diagnosed as having thalassemia *intermedia* (which often has a milder course and is believed to respond better to thalidomide/ hydroxurea treatment). The differences in types of thalassaemia and pros and cons of the new treatment were explained to him. Rajan and I were shown the notebook they had been given. It was in English with hand-written translation in Hindi and explained in detail how to take the medicines daily, monitor pulse and other signs and a schedule for regular blood tests.

The first batch of medicines was provided for four months and the family were hopeful of the treatment being effective since Papu and Hansa were weaned off transfusions. On their second visit, the doctor was a bit brusque when Rajesh raised the issue of not having enough cash on him. He was told in no uncertain terms, "You can either take these medicines or go back to transfusions." Eventually, the clinic administrator agreed to an electronic transfer of money so that medicines would be couriered to the family. By the time of their third visit, he had spent a substantial sum of nearly 3.5 lakh (350.000) rupees and he realised that spending 20.000 rupees a month, with additional costs for regular blood tests for both the children, was not sustainable in the long term. Hoping that this treatment would work, he had taken out a loan from the bank. Unfortunately, that year, the harvest had been disappointing, followed by COVID-19 a couple of years later, making it difficult for him to repay his loan.

Like most parents, Prakash was desperate to try any new treatment for his children. He believed that stem cell transplants carried an 80 percent risk of death, even though it promised a cure. It was a difficult choice for him to discontinue the treatment, given that both the children had benefitted from it for 18 months. Prakash speculated, "If only the doctor had specified that these medicines were to be taken for 2–3 years, I would have managed the finances". We do not know what the potential treatment outcomes might have been, had the family had enough money to persevere with the treatment. On a positive note, in May 2022, I learnt that the blood separating machine at the local hospital was finally operational, making the treatment routine emotionally and financially less challenging for Prakash and other parents like him.[6]

## Reflections on other potential endings, limits of hope

Meanwhile, doubts about the long-term benefits of *jhanduwalla ilaj* had surfaced in the group, as one of the patients suffered an adverse reaction and had to revert to transfusions. Such incidents had an impact across families who shared a treatment routine and were bound by a kinship of caring (see Unnithan et al. 2023). Ravi's parents, for instance, said that they had discontinued the treatment due to concerns about side effects. Ravi, a frail young man in his 20s, however, added that the treatment was "too expensive anyway". Given their lower-middle class background, it is not clear to what extent their decision might also have been related to competing financial commitments. It is an important aside that, whilst Ravi struggled with his studies at college due to his poor health, his sister was being coached privately to sit for the highly competitive, examination for entry into a medical school. Families with limited resources had to prioritise their needs, often resulting in subtle differences in caring practices. In both Papu's and Ravi's family, education of the healthier/brighter sibling was the focus. When I asked how they made such ethical choices, middle class parents usually claimed that they treated both/ all their children the same.

What we can say with some confidence, however, is that access to cash or the ability to take a loan, often informally from kin or from a bank, rather than severity of the illness *per se,* played a significant part in decisions related to starting and discontinuing the novel treatment. For instance, in contrast with Prakash's situation, Pawan, who was in his late 20s and training to be a teacher when I met him in 2019, came from a relatively better off farming family. He had been pursing *Jhanduwalla* treatment for over a year, even though he had milder form of thalassaemia (intermedia) needing intermittent transfusions. When asked how he was doing, Pawan replied, "Ab me theek hun" ("I am fine now/at the moment"). I asked him what he meant by the term *theek hona* since, in Hindi, it can mean both getting better or being cured. He was clear that in his case cure meant not needing blood. He did not have any concerns about the safety or the expenses related to the treatment and wanted to continue as long as it worked, and his father supported him financially, whilst he invested in his training.

Vibha's father was the only parent of the five families that we followed who had access to scientific papers on clinical trials and new medical interventions, having

---

6 Some of the accounts of the second/ third visit to the family are reconstructed after I had interviewed Dr Dev in 2018.

worked in the pharmaceutical industry. They shopped around online to save money on the prescription each month and maintained regular contact with the doctor online and by phone during the pandemic. Her family had the added advantage of cultural capital that helped in better communication with the doctor, greater confidence in knowing the pros and cons of the medicines and better resources for addressing their doubts. Even he did not broach the subject of the scientific controversy regarding the use of thalidomide, despite mentioning the research he had been following in the field. Vibha's parents were protective gatekeepers and did not want any negative information being filtered to her. On both the occasions, contact was mediated through parents who sat in on both the interviews. What mattered to Vibha and her parents was that her condition was well controlled since she started *Jhanduwalla* treatment. In Spring of 2022, it had been four years without any adverse effects. Vibha had since finished her studies and moved on in life.

Vibha's family were different from the other four in that their cultural capital enabled them to seek information and exercise choice about the potential risks of the novel treatment, economising on costs by looking for safe but cheaper brand of the same medicine in the market. Using Pierre Bourdieu's concept of cultural capital, we can understand the significance of embodied, objectified, and institutionalised forms of cultural capital (e.g., dispositions, values, knowledge, books, technology and educational qualifications) as being central to the perpetuation of class based, structural inequalities (1986: 17–20). The role of cultural capital has been central to debates on the complex intersections between structural inequalities underpinning vulnerability to ill-health, health seeking behaviour and outcomes of care (see Baru and Murugan 2016; Abel 2008).

Whilst these social determinants do not impact on who inherits thalassaemia, the inverse relation between social class and the susceptibility to ill-health and adversity in general have a cumulative impact over time. This was more visible in Sabiha's case who unfortunately died while still in her mid 20s, following an illness caused by dengue, a common infectious disease. The last time I talked to Sabiha on phone was in Summer 2021. She sounded quite cheerful and said that since she was continuing with *Jhanduwallah* treatment and had not had transfusions for two and a half years. She had had two-three serious events resulting in emergency care that she did not consider significant. When I first met her in 2018, Sabiha looked and felt quite ill. Her iron overload was very high, her tummy was swollen due to an enlarged spleen, and she had little appetite. What she described were signs of a poorly managed thalassemia as a child. She spent most of her time in her room barely having the strength to move, until it was time for her next transfusion in two weeks. Even though her mother complained about the *Jhanduwalla ilaj* being expensive, the family owned a small business and managed to chip in.

In Spring 2022, I learnt that Sabiha had developed dizzy spells and fever [dengue] in Autumn 2021. She was critically ill and admitted to the Intensive Care

Unit for a few days, and never returned home. I went to commiserate with the family. It was *iftiari*, the evening time to open the fast during the holy month of Ramazan. Her mother was in the kitchen and did not come out to meet me, her silence marking her mourning. Her brother described the events preceding her death and kept repeating, "[...] she was doing well (*who achi thi*) until she developed fever [...]. It was our oversight (*hamse bhool ho gayi*)." It took the family a few days to realise that she could be seriously ill with dengue (given her thalassemia). They should have rushed her to the hospital earlier. He would always regret that she did not live to see his wedding—an event that she had told me, she was so looking forward to. In taking on the blame for what he saw as a lapse of judgement on their part, we are reminded that better educated parents or siblings might have read the critical signs in relation to her underlying condition serious or sought clinical advice from a network of friends to evade her death.

Given a better sense of what this *Jhandhuwalla ilaj* entailed, I was ready to meet Dr Dev at his clinic in Spring 2018, to find out more about his perspective and practice.

## Therapeutic innovation, private market and the role of medical pioneers

Dr Dev's online profile highlighted that he was an established specialist in his field, affiliated with several national and international clinical bodies. He had already published several papers based on his clinical practice, ranging from leukaemia to sickle cell and thalassemia. His clinic was in a busy part of the old city, in a building that housed other clinics, a courier service as well as a furnishing house. Given that 70 percent of healthcare is provided in the private sector, these are familiar sights across India. The clinic was custom-built and well organised with rows of patients waiting to be seen. I started by asking Dr Dev about his training and interest in thalassaemia. He responded:

> In fact did my first transplant in 2006 [...]. We have done identical, haplo transplants for thalassemics. We have done cord [blood] and all of them have unique challenges. And what I feel is that they are not the perfect option. Why do I feel so? There are ten thousand children who are born every year [with thalassaemia]. Around eight thousand three hundred are dying every year because of lack of transfusion or lack of chelation. [...] we are doing some two or three hundred transplants a year. How can that be an ideal treatment? The standard of care should be something which will cater to majority of the population.

A conjectural estimate of children dying of thalassaemia each year appears as a rhetorical device in aid of his case for a novel treatment, as revealed later. Apparently, thalassaemia was common in his community and the death of a child in the extended family (a decade ago) made him think:

> [...] that we should have a solution for somebody who cannot have a transplant. And talking about ideal things (protocols), about transfusions, in this country is probably talking about a bullet train [...] (next to impossible).

So, what would an ideal treatment protocol look like, in his view, I asked. Dr Dev was critical of any notion of universal protocols premised on the scenario in Italy or the UK. He showed me a diagram demonstrating the progression of the disease and the treatment scenarios, and explained:

> [...] This whole pharmacological induction of fetal hemoglobin comes in and that's how I started in 2009, with an interest with hydroxyurea. And then we had this graft failures with our transplants, thirteen of them, whom I wanted to pull out of transfusion, and that's how I stumbled upon thalidomide. It is not my innovation [...]. Eglar Lopez has already done [...] and it's just that our doctors are blind to it. They just want to talk about the phocomelia (rare foetal anomaly of limbs) which occurred in 1960s to pregnant ladies. Our kids are not going to get pregnant? If they are going to get pregnant, we have [...] women, [options] by stopping the medicine and have got normal pregnancies.
> So we are mixing up two issues. The issue today in India or in the world for thalassaemics is that: a) transfusion is not free, b) it is not safe, and c) it leads to iron deposition, ultimately leads to all this [complications and organ failure—pointing to the diagram on his desk]. After the age of ten years you get all this. This is a British diagram but in India I feel this curve is here [...]. And by twelve to fourteen years of age we have cardiac events and kids have just died [...]. So what it means is that India has a bigger problem.

Due to these premature complications caused by poor clinical management, Dr Dev said that the outcomes of stem cell transplants were also poor and that the aim of clinicians should be to improve their lifespan and quality of life rather than a cure. On a more philosophical note, he later added, "cure is always operational", an important statement to which I shall return.

The pace of the interview was set by his swift thinking and counter questioning, highlighting the scale of the problem and potential solutions that cater to the maximum number of people (principle of equity of care) and are sustainable economically. He went on to criticise the "tunnel vision" of established clinicians who are not willing to take any risks:

> [...] Today we have more than, we have stopped counting them (patients)...more than the number in England [...] *here in one single centre.* So that's what I feel that

going forward [...] we need to understand the needs of the patients. Idealism has to be kept away from practicality because we need to know [...] for example, we were calculating the economic impact of thalassaemia on Indian economy. My rough estimate, which maybe exaggerated, [...] approximately *two billion dollars* (his emphasis).

Steering the conversation away from the neoliberal logic of how much each patient costs the state, I asked him, what he considered to be an ideal regimen with a view to preventing iatrogenic effects of standard treatment. His rehearsed response sounded like a perfect marketing pitch for his new treatment:

There is nothing ideal. Everything is imperfect. The transplant is imperfect, the transfusion is imperfect, the Chelation is imperfect because chelators also cause renal failure, eye, ear toxicity[...]. why do I choose this (thalidomide) [...] here in my clinic?: a) This you can take at home, b) [...] you can treat a larger pool of patients.

Towards the end of the interview, I was brave enough to finally broach the subject of his thalidomide/ hydroxyurea prescription. He reminded me, again, that he did not invent the combination of these drugs, others had published their results from Italy and elsewhere. This provided a certain legitimacy for the scientific rationale in the absence of a clinical trial, even if reinforcing the Eurocentric epistemic prejudice of credibility of science. The following excerpt from his interview captures Dr Dev's rationale:

*S:* Yeah, but they are always very small numbers (referring back to the studies from outside India). One patient here and a case-study there and that's why there is a lot of scepticism about the use of Thalidomide.

*Dr Dev:* [...] You look at the Elgar-Lopez's (paper) [...] and 17 years of her use [...] (publication). So, moral of the story is that it may not be a policy today, it may become a policy tomorrow. When I started in 2009 with Hydroxyurea, people said, "Don't use Hydroxyurea". Now they are saying that everybody is happy using Hydroxyurea in this country [commonly prescribed in treating sickle cell disorders]. It's just passage of time [...]. See, data has to be accumulated. If we just sit on the side-line, nothing is going to be done. Somebody has to jump in and do the thing. Now you will say, "Start a clinical trial". See off-label drug use, you know it [is used] in England, you know it in USA. Pediatricians do it. So this is one of the off-label drug uses.[7] [...] from my limited data, I can see, it is benefitting the patients. So [...] why should I put them at risk of HIV, Hepatitis B, Hepatitis C and

7 It is not uncommon in India for a drug to be prescribed by clinicians which might still not be approved by the state regulatory authority. For example, at the time, Hydroxyurea was

iron overload by giving transfusions? Leave alone the pain, the cost and everything else.

One can certainly not fault Dr Dev's theoretical logic about the scale of suffering and the iatrogenic effects of transfusions within the Indian context. His concerns aligned closely with the motivations reflected in the therapeutic journeys of the parents/ patients we met in the previous section. Strictly speaking, he sought informed consent in principle by explaining risks in relation to the type of thalassaemia, the costs of each treatment cycle and laboratory investigations. Equally, the written instructions provided to the family highlighted signs of critical events needing medical attention from a doctor. The geographical distance from the clinic meant that follow up consultations were arranged on phone, while medicines were delivered by post—far from an ideal situation. There is a certain *laisse-faire* attitude to managing risk on both sides, the doctor, and the patients/families, that is best encapsulated in the spirit of *jugaad* (making do/innovating with little to hand). *Jugaad* has been defined as "disruptive innovation", finding solutions for seemingly insurmountable problems that are far from ideal, which might be considered unsafe or even unethical in other healthcare settings (see Kaur 2016; Birtchnell 2011). Indeed *jugaad* is, "[...] often celebrated as an almost national trait and Indians often pride themselves in being able to navigate suboptimal contexts and marshal available resources, in order to find compromise and solutions that somehow work" (Broom et al. 2020: 24).

Going back to my initial scepticism, I wanted to know what motivated clinicians like Dr Dev to face a reputational risk and criticism from peers in practicing, what Bhardwaj critiques as *badnam* (bad/unethical) science (Bharadwaj 2015). What I had not considered was that they might consider themselves to be moral pioneers with a vision, rather than simply exploiting a gap in the market (see Rapp 1988). This is not to deny the role of the market and profit underpinning Dr Dev's thriving private practice. He was not providing the treatment free of cost to patients who struggled, as we learnt from Prakash's account. Nor was he promising a mass cure. In fact, analytically, what is fascinating in his approach is that he defines all cure as operational (provisional) and both risk and treatment protocols as being relative to a therapeutic milieu.

## Concluding reflections

In contrast with the post-modern notion of risk as colonising the future (Giddens 1991), precarity draws our attention to the "ethics of immediacy" (Mittermaier 2014,

still awaiting approval, even though doctors were able to prescribe the medicine subsidised by the state.

as in Hyde and Willis 2020: 299). In the narratives of families seeking *Jhanduwalla ilaj*, we saw the complex intersection of the materiality of the disease and the socio-structural factors (financial and cultural capital) determining the potential outcomes that unfold in time. The uncertainty of what the novel treatment entailed, both in terms of its composition and outcomes, left the door ajar for hope of, what Dr Dev called, a "functional cure".

However, none of these patients or family carers appeared as passive victims of exploitation at the hands of a "guileful maverick" to borrow Bharadwaj's phrase (for a critique, see Bharadwaj 2018: 15; 2015; Sleeboom-Faulkner and Patra 2011). They had actively chosen to try this treatment without a clinician's referral. We had a glimpse of how patients and family carers struggled to access safe care, moving between hospitals, across cities, changing doctors, pursuing unknown treatments remotely. Irrespective of their level of literacy or lack of knowledge about the medicines, they were not pursuing a miraculous cure. What they were aiming for was freedom from the relentless transfusion routine and the known dangers of iron overload, hoping to prolong life. They were not engaged in the wider processes of knowledge production (research) or governance of thalassaemia and, instead, operated within a very different political economy of hope than envisaged by Novas and others (op cit: 291).

It is fair to say that, arguments for democratisation/decentring of knowledge production and sharing, so well represented in the collection edited by Bharadwaj (2018), for instance, reflect a middle class bias in research. To engage with the clinical/scientific knowledge on trials, risk, and evidence in order to make informed choices about treatment or cure with uncertain outcomes, requires cultural and financial capital. The lives and journeys of the families shared here remind us that most of these parents and patients were unaware of the historical controversy surrounding thalidomide and the potential risk of infertility due to the use of hydroxyurea. They weighed the known, often irreversible, iatrogenic effects of standard treatment and an (perceived) imminent risk of death against the hope of an "operational" cure. The significant financial hardship and potential adverse health outcomes were balanced by the safety-net of state healthcare. If they had to revert to transfusions, they would simply go back to their state hospital and continue receiving free care.

Given the Indian context above, Dr Dev's critique of idealism and universal treatment protocols makes perfect sense, carving a space for therapeutic novelty as "pragmatic improvisation" that he considered to be "frugal, flexible and inclusive" (see Prabhu and Jain 2015: 3). Even though he did not claim credit for developing it, the innovation was embedded in how he practiced it so that it reached patients living hundreds of miles away, without regular follow up visits. The families were responsible for monitoring the treatment, getting the tests done and communicating the results to the doctor either on phone or electronically, unless they lived locally. It was left to them to understand the script of signs signalling an impending health event and seek immediate medical care closer home. There was something common to this *ad hoc* attitude to risk on both the sides. It resonates with what Veena Das, in her study of the urban poor in Delhi, so eloquently describes as the expectation of things going wrong or failing that is seen as being "normal". She writes, "The lives of the poor are strongly defined by living this normal—yet remaining attentive to the critical" (Das 2017: 222; also see Miller 2014). Even though Sabiha's brother regretted that they had not initially taken Sabiha's fever seriously, she was eventually admitted to the ICU.

Finally, as Dr Dev had predicted, there have since been other publications on the use of thalidomide from India, some from researcher-clinicians in the state sector. It is likely, that the novelty will be routinised, as better markers for risk assessment and safer protocols emerge. Whether and to extent such treatments actually helps address the scale of structural inequities in health across India, remains open to discussion.

## References

Abel, Thomas. 2008. Cultural Capital and Social Inequality in Health. Journal of Epidemiology and Community Health, 62(7): e13 (http://jech.bmj.com/cgi/content/full/62/7/e13).

Allison, Anne. 2013. Precarious Japan. Durham, N.C.: Duke University Press.

Baru, Amanti, and Murugan Padmanabhan. 2016. Social Determinants of Vulnerability to Ill Health: Evidences from Mendi Town, Western Ethiopia. Journal of Health and Social Sciences 1(3): 263–278.

Bharadwaj, Aditya. 2015. Badnam Science? The Spectre of the 'Bad' Name and the Politics of Stem Cell Science in India. South Asia Multidisciplinary Academic Journal [Online] 12: 2015 (http://samaj.revues.org/3999; https://doi.org/10.4000/samaj.3999)

Bharadwaj, Aditya, ed. 2018. Global Perspectives on Stem Cell Technologies. Cham: Palgrave Macmillan.

Birtchnell, Thomas. 2011. Jugaad as Systemic Risk and Disruptive Innovation in India. Contemporary South Asia 19(4): 357–372.

Bourdieu, Pierre. 1986. The Forms of Capital. *In* Handbook of Theory and Research for the Sociology of Education. John G. Richardson, ed. Pp. 241–258. New York: Greenwood Press.

Broom, Alex, Katherine Kenny, Emma Kirby, et al. 2020. Improvisation, Therapeutic Brokerage and Antibiotic (Mis)use in India: A Qualitative Interview Study of Hyderabadi Physicians and Pharmacists. Critical Public Health 30(1): 16–27.

Brown, Nik. 2003. Hope Against Hype—Accountability in Biopasts, Presents and Futures. Science Studies, 16(2): 3–21.

Centellas, Kate M., Emma Willoughby and John Green. 2019. Epistemic Prejudice and Geographies of Innovation: Health Disparities and Unrecognized Interventions in Mississippi. Medicine Anthropology Theory 6(4): 1–28.

Chandra, Jagdish, Nupur Prakash, Neha Singh Sidharth, et al. 2021. Efficacy and Safety of Thalidomide in Patients with Transfusion Dependent Thalassemia. Indian Pediatrics 58 (July 15): 611–616.

Chattoo, Sangeeta. 2018. Inherited Blood Disorders, Genetic Risk and Global Public Health: Framing 'Birth Defects' as Preventable in India. Anthropology & Medicine 25(1): 30–49.

Das, Veena. 2015. Affliction: Health, Disease, Poverty. New York: Fordham University Press.

Das, Jishnu, and Mohpal Aakash. 2016. Socioeconomic Status And Quality Of Care In Rural India: New Evidence From Provider And Household Surveys. Health Affairs 35(10): 1764–1773.

Ford, Andrea. 2019. Advocating for Evidence in Birth: Proving Cause, Effecting Outcomes, and Making the Case for 'Curers'. Medicine Anthropology Theory 6(2): 25–48.

Giddens, Anthony. 1991. Modernity and Self-Identity: Self and Society in the Late Modern Age. Cambridge: Polity Press.

Good, Mary-Jo DelVeechio. 2010. The Medical Imaginary and the Bioethical Embrace: Subjective Experiences of Clinical Scientists and Patients. *In* A Reader in Medical Anthropology: Theoretical Trajectories, Emergent Realities., Byron J. Good, Michael Fischer, Sarah S, Willen and Mary-Jo DelVecchio Good, eds. Pp. 272–283. Oxford: Wiley-Blackwel.

Good, Mary-Jo DelVeechio, Byron J. Good, Cynthia Schaffer, and Stuart E. Lind. 1990. American Oncology and the Discourse of Hope. Culture, Medicine and Psychiatry 14(1): 59–79.

Hinton, Denise, and Susan Kirk. 2017. Living with Uncertainty and Hope: A Qualitative Study Exploring Parents' Experiences with Childhood Multiple Sclerosis. Chronic Illness 13(2): 88–99.

Hyde, Sandra Teresa, and Laurie D. Willis. 2020. Balancing the Quotidian: Precarity, Care and Pace in Anthropology's Storytelling. Medical Anthropology 3(4): 297–304.

Kalra, Manas, Virender K. Khanna, and Amita Trehan. 2017. Thalidomide in Transfusion Dependent Thalassemia: Hype or Hope. Journal of Paediatric Haematology and Oncology 39(6): 485.

Kaur, Ravinder. 2016. The Innovative Indian: Common Man and the Politics of Jugaad Culture. Contemporary South Asia 24(3): 313–327.

Miller, Kathleen M. 2014. The Precarious Present: Wageless Labour and Disrupted Life in Rio de Janerio, Brazil. Cultural Anthropology 29(1): 32–53.

Mittermaier, Amira. 2014. Bread, Freedom, Social Justice: The Egyptian Uprising and a Sufi Khidma. Cultural Anthropology 29(1): 54–79.

Prabhu, Jaideep, and Sanjay Jain. 2015. Innovation and Entrepreneurship in India: Understanding *Jugaad*, Asia Pacific Journal of Management 32(4): 843–868.

Novas, Carlos. 2006. The Political Economy of Hope: Patients' Organizations, Science and Biovalue. BioSocieties 1(3): 289–305.

Parmar, Lalith, Amit Sedai, Kumari Ankita, Rakesh Dhanya, et al. 2017. Can Inequity in Healthcare Be Bridged in LMICs: Multicentre Experience from Thalassemia Day Care Centres in India. Pediatric Hematology Oncology Journal 2(4): 88–93.

Povinelli, Elizabeth A. 2011. Economies of Abandonment: Social Belonging and Endurance in Late Liberalism. Durham, N.C.: Duke University Press.

Rapp, Rayna. 1988. Moral Pioneers: Women, Men and Fetuses on a Frontier of Reproductive Technology. Women and Health 13(1-2): 101–17.

Ramanan, Vijay, and Ketki Kelkar. 2017. Role of Thalidomide in Treatment of Beta Thalassemia. J Blood Disord Med 3(1): http://dx.doi.org/10.16966/2471-5026.119.

Shah, Sandip, Radhika Sheth, Kamlesh Shah, and Kinnari Patel. 2020. Safety and Effectiveness of Thalidomide and Hydroxyurea Combination in b-Thalassaemia Intermedia and Major: A Retrospective Pilot Study. Br J Haematology 188(3): e18-e21. https://doi.org/10.1111/bjh.16272.

Simpson, Bob. 2007. Negotiating the Therapeutic Gap: Prenatal Diagnostics and Termination of Pregnancy in Sri lanka. Journal of Bioethical Inquiry 4(3): 207–215.

Sleeboom-Faulkner, Margaret, and Prasana K. Patra. 2008. The Bioethical Vacuum: National Policies on Human Embryonic Stem Cell Research in India and China.Journal of International Biotechnology and Law 5(6): 221–234.

Taussig, Karen-Sue, Klaus Hoeyer, and Stefan Helmreich. 2013. The Anthropology of Potentiality in Biomedicine: An introduction to Supplement 7. Current Anthropology 54(S7): 3–14.

Unnithan, Maya, Chhaya Pachauli, Sangeeta Chattoo, and Karl Atkin. 2023. Only Parents Can Understand the Problems and Needs of Children with Thalassaemia: Parental Activism for Thalassaemia Care in Northern India. Anthropology and Medicine 30(1): 48–63.

# 5 Between Uncertainty and Routinization

## Accounting for Non-Invasive Prenatal Genetic Testing in Germany

*Stefan Reinsch*

## Introduction

Non-invasive prenatal testing (NIPT) for genetic conditions such as Down syndrome (DS) as early as the 9th week of pregnancy became available in 2012 to German women. In contrast to the current gold standard procedure, amniocentesis, which brings a small procedure-related risk of miscarriage, NIPT is promoted by pharmaceutical companies as a safe alternative requiring "only a blood sample from the mother". The advent of NIPT in Germany presents a special case of the broader issue of how to account for the social dimensions and implications of new biomedical technologies (Franklin and Roberts 2006).

In her book *Imperfect Pregnancies*, the biologist and science historian Ilana Löwy (2017) showed how the search for fetal abnormalities, once reserved for older women and those with a family history of birth defects, has emerged since the 1970s as a routine part of prenatal care in Western health care systems. In a follow-up book, Löwy (2018) pointed out that prenatal testing has become primarily a risk management technology aimed at preventing the birth of children with congenital impairments, ideally through interventive therapies, but in practice mainly through abortion. She had argued that, with the advent of relatively risk-free NIPT, serum testing for DS has become so commonplace that many women equate it with being a "good" mother and therefore consent to it without reflection (Löwy 2017).

Social scientists have highlighted the ambivalent medico-ethical features of such predictive genetic testing (Konrad 2005; Hadolt and Lengauer 2009). Among some recent examples of such ambivalence, Guell (2011) has shown that the emergence of genetic tests predictive for diabetes is creating new biosocialities that are at once exclusionary and emancipatory. Lock (2005) has argued that in the case of Alzheimer's disease, claims of predictability and control are coming to resemble a modernized form of fortune telling. Considering the well-known example of testing adults with a family history for Huntington's Disease, cultural studies scholar Katrin

Solhdju (2018) has argued that predictive genetic tests create a "temptation to know" that is generated by the very existence of the test, and by a need for reassurance. These cases of ambivalence of predictive genetic testing, which both exclude and emancipate, claim predictability and yet distance themselves from those claims, and create uncertainty while promising reassurance, can only exacerbate existing ethical conflicts in the context of pregnancy (Löwy 2017). Some social scientists speculate that NIPT might contribute to a further routinization of screening and genetic testing, thereby disempowering women and further excluding people with disabilities from existence and integration in society (Thomas and Rothman 2016).

## "A safe test that may relieve your concerns"

NIPT is based on the detection of fetal cell-free DNA (cfDNA) circulating in the mother's blood. The assay can detect variations in the number of chromosomes (aneuploidy) in the fetus—trisomy 13, 18, and 21 (Patau syndrome, Edwards syndrome and DS, respectively). Some tests also detect sex chromosome aneuploidies and other chromosomal microdeletions and duplications. In Germany and other countries, laboratories already offer tests for monogenetic disorders such as sickle cell disease, Huntington's disease, and cystic fibrosis. Thus, the debate about routinization is poised to assume a broader aspect. However, since most of the controversy surrounding NIPT hitherto centers on the detection of DS, I will focus on this in the present article.

NIPT is a technically simple procedure that requires "just a blood sample"[1] collected from the mother. It is non-invasive and therefore does not carry the risk of miscarriage associated with amniocentesis and chorionic villus sampling (CVS). The amniocentesis approach has a procedure-related pregnancy loss rate that is generally reported as 1/200, but can be as low as 1/1000 when corrected for spontaneous miscarriage and practitioner expertise in the procedure (Salomon et al. 2019).[2] NIPT has varying rates of false-positive and false-negative results, depending on the condition being tested for. However, as a screening test for DS, NIPT is highly accurate, with sensitivity and specificity[3] both exceeding 99 percent, and reaching 100 percent in one industry-sponsored study (Flöck et al. 2017). Taken together, NIPT presents

1 Quote from official information provided by the pharmaceutical company Lifecodexx.

2 Amniocentesis requires puncturing the belly of the mother and passing a needle into the amnionic fluid, which brings inherent risks that are moderated by the degree of expertise of the practitioner. However, in the large meta-analysis by Salomon et al. (2019), which controlled for expertise by only including studies with >1000 cases, the corrected rate for procedure-related loss of pregnancy was 0.12%, or roughly 1/1000.

3 Sensitivity is the proportion of cases detected among the total of those affected, and specificity is the proportion of detected cases that are correctly identified.

three main advantages over previous predictive tests for prenatal screening: it can be used earlier in pregnancy, is less invasive, yet more accurate. There are some caveats to all three aspects, but NIPT is typically pitched to the expectant mother as yet another reassuring tool, providing knowledge that "may help alleviate your concerns and worries about possible health problems in your child".[4]

## "Reassuringly routinized" technologies of pregnancy care

Social scientists have repeatedly expressed concerns that the adoption of routinization of NIPT might lead to the disempowerment of patients and the further marginalization of disabled people by yet another biomedical technology (Clarke et al. 2003) and the relentless marketing of health by pharmaceutical companies (Dumit 2012), These authors present the adoption of "routine" as part of a negative power relationship. However, rather than assuming *a priori* that "routinization" is negative, I would like to unpack and discuss its different meanings.

Routinization in the context of prenatal testing has distinct meanings at the level of the health care system—possibly involving public funding—and for the individual. At the level of health systems, the routinization primarily refers to a transition from NIP testing to NIP screening, where the practice becomes routinized as a first-tier method replacing conventional biochemical and genetic screening in the first/second trimester. At the time of this study (2017–2020), the debate in Germany, driven in part by requests for insurance coverage of NIPT, is an example of partial rather than complete routinization. For example, if NIPT were to be covered by German health insurance but still offered only to "high-risk pregnancies", it would constitute routinization at the level of health insurance, but not in regard to population screening.

Routinization can also refer to the private, personal level: that of the pregnant woman who elects to take the test because of its "tempting features", and then participates in an "automatic, routinized" way, perhaps without thorough reflection on its meaning and possible implications. In the ethical and psychosocial literature, routinization at the personal level is considered to negatively affect three areas: informed choice, freedom of choice, and the lives of people with a disability (Kater-Kuipers et al. 2018). First, there is apprehension that broader adoption of NIPT will lead to uninformed choice, meaning that couples may not reflect upon their choice and thus be aware of the possible consequences of testing (Gottfreðsdóttir and Arnason 2011). Second, there are concerns that NIPT could become taken for granted as "just another blood test" (Griffin et al. 2017), which would lead to increased participation, heightened social pressure to test, and proliferating termination of affected

4 Quote from official information provided by the pharmaceutical company Lifecodexx.

pregnancies (de Graaf et al. 2017). Third, the total number of people born with a disability could well decrease, leading to reduced healthcare expertise, but correspondingly increased discrimination against people living with a disability. In turn, declining healthcare requirements for people with DS and/or a negative public image of DS could pressure women to opt for prenatal screening and terminate affected pregnancies (van Schendel et al. 2017; Kater-Kuipers et al. 2018). By negatively affecting informed choice and freedom of choice, "routinization of NIPT" could undermine "procreative autonomy", which is seen by some as the only legitimate aim of prenatal testing (Dondorp et al. 2015).

Social scientists have shown how interactions occur for the various concerns arising under the umbrella term of routinization: the uninformed choice, the lack of deliberation, as well as the social pressure to test and terminate a pregnancy upon discovery of a lifelong disability. In his book *Down's Syndrome Screening and Reproductive Politics*, sociologist Gareth Thomas (2017) argues that the routinization of DS screening is fueled by "downgrading" of the procedure and its framing as "just another test". Drawing on ethnographic research in two UK fertility clinics, he describes how clinicians were able to "downgrade" screening in the clinical hierarchy. Because DS screening was, for many reasons, seen as a routine and "simple" test, responsibility for its implementation was assigned to midwives and sonographers. Thomas argues that framing ultrasound screening to parents as "just another simple test" —either explicitly, such as by describing the screening as a "simple test", or implicitly, such as by leaving open the door of the consultation room—may have led some women to passively opt in.

This consideration takes up a line of argument formulated in the book *The Tentative Pregnancy*, by the sociologist Barbara Katz Rothman (1986), who showed from her interviews with women who had undergone amniocentesis that the risk of miscarriage then gave women a "good" reason to refuse prenatal testing. The risk to the life of the child is a strong and rational argument for a woman inclined to refuse the test, whereas it is much more difficult to articulate emotional concerns about her "temptation to know more" about the unborn child. Over 30 years ago, Rothman (1986: 82) predicted that the eventual availability of a blood test for early pregnancy would strip the issue down to its bare bones and confront us with the essential moral issues: "When the risk is removed, the last completely socially acceptable reason for not wanting to know about fetal defects will be gone".

Prenatal diagnosis (PND), of which NIPT is a part, is presented by health care providers as a simple choice for or against undergoing a test. At the same time, PND is embedded in a complex system of medical diagnosis and pregnancy monitoring. This combination raises concerns about increasing routinization that is described as being at once reassuring and frightening. This view of the dual nature of routinization resonates with what anthropologist Rayna Rapp (2000: 23) wrote in her book *Testing Women, Testing the Fetus*: "The technologies of prenatal diagnosis that pregnant women encounter appear reassuringly routinized". Rapp (2000: 40–41) thus reminds us that the development and routinization of prenatal diagnosis in the US depend upon a complex intersection between biomedical scientific research, social policies affecting abortion, social movements influencing the cultural climate, and a specific history of litigation pressuring health care providers to improve standards of care.

In this article, I attempt to unpack the umbrella term routinization by empirically investigating how women pragmatically use and make sense of medical technology (Lock and Kaufert 1998). My central argument is inspired by the sociologist Annemarie Mol's (2008) book *The Logic of Care*, in which she argues that modern health care posits two logics: a "logic of choice" and a "logic of care". The "logic of choice" is based on an understanding of people as rationally acting agents, citizens or customers. Here, the ideal agent is an autonomous, informed patient who uses specifically adapted and predetermined tools for solving a problem. Conversely, in the "logic of care", health care is an evolving practice that is concerned less with decision-making than with "tinkering" and "doctoring" (Mol et al. 2010). In this view, tinkering means "making do with what you have in non-ideal circumstances" and adapting it on the spur of the moment. My aim is to problematize and reconstruct the two logics (care and choice) not as a dichotomy, but as complementary analytical axes that encompass a spectrum of cognitive and behavioral strategies. In explicating this analytical "space" between the two logics, I shall show how women's agency is expressed, and how its degree of freedom is limited by existing or developing attachments to a child, or by the decision to take a test under pressure from pre-existing attachments to a child or family.

## Pregnancy care and the debate around NIPT in Germany

Germany is the forefront of modern Western technology, which enshrines a specific set of professional cultures, regulations, and policies regarding reproductive medicine and the safety net for children born with a disability. As distinct from the USA, the source of a considerable body of research on genetic testing during pregnancy, Germany has universal health insurance. While the German Health Care System generally provides good medical coverage, it is also criticized for not meeting the needs of families with disabilities (Blümel et al. 2020). While there is an abundance of early intervention services for people with disabilities in large urban centers, such support has been inadequate in rural areas (Thyen et al. 2003). Better recognition of disability in the first years of life has led to improved financial support in recent years (Pflegestärkungsgesetz 2015). For example, parents of children with DS in Germany receive care allowance which enables them to work fewer hours during the child's infancy. While the situation is improving, a focus on the whole family system and its social integration is still lacking (Vonneilich et al. 2016). As long as there remains a gap between living conditions for families with and without a child with DS, there will be ongoing discussions about testing and funding.

Preventive care during pregnancy and the perinatal period in Germany is described in detail in the binding *Motherhood Guidelines* published by the Federal Joint Committee, the self-governing body that decides on issues of insurance coverage (G-BA 2023). Coverage by universal health insurance has included prenatal diagnosis (PND) and newborn screening (NBS) since the 1970s. Free PND in Germany includes an ultrasound scan during weeks 6–12 of pregnancy to estimate gestational age and determine the number of fetuses, and a basic ultrasound scan of fetal anatomy in weeks 19–25. In Germany, further ultrasound scans, amniocentesis, chorionic villus sampling and umbilical cord sampling are covered if medically indicated. Medical indications include known genetic abnormalities in the family, suspicious ultrasound findings, but also maternal age over 35, which is considered "high-risk pregnancy" by the *Motherhood Guidelines*. At the time of the interviews for this article, specific tests for disabilities such as DS or spina bifida, including the first-trimester scan (FTS), ultrasound without specific indication, the triple test, and NIPT, are mainly paid out of pocket by patients.

Since its 2012 introduction in Germany, NIPT has become a matter of public controversy, more so than in many other countries (Braun and Könninger 2018), with concerns being raised about its fundamental social and ethical issues (Deutscher Bundestag 2019). This debate intensified in 2016 after the National Association of Statutory Health Insurance Funds, the Association of Statutory Health Insurance Physicians, the impartial Chair person, and other impartial members of the Federal Joint Committee requested the inclusion of NIPT in the *Motherhood Guidelines*, and the reimbursement of test costs. In September 2019, the G-BA decided in favor of the 2016 application, but limited to high-risk pregnancies (G-BA 2019a). From the end of 2020, "NIPT can be used and covered by statutory health insurance if the question of whether a fetal trisomy might be present arises during medical prenatal care and this possibility represents an unacceptable burden for the pregnant woman" (G-BA 2019b: 2, translation by the author). Aspirationally, a negative NIPT result will make amniocentesis unnecessary, such that the new regulation should help to reduce the number of invasive tests and consequent miscarriages.

Some see insurance coverage of NIPT as a necessary step towards comprehensive reproductive justice, since NIPT has had to be paid for out-of-pocket, even though amniocentesis is covered for high-risk pregnancies (Buyx 2019). Others argue that insurance coverage serves those who favor increased NIPT use, particularly pharmaceutical companies (Rüffer 2019), calling it the "beginning of the expansion" of these tests (Achtelik 2019), and warning that NIPT coverage puts pressure on women to use the test. Others characterize the expected effect of introducing NIPT in terms of an expected significant reduction in miscarriage rates, which has not yet been demonstrated (Malan et al. 2018). There are also concerns that the G-BA's decision will reduce the use of more comprehensive ultrasound screening, which will in turn create a false sense of reassurance among women, insofar as NIPT sensitivity and specificity estimates convey a spuriously higher validity than the test actually possesses for some patient groups (BVNP 2020). In Germany, these debates about the pros and cons of NIPT have occurred in the public sphere, but there has been no systematic investigation of women's lived experiences and views on their decision to use or refuse NIPT. In this exploration of women's experiences and practices of NIPT, I aim to bring a better understanding of the meaning and social implications of this new technology.

## Methods

This article derives from the 2017–2020 project "Meanings and Practices of Non-invasive Prenatal Genetic Diagnostics in Germany and Israel (PreGGI)", which combined perspectives from philosophy, sociology and clinical medicine. A selection of the project results is published as a book (Schües 2022). The project included a qualitative study in which narrative interviews were conducted following an interview guide. The interviewees were intentionally selected to capture social groups identified as being relevant (Patton 2001: 238). The project team interviewed 48 people in Germany for the study. The interviewees included 21 women who chose NIPT and 15 who did not, 16 women and men with family members affected by DS or another disability, four health professionals, and eight experts on disability and/or genetic testing, with the total (64) exceeding 48 because some respondents met more than one category. Interviews were audio-taped and fully transcribed; the transcribed interviews were anonymized and analyzed using the method of constant comparison (Corbin and Strauss 2008). A comprehensive report of the entire cohort can be found in a previous publication (Reinsch et al. 2021). Uncertainty and routinization emerged as useful analytical concepts during the process of analysis, and the two narratives that were chosen for this article were exemplary of a central dichotomy emerging from the study.

## Accounting for Non-Invasive Prenatal Genetic Testing in Germany

The temptation to test and know more about their unborn child, on the one hand, and the concern to decide in advance what to do with the test result, on the other hand, emerged as the core social and moral tension among women who used or refused NIPT in Germany. This ambiguity reflects a dilemma for women in neoliberal, techno-scientific societies, where the elimination of risk and the temptation to know are powerful cultural narratives. I aim to disentangle this coexistence of the temptation to know more and the urge to know how to handle the results. Two personal vignettes serve to illustrate broader narratives and the range of choices that women have. The use of personal vignettes allows for a presentation of findings that are embedded in the lifeworld [Lebenswelt] of the informants. I present and juxtapose the selected stories sequentially, illustrating different aspects of the complex negotiations of meanings and practices of NIPT within the whole spectrum of prenatal testing practices. Sabrina's story shows how she urges women to reflect carefully about whether to test, considering that the subsequent situation is not straightforward, but "always different after the test". Sabrina's story is contrasted with that of Dorothee for whom NIPT functions as a specific tool in a routinized "logic of testing" that allows her to take responsibility for her family.

## Dealing with uncertainty: "It's always different after the test"

Sabrina is a 42-year-old former police officer. After three previous miscarriages she gave birth to a child with DS. I found out about the child's status indirectly during the interview, and remember that this situation was as revealing to me as the content of our conversation. When she contacted me, Sabrina wrote that she had taken NIPT "because some soft markers were positive". I met her in her flat in the south of Berlin, greeted at the door by Sabrina and her 2-year-old child. She and I sit down in the tidy, spacious, and bright living room, and I am offered a cup of tea. The tea cup, decorated with, as I later learn, the child's name, and my observation of a large gap between the first and second digit of the foot (a medical telltale sign of the condition that has been adopted by DS families) confirms that the child has trisomy 21. This positive affirmation was a nice way to learn the diagnosis. Sabrina's manner is "show, don't tell". During the interview, the child enters the room several times, sits on my knees, and wants to draw. Apart from a specific sign language used by mother and child, nothing would distinguish this child during our interview.

Sabrina remembers having felt very positive when she went for her first trimester screening. She was relieved to have avoided the risk of early spontaneous abortion, and saw herself as a normal, healthy mother-to-be. After all, "what could possibly happen now that I had reached 12 weeks?" When I asked her why prenatal diagnosis had not been an option at that point, she replied, "I wouldn't have known why [that would be necessary]". But when her gynecologist remarked, "Do you want to have the finediagnosis—after all, you are older", the then 39-year-old woman agreed. Looking back, she considers herself "naive to have thought that nothing could go wrong". During the ultrasound scan, the prenatal diagnostician said, "We need to talk", which was her first hint that something might be amiss.

She then received advice about the implications of shortened nasal bone and heart malformation, which she recalled as being "non-directive":

> I was told that I could choose to do nothing or have an amniocentesis, and that the latter carried a risk of miscarriage. At that point, I interrupted the prenatal diagnostician and said, "This is a risk I am not prepared to take".

She had heard about NIPT from a friend and suggested it herself because the test was advertised as being risk-free. Only after getting the result did she learn what the test meant in terms of probabilities and certainties. Before taking the test, she had thought, "whatever the test result is, that's what it will be". She believed that the test would be 100 percent accurate and that she could accept the result. However, until she received the NIPT result, she had "hoped that the prenatal diagnostician was wrong". She vividly remembers receiving the result over the phone:

> The ground beneath my feet disappeared. A Saturday three years ago. The day before Christmas. I ate spinach pizza. I have not been able to eat spinach pizza since. I knew that from that moment forward everything would be different.

The effect of the test result on her pregnancy was a psychological "divorce from the child", until weeks later she felt the child's movements. She did not fully embrace having the child again until it was born. "I remember finding a box of maternity clothes some time ago, all black". Looking back on her pregnancy experience, she wishes she had "never known". Sabine's statement about whether she would recommend NIPT to another woman was therefore very nuanced:

> Not in general. For women who are afraid of amniocentesis and who have an increased likelihood [of genetic abnormalities]. They should think in advance about what they would do, how they would deal with the result. Although, as in my case, it is always different after the test.

Sabrina was somewhat unprepared for the ultrasound scan, because she had not thought herself at risk and in particular need of prenatal diagnostics. When it became clear that she was at risk, she opted for NIPT rather than amniocentesis, which posed a lesser risk to her fetus. However, she was reluctant to accept the logic of prenatal testing, still clinging to hope that the clinicians were wrong. Her strong statement on receiving the result, and her subsequent emotional divorce from the child in utero, the child she had hoped the test would protect, led her to say that she wished she had not known. For her, testing practices such as NIPT have ill-framed assumptions and ponderous consequences:

> I currently know of two women who are pregnant again after having a child with DS, and both chose not to have skin fold translucency measured on ultrasound or a fine diagnosis ultrasound later in pregnancy. I would do the same. A test against [DS like NIPT] would not be possible for us. You can't first decide for and later against. It would also be a sign to him [her child], and that is unthinkable.

Sabrina's way of responding to her urge to know is embedded in a logic of "caring". It is centered on the expectation of an unburdened pregnancy, in which the woman, not the clinician, is the expert. Within this logic, NIPT introduces "one more uncertainty" about what to do with the test result and burdens the pregnancy with negative emotions. Sabrina, again concurring with some of the other women I interviewed, said: "Many might not reflect upon implications of NIPT because it is 'just a blood test', with no direct risk to the baby". By this, Sabrina is suggesting that the pharmaceutical company's slogan, which presents NIPT as "an alternative to amniocentesis without the risk (of miscarriage)"[5], misleads women because it obscures the implications of a result. This shows that while NIPT may present the advantage of being clinically non-invasive, the test had multiple personal, social, and medical consequences, and could thus be considered highly invasive.

## Testing against uncertainty: "A safe enough test"

37-year-old Dorothee is in her 15th week of pregnancy at the time of our interview. She undertook NIPT to be extra sure that she would not have a child with DS—this would not have been compatible with her own and her partner's ideas of family life, as informed by her sister-in-law's DS. For Dorothee, the outcome was a relief: "One less problem to look after".

Dorothee is in many respects a modern cosmopolitan German woman. Like most of our highly educated respondents, she has a university degree and lives in a densely populated urban area of Berlin. The interview takes place in the open-plan kitchen of a spacious flat, while her partner works in his home office in the adjacent room. Dorothee had her first child 12 years ago, a girl, followed six years later by separation from her first partner, whereupon she moved into a flat next door with a new partner. The responsibilities for the daughter are shared between the two biological parents. Dorothee emphasizes several times that she has a very close, sharing relationship with her 12-year-old daughter and that she considers herself a very good mother when she is herself happy.

Three months before her current pregnancy, Dorothee had an early spontaneous abortion. "Did the loss change your experience of pregnancy?", I asked. "Yes. Now I try not to be too happy, and worries and thoughts are much more present". After

5 Quote from the official information of the pharmaceutical company Lifecodexx.

the miscarriage, she and her partner had a conversation about disability and what kind of child they wanted. Dorothee remembers that it occurred during an underground train ride to the opera, and that the discussion was relatively brief because they both agreed that disability would not be compatible with their mutual aspirations of family life: "My understanding of family life is a partnership, where you are together—independently, participating and sharing in the life of the other family members". Family and loss are an important theme throughout our conversation. Her own parents lost a severely disabled infant at the age of five days. Her brother had died of cancer 15 years ago and her mother died prematurely ten years ago. Of her biological family, only her father and her own daughter remain.

For Dorothee, it was a "relief" to have this conversation on the underground train and to hear her partner say that he would not want his child to have a life like his sister's. "After all, he might have had reservations because of his sister". Nor would the partner want Dorothee to live the life of his mother, who is the sole carer for his 38-year-old disabled sister. Dorothee explains carefully:

> I've had never been in contact with a person with trisomy 21, like my sister-in-law, and [...] it's a pretty severe trisomy 21. She can't communicate and she's 38 years old and she lives in Chile with her mother, and [...] yes, that had an enormously big influence, since I've known her the past five years now. Influenced by seeing a life that I wouldn't want for myself, wouldn't want for my child. [...] Yes, I think my sister-in-law is quite happy in her world, but her world is not connected to our world. [...] Well, she really can't, she can't communicate, she can't go to the toilet by herself, and of course that's an extreme case, but [...] my partner and I [...] can't imagine having a child with trisomy 21, and we would like to rule that out if it's possible.

Dorothee has a clear idea of "what a family should be like": without disability. She wanted to spare her family the hardship of bringing up a disabled child. She reminds me of the attachment to family that women care the most about when considering whether to take this particular test. I use her example because it helps us to understand that thinking in a "logic of testing" is not about choosing an isolated, specific test, NIPT or any other. Rather, testing is part of an ecology of practices that involves thinking in terms of probabilities, a very specific kind of certainty that one must accept. I am not suggesting that Dorothee is representative of "German" women, although I have noted her way of thinking, and of confronting uncertainty by seeking knowledge many times among German women.

In a different part of the interview, Dorothee also points to the common critique of the insufficient supportive care or "safety net" for families of children born with DS:

> Every time I'm [with my family-in-law] I realize that this is not the life I want. And what I want for my child, and [...] so, of course, a child accompanies you for life, but not really like that, not in the way that until the child dies, um, how shall I put it, that you must take care of everything.

This critique was also raised by respondents from rural areas, some of whom had to travel two hours to see a specialist. For people like Sabrina, who takes her child to early intervention four times a week, this would be a full-time job if she lived in a rural area.

Dorothee is an exemplary informant because she has a relative with DS and has previously miscarried. She and her partner knew that they did not want a child with DS long before they found out about NIPT. In this sense, Dorothee meets all of Sabrina's stated requirements for testing. Dorothee found "reassurance" in NIPT because of the negative result, but also because in the event of finding of an abnormality she would have been able to opt for an abortion, thus "sparing" her family "a life of hardship". I think that because of her previous experiences, NIPT functions for Dorothee as a specific tool in a routinized "logic of testing". DS, but not disability in general, was something to be avoided; not because it was a frightening unknown, but because her sense of obligations to her family made DS incompatible with "family life where you are together, independent and sharing each other's lives".

Within the logic of eliminating unpredictability, NIPT offers itself as a medico-technological tool with an understanding that is co-inscribed in the tool and its users. This anticipated interdependence (Prout 1996) can also be seen in Dorothee's case. She wanted to avoid the outcome that the test was designed to reveal, and was prepared to face the consequences, and if necessary, terminating the pregnancy. She saw this from the biomedical perspective, thus it was not problematic for her that the clinicians were the experts. At the antenatal clinic she was told that they would usually order a triple test first, and then, if there was a suspicion, be advised to undergo NIPT for "extra" certainty. However, Dorothee wanted NIPT straight away, to be "extra sure" about DS. She had been told about the residual risk of a false result in NIPT, but thought it was "much more minimal" compared to the triple test. She also thought a 98 percent chance was "safe enough" for her, so there was no need for an even more accurate test like amniocentesis.

## Discussion: Ways of caring while facing an uncertain future

I sought to understand how a new predictive genetic test, NIPT, is becoming routinized in prenatal diagnosis, while at the same time introducing uncertainty and the potential for women to gain more agency within the complex relationship between pregnancy, disability, and family life. My aim was to show how, far from being prey to technology, some women make pragmatic use of NIPT as a resource or tool for gaining knowledge, while others reject the demands and obligations of testing practice by embracing the uncertainty of an unfolding pregnancy as an alternative logic.

I have selected two case narratives that represent distinct ways of responding to the urge to "know what you would do", which are embedded in different logics: First, the story of Sabrina, the mother of a child with DS, describes the complex negotiations of meanings and practices of NIPT within the spectrum of prenatal testing practices. Sabrina invites other woman to "know what you would do if you had a positive result" before deciding to test. Her advice is based on the difficulty of resisting the "temptation to know more" as she moves along the spectrum of PND. These difficulties increase with each successive test, in what is often described as a diagnostic spiral. Sabrina understands NIPT as potentially leading to a decision to abort. Her own experience has led her to urge others to reflect carefully about what it means to abort or to live with a disabled child. When Sabrina asks women to consider the consequences of knowing they are carrying a disabled fetus, which includes the prospect of choosing abortion, she is asking them to be informed consumers. At the same time, the choice and deliberation are, as Sabrina points out, complex and call for being "very, very, very careful", in line with the logic of care.

In contrast, Dorothee has a relative with DS and, like Sabrina, had previously lost a fetus due to miscarriage. She and her partner knew they did not want a child with DS before they found out about NIPT. Dorothee found "reassurance" in NIPT—because of the negative result, but also because she would have been able to undergo an abortion in the event of finding an abnormality, thereby sparing her family "a life of hardship". For Dorothee, NIPT becomes a medical technology that functions as a specific tool in a routinized "logic of testing". In this logic, women seek medical reassurance with the help of clinical experts and the NIPT, which offers itself as a medico-technological tool with an inscribed logic (Prout 1996): that of eliminating unpredictability, which is itself based on a "trust in numbers" (Porter 1995).

Sabrina and Dorothee both used NIPT in search of certainty. They are similar in that they have had previous spontaneous abortions, which led them to embrace NIPT as a safe alternative to riskier amniocentesis. However, they both seek reassurance in different ways. Risk and certainty, safety and security are different from the peace of mind that can be found in not knowing (Schües et al. 2022). Whether the prenatal specialist offers relative certainty or complete certainty does not matter to a woman like Sabine, who is looking for knowing in the body, a knowing that is embodied and cannot be abstracted from the knowing body of women (Mol 2014).

I argue that women like Sabine challenge the imperative to know and act based on probabilistic knowledge, refusing self-management, and the privatization of risk by continuing with testing and, if need be, terminating the pregnancy. Instead, the uncertainty of her unfolding pregnancy occupies center stage. Certainty herein lies an embodied practice of knowledge. Sabine cannot even speak of testing without referring to her child, who might have been aborted. Women like Sabine have become acutely aware of NIPT as a matter of "testing and avoidance". If the experience of an unburdened pregnancy is at the forefront, NIPT adds the uncertainty of the possible decision to keep or abort a (handicapped) child. There are other narratives of women saying they wanted to know in order to prepare themselves, but the more common view of NIPT as an element in an ecology of testing practices leading to abortion is also based on estimates from experts that nine out of ten fetuses with DS in Germany are indeed aborted (ÄrzteZeitung 2017). In Germany, under certain circumstances, abortion is permitted throughout the pregnancy, and is covered by insurance. Abortion is tolerated in Germany for the sake of the physical and psychological integrity of the pregnant woman, which could be endangered by a disabled child. In other words, disability is used as an indirect justification for abortion.[6]

Within a logic of caring for the ongoing pregnancy, NIPT introduces uncertainty and burdens pregnancy with negative emotions. The finding that highly educated women did not "understand" the "probabilistic" nature of NIPT could be interpreted as reflecting poor counselling. However, drawing such a conclusion would fall short of my aim to understand NIPT in constructivist terms, i.e., to reject scientific claims and understandings as the only rational and objective "truth", whereas all other discourses are based on false "belief". If we treat scientific and experiential claims symmetrically, and seek to understand each claim in the specific context of its actual, concrete practices, we could also argue that women are required to "de-script" (Akrich 1992) the meaning of NIPT, untie it from its intended use, and re-inscribe a new meaning.

By answering "you know what you are going to do", but warning that "it is always different" after receiving the test result, women like Sabrina remind us of the very complex nexus of life plans, ideas and ideals of family life, expectations of a healthy child, of what the parents think is desirable, and what is possible for them in society. Pregnancy, these women remind us, cannot be thought of in isolation, abstracted from the real world in which the test is available. Nor can NIPT be considered in isolation from the world in which the child might live. NIPT and its milieu interfere with each other, obliging practitioners to engage in certain other testing or caring practices.

For Sabrina, having a child with DS obliges her to see NIPT as a test that would deprive her existing child of legitimacy, dignity, and the right to live. Testing prac-

6 In Germany, abortions are formally prohibited without medical indication (§218 SGB). However, they are not punishable and are tolerated under the caveat of compulsory counselling, and if they are carried out within the first 12 weeks of pregnancy, which accounts for 96% of the abortions recorded between 2012 and 2022 (DESTATIS 2023). Abortions on medical grounds are covered by health insurance and are permitted throughout pregnancy.

tices, as I have argued, are not just about actions, but also about values and relationships. Because of the commitment to a child that progressively affirms itself, the timing of testing with NIPT is a matter of concern for Sabrina. Early testing would not allow a child to affirm itself.

Expectant parents must position themselves for a possible future that has not yet been mapped out. Choosing uncertainty does not mean that they deliberate less carefully, but that they have different attachments and obligations than in their previous actions. For Dorothee and Sabrina, the attachment is to an already born child and to their existing family. For both women, NIPT, with its probabilistic certainty and clinical non-invasiveness, forms a different element in their respective ecologies of care. The two women profer different responses to the offer of "knowing more" through NIPT and the routinization of testing during pregnancy. However, if we agree with Mol (2008: 75) that what constitutes "good", "worse", or "better" care does not precede practice but is rather an integral part of it, something to be negotiated within the situation or tinkered with as contingencies arise, then both logics are equally valid ways for women to care for the child to be born and the family into which it is to be born.

In some respects, the test for DS might be seen as more than just "seeing what is about to be born" (Löwy 2018). Parents are required to evaluate NIPT in the context of the world into which their child will be born, which are altogether different for Sabine and Dorothee. In this sense, women are more than just "moral pioneers" (Rapp 2000): they are field testing NIPT—with all its implications and obligations—for a society in which technological advances are continuously outpacing ethical and practical considerations.

## Acknowledgements

The project *Meanings and Practices of Non-Invasive Prenatal Genetic Diagnostics in Germany and* Israel *(PreGGI)* was funded by the German Research Foundation, DFG, grant RE2951/3-1 for 2017–2020. I would like to thank the project team: The PIs Christina Schües and Christoph Rehmann-Sutter, Anika König, who developed the interview guide and conducted the first half of the interviews, and Hannes Foth, Tamar Nov-Klaiman, Yael Hashiloni-Dolev and Aviad Raz for discussions and comments on ideas and drafts that led to this article. Most importantly, I am grateful to all the women and men who shared their stories with us.

## References


Achtelik, Kirsten. 2019. Anfang der Ausweitung. Gen-ethischer Informationsdienst (GID) 35(251): 32–33.

Akrich, Madelaine. 1992. The De-Scription of Technical Objects. *In* Shaping Technology. Weibe Bijker and John Law, eds. Pp. 205–224. Cambridge, MA: MIT Press.

ÄrzteZeitung. 2017. Trisomie-21-Diagnose führt meist zur Abtreibung, published 21.03.2017 Online https://www.aerztezeitung.de/Politik/Trisomie-21-Diagnose-fuehrt-meist-zur-Abtreibung-295904.html

Blümel, Miriam, Anne Spranger, Katharina Achstetter, Anna Maresso, and Reinhard Busse. 2020. Germany: Health system review. Health Systems in Transition 22(6): 1–272.

Braun, Kathrin, and Sabine Könninger. 2018. Realizing Responsibility: Institutional Routines, Critical Intervention, and the "Big" Questions in the Controversy Over Non Invasive Prenatal Testing in Germany. New Genetics and Society 37(3): 248–67.

Buyx, Alena. 2019. Kostenübernahme für pränatale Bluttests: Pro und Contra. Pro. Deutsches Ärzteblatt 115(44): A1988.

BVNP (Berufsverband niedergelassener Pränatalmediziner e.V.). 2020. NIPT als Kassenleistung: Pränataldiagnostiker sehen gravierende Mängel in G-BA Beschluss. In. Hürth: BNP.

Clarke, Adele E., Janet K. Shim, Laura Mamo, Jennifer Ruth Fosket, and Jennifer R. Fishman. 2003. Biomedicalization: Technoscientific Transformations of Health, Illness, and US Biomedicine. American Sociological Review 68(2): 161–194.

Corbin, Juliet and Anselm Strauss. 2008. Basics of Qualitative Research (3rd ed.): Techniques and Procedures for Developing Grounded Theory. Thousand Oaks, CA: Sage Publications, INC.

De Graaf Gert, John JM Engelen, Antoinet CJ Gijsbers, et al. 2017. Estimates of Live Birth Prevalence of Children with Down syndrome in the Period 1991–2015 in the Netherlands. J Intellect Disabil Res. 61: 461–70.

DESTATIS. 2023. Schwangerschaftsabbrüche. online https://www.destatis.de/DE/Themen/Gesellschaft-Umwelt/Gesundheit/Schwangerschaftsabbrueche/Tabellen/03-schwangerschaftsabbr-rechtliche-begruendung-schwangerschaftsdauer_zvab2012.html (accessed 18.09.2023)

Deutscher Bundestag. 2019. Plenarprotokoll 19/95 vom 11.4.2019. Berlin.

Dondorp, Wybo, Guido de Wert, Yvonne Bombard, et al. 2015. Non-invasive Prenatal Testing for Aneuploidy and Beyond: Challenges of Responsible Innovation in Prenatal Screening. Eur J Hum Genet. 23: 1438–50.

Dumit, Joseph. 2012. Drugs for Life: How Pharmaceutical Companies define our Health. Durham: Duke University Press.

Flöck, Anne, Ngoc-Chi Tu, Anna Rüland, et al. 2017. Non-invasive Prenatal Testing (NIPT): Europe's First Multicenter Post-market Clinical Follow-up Study Validating the Quality in Clinical Routine. Arch Gynecol Obstet 296: 923–928.

Franklin, Sarah, and Celia Roberts. 2006. Born and Made: An Ethnography of Preimplantation Genetic Diagnosis. Princeton: Princeton University Press.

G-BA. 2019a. Beschluss des Gemeinsamen Bundesausschusses über eine Änderung der Mutterschafts-Richtlinien (Mu-RL): Nicht-invasive Pränataldiagnostik zur Bestimmung des Risikos autosomaler Trisomien 13, 18 und 21 mittels eines molekulargenetischen Tests (NIPT) für die Anwendung bei Schwangerschaften mit besonderen Risiken. In BAnz AT 20.12.2019.

G-BA. 2019b. Nicht-invasiver Test zum Vorliegen von Trisomien als mögliche Alternative zu invasivem Eingriff. Berlin: Gemeinsamer Bundesausschuss (G-BA).

G-BA. 2023. Richtlinien des Gemeinsamen Bundesausschusses über die ärztliche Betreuung während der Schwangerschaft und nach der Entbindung ("Mutterschafts-Richtlinien") In BAnz AT 29.06.2023.

Gottfreðsdóttir, Helga, and Vilhjálmur Arnason. 2011. Bioethical Concepts in Theory and Practice: An Exploratory Study of Prenatal Screening in Iceland. Med Health Care Philos 14: 53–61.

Griffin, Blanche, Samantha Edwards, Lyn S. Chitty, and Celine Lewis. 2017. Clinical, Social and Ethical Issues Associated With Non-invasive Prenatal Testing for Aneuploidy. J Psychosom Obstet Gynaecol 8: 1–8.

Guell, Cornelia. 2011. Candi(e)d Action: Biosocialities of Turkish Berliners living with Diabetes. Medical Anthropology Quarterly 25(3): 377–394.

Hadolt, Bernhard, and Monika Lengauer. 2009. Genetische Beratung in der Praxis: Herausforderungen bei präsymptomatischer Gendiagnostik am Beispiel Österreichs. Frankfurt/Main: Campus.

Kater-Kuipers, Adriana, Inez D. de Beaufort, Robert-Jan H. Galjaard, and Eline M. Bunnik. 2018. Ethics of Routine: A Critical Analysis of the Concept of 'Routinisation' in Prenatal Screening. J Med Ethics 44: 626–631.

Konrad, Monica. 2005. Narrating the New Predictive Genetics: Ethics, Ethnography and Science. Cambridge: Cambridge University Press.

Lifecodexx. official website http://lifecodexx.com/en/expectant-mothers/ (accessed 15.05.2019).

Lock, Margret. 2005. Eclipse of the Gene and the Return of Divination. Current Anthropology 46(5): 47–70.

Lock, Margret, and Patricia Kaufert, eds. 1998. Pragmatic Woman and Body Politics. Cambridge: Cambridge University Press.

Löwy, Ilana. 2017 Imperfect Pregnancies: A History of Birth Defects and Prenatal Diagnosis. Baltimore: Johns Hopkins University Press.

Löwy, Ilana. 2018. Tangled Diagnoses: Prenatal Testing, Women, and Risk. Chicago: University of Chicago Press.

Malan, Valérie, Laurence Bussieres, Norbert Winer, et al. 2018. Effect of Cell-Free DNA Screening vs Direct Invasive Diagnosis on Miscarriage Rates in Women With Pregnancies at High Risk of Trisomy 21: A Randomized Clinical Trial. JAMA 320(6): 557–565.

Mol, Annemarie. 2008. The Logic of Care: Health and the Problem of Patient Choice. London: Routledge.

Mol, Annemarie. 2014. Language Trails: 'Lekker' and Its Pleasures. Theory, Culture & Society 31(2-3): 93–119.

Mol, Annemarie, Ingunn Moser, and Jeanette Pols, eds. 2010. Care in Practice. On Tinkering in Clinics, Homes and Farms. Bielefeld: transcript.

Patton, Michael Quinn. 2001. Qualitative Research and Evaluation Methods (2nd Edition). Thousand Oaks, CA: Sage Publications.

Pflegestärkungsgesetz. 2015. Zweites Gesetz zur Stärkung der pflegerischen Versorgung und zur Änderung weiterer Vorschriften (Zweites Pflegestärkungsgesetz – PSG II) Vom 21. Dezember 2015 Bundesgesetzblatt Jahrgang 2015 Teil I Nr. 54, ausgegeben zu Bonn am 28. Dezember 2015.

Porter, Theodore M. 1995. Trust in Numbers: The Pursuit of Objectivity in Science and Public Life. Princeton: Princeton University Press.

Prout, Alan. 1996. Actor-network Theory, Technology and Medical Sociology: An Illustrative Analysis of the Metered Dose Inhaler. Sociology of Health & Illness 18: 198–219.

Rapp, Rayna. 2000. Testing Women, Testing the Fetus: The Social Impact of Amniocentesis in America. New York and London: Routledge.

Reinsch, Stefan, Anika König, and Christoph Rehmann-Sutter. 2021. Decision-making About Non-invasive Prenatal Testing: Women's Moral Reasoning in The Absence of a Risk of Miscarriage in Germany. New Genetics and Society 40(2): 199–215.

Rothman, Barbara Katz. 1986. The Tentative Pregnancy: How Amniocentesis Changes the Experience of Motherhood. New York: Norton.

Rüffer, Corinna. 2019. Kostenübernahme für pränatale Bluttests: Pro und Contra. Kontra. Deutsches Ärzteblatt 115(44): A1989.

Salomon, Laurent J., Alexandros Sotiriadis, Camilla Bernt Wulff, Anthony Odibo, and Ranjit Akolekar. 2019. Risk of Miscarriage Following Amniocentesis or Chorionic Villus Sampling: Systematic Review of Literature and Updated Meta-analysis. Ultrasound Obstet Gynecol 54: 442–451.

Schües, Christina, Ed. 2022. Genetic Responsibility in Germany and Israel: Practic es of Prenatal Diagnosis. Bielefeld: transcript.

Schües, Christina, Stefan Reinsch, Aviad Raz, and Christoph Rehmann-Sutter. 2022. Can Not Wanting to Know be Responsible? Conceptual Analysis and Meanings of Not-knowing in Israeli and German Prenatal Genetic Practices. *In* Genetic Responsibility in Germany and Israel. Christina Schües, ed. Pp. 307–352. Bielefeld: transcript.

Solhdju, Katrin. 2018. Die Versuchung des Wissens: Vorschläge für einen gemeinschaftlichen Umgang mit prädiktiver Gen-Diagnostik. Bielefeld: transcript.

Thomas, Gareth M. 2017. Down's Syndrome Screening and Reproductive Politics: Care, Choice, and Disability in the Prenatal Clinic. New York: Routledge.

Thomas, Gareth M., and Barbara Katz Rothman. 2016. Keeping the Backdoor to Eugenics Ajar?: Disability and the Future of Prenatal Screening. AMA Journal of Ethics 18(4): 406–15.

Thyen, Ute, Jürgen Sperner, Matthias Morfeld, Christiane Meyer, and Ulrike Ravens-Sieberer. 2003. Unmet Health Care Needs and Impact on Families With Children With Disabilities in Germany. Ambulatory Pediatrics 3(2): 74–81.

Van Schendel, Rachel V., Adriana Kater-Kuipers, Elsbeth H. van Vliet-Lachotzki, et al. 2017. What Do Parents of Children With Down Syndrome Think About Non-Invasive Prenatal Testing (NIPT)? J Genet Couns 26: 522–31.

Vonneilich, Nico, Daniel Lüdecke, and Christopher Kofahl. 2016. The Impact of Care on Family and Health-related Quality of Life of Parents with Chronically Ill and Disabled Children. Disabil Rehabil 38(8): 761–767.

# 6 "Being a Little Bit Pregnant"
## Temporality and the Pragmatics of Uncertainty and Hope in In-Vitro Fertilization

*Bernhard Hadolt*

> Auch Hoffnung existiert nicht in einem sozialen und historischen Vakuum, sie hat immer eine Geschichte, und die Tragfähigkeit jeder Hoffnung hat viel mit dem Konsens zu tun, der über diese Geschichte herrscht und im Austausch und Gespräch weiterentwickelt wird.
>
> Hope too does not exist in a social and historical vacuum, it always has a story/history, and the bearing of any hope has a lot to do with the consensus that prevails about this story/history and is advanced in exchange and discussion.
> *(Kinsky 2023: 34, my translation)*

### Introduction

When my colleague Monika Lengauer and I were deeply immersed in ethnographic fieldwork for our study on how users of assistive reproductive technologies (ART) deal with these technologies in Austria (Hadolt and Lengauer 2003; Hadolt 2005), we always felt the urge to tell each other about the things that had just happened. Whether accompanying our informants to a medical appointment or talking to them about past events and future plans, we felt this need to share experiences whenever one of us left the field. We met at the hospital's café after saying goodbye to our informants or talked on the phone later in the evening, marvelling about the amount of work, suffering, and money users of In-vitro fertilization (IVF) put in. We were struck by the determination and dedication with which the couples we worked with worked through all required medical procedures over and over again, enduring pain and failure while pursuing their ultimate goal of having a baby and starting a family. They often invested their entire vacation time and all their savings and often risked the breakup of their partnership, all the while knowing all too well that the outcome was uncertain. Through dramatic ups and downs, pondering upon what might be the case medically speaking, pragmatically weighing up the options and imagining the—hoped for or feared—outcome of these options, for better or worse and sometimes against all odds, they maintained hope that all would turn out fine as they underwent another IVF treatment. In the one and a half years in which we followed these couples in their engagement with ART treatment, this hope has been fulfilled for some, but not for others.

Among the well-known ethnographies in medical anthropology that deal with such predicaments of suffering and uncertainty is Susan R. Whyte's (1997) *Questioning Misfortune.* Based on long-term ethnography, Whyte explores the ways how the Nyole people in eastern Uganda make sense and deal with misfortunes, such as sickness, marital problems, and death. Drawing on the work of John Dewey and other proponents of American pragmatism, she contends that Nyole respond to misfortune and the associated uncertainty with a pragmatist stance, prioritizing the actions taken to alleviate misfortune and the consequences of doing so over convictions. "For acting subjects," Whyte concludes more generally, "dealing with misfortune is a process of apprehending uncertainty, questioning experience, considering terms of action, implementing ideas, and looking to the results"; she continues: "You try, consider consequences, doubt, reconsider, revise your purpose perhaps, hope, and try again. In the process, you may never achieve certainty, though you may gain some degree of security" (ibid.: 224)—our informants could have expressed their experience in their quest for a baby in a similar way.

The situatedness and intentionality that define such pragmatics of uncertainty are also recognized in in the above epigraph. In her poetic essay *Gedankenspiele über die Hoffnung* (*musings about hope*) German writer and translator Esther Kinsky (2023) explores hope through five motions. They range, among others, from her father's induced coma after a failed heart surgery, a state "without hope", thirty years ago, to an analysis of Emily Dickinson's poem *Hope is the thing with feathers* "that perches in the soul", to a contemplation of *Hoffnung* (*hope*), the title of a poem by Friedrich Schiller. In the fourth motion—from which the introductory quote is taken—Kinsky examines Homer's Odysseus' hope for returning home when he recounts his odyssey at King Alcinous' banquet. In telling his story, Kinsky argues, Odysseus formulates a past through a retrospective present that engenders a hopeful, if uncertain, future. Significantly, Kinsky uses the German word *Geschichte* which has a double meaning, in the sense of an individual story to be told, but also in the sense of a more general history, perhaps best translated as *narrative*. The bearing of hope, Kinsky asserts, rests on the bearing of such a double-faced *Geschichte*, which is to be socially shared and advanced as time passes to become real.

In this chapter[1], I set out to explore the stories/narratives, unfolding over time, in which IVF users (and their medical professionals as well as ethnographers) are enmeshed as situated and purposeful actors and participants in social practices related to ART along the lines of the pragmatics of uncertainty and hope. For reasons of space, I focus on the final phases of IVF treatment, embryo transfer and implantation, and leave out how hope and uncertainty play out in earlier IVF phases and outside the clinic in the homes of IVF users, in media reports, on IVF clinics web pages, in self-help groups, in ART medical tourism advertising, and in policy-making.

I start from the assumption that affects and emotions are to be understood as happening relationally between people (and between people, non-human organisms, more-than-human beings, and things) and as an intrinsic part of the social, rather than as private mental or somatic states of feeling (e.g. Ahmed 2004; Collu 2019; Reckwitz 2016; Wetherell 2012). From a praxeological perspective (Schatzki 1996; 2002), I argue that hope, as a feeling and as a power technique that makes things happen, plays a crucial role in holding together and co-ordinating the manifold doings and sayings (and by extension the involved human and non-human participants) that constitute IVF as a social practice.

## A note on the study and its participants

The empirical material discussed in this chapter comes from ethnographic fieldwork that Monika Lengauer and I carried out between spring 2000 and autumn 2002 as part of the above-mentioned research project (Hadolt and Lengauer 2003; Hadolt 2005). The bulk of our data relates to eight case studies of involuntary childless couples whom we followed over a period of 18 months in their quest for a child of their own by using ART. During this time, we accompanied them to their clinical appointments at the IVF outpatient clinic of a university hospital in Vienna and at other private ART clinics and visited them at home for regular interviews. My analysis in this chapter draws heavily on the analysis we conducted in this research project. It is an effort to deal with this material with a fresh look.

The female participants were between 27 and 42 years old, and the men were between 30 and 52. Apart from one couple from Belgium, all participants had Austrian

1 An early version of this chapter was presented at the XI Medical Anthropology at Home (MAAH) Conference, held at the Schüttkasten Geras, Austria, in 2021. I am grateful to the participants and especially to Andrea Stöckl for their insightful comments. The study was funded by the Austrian Federal Ministry of Education, Science and Culture (BMBWK).

citizenship. All couples had been married for at least four years. One woman and one man already had an adult child from a previous marriage; all the other people were childless and, except for one woman, had never been pregnant. The diagnosis of medical infertility varied between couples, but also over the course of ART treatment for the same couple. The informants who—among others—play the main role in this text are as follows (in the order of first appearance):

At the time of our study, *Mrs Marek*[2] is 29 years old, *Mr Marek* is 34. Both come from eastern Lower Austria, where they live in a newly built house near Mr Marek's parents' house. Mrs Marek commutes to Vienna for her job in an office. Mr Marek works as a driver for a transport company. They have been married for nine years and have been trying to conceive a child for seven years. Six years ago, Mrs Marek talked to her gynaecologist for the first time about her "Kinderwunsch" ("wish for a child"), as wanting to have a child is called in Austrian discourse. After the couple had undergone four unsuccessful inseminations at a private ART clinic, they switched to the IVF outpatient clinic at the university hospital in the fall of 2000, where they completed an unsuccessful IVF cycle. Due to financial reasons, the couple switched back to the private clinic, where they underwent another two unsuccessful IVF cycles. The couple then decided to take a longer break from treatment. During this time Mrs Marek surprisingly becomes pregnant without medical intervention.

*Mrs Koller* is 33 years old; her husband is 32. Mrs Koller grew up in Vienna, where she also lives and works as a university teacher. Mrs Koller has been married for about six years and had been trying to get pregnant for four years. As her gynaecologist's advice to have "gezielten Geschlechtsverkehr" ("targeted intercourse") did not work, the gynaecologist referred her to the IVF outpatient clinic, where she underwent three unsuccessful IVF cycles before the fourth cycle results in a pregnancy. In contrast to most other couples, Mrs Koller underwent IVF treatment "single-handedly" in that her husband only came to the clinic for those appointments where his presence was absolutely necessary (for the initial consultation and for the sperm donation before the puncture).

*Mrs Salzer* is 36 years old, and *Mr Salzer* is 43. They both graduated from grammar school and work as clerks at various companies in Vienna. The couple lives in a newly built house to the west of Vienna, which they planned and built with a future child in mind. They have been married for thirteen years and have wanted a child for just as long. About seven years ago, during a routine gynaecological examination, Mrs Salzer approached a gynaecologist for the first time concerning her "Kinderwunsch." As Mr Salzer was diagnosed with "severely reduced sperm quality," several doctors recommended IVF treatment. For financial and organizational reasons, the Salzers turned to the IVF outpatient clinic, where they underwent their first IVF cycle in the spring of 2000, which was unsuccessful. The couple had two more unsuc-

2 All names are pseudonyms.

cessful IVF cycles before an ultrasound examination of Mrs Salzer revealed first a polyp and then a fibroid. Because the Salzers found the treatment at the IVF outpatient clinic very unsatisfactory, they switched to a private clinic, where they underwent their fourth IVF cycle at the beginning of 2002. This also failed. Further examinations were carried out at the private clinic, which ultimately led to the conclusion that successful IVF treatment was "very unlikely." The couple then decided not to continue with IVF treatment.

## IVF dramaturgy and temporal horizons

IVF users—women as well as men—often describe their engagement with IVF treatment as something of an emotional rollercoaster that indexes the drama of their stories about having a child. Here are some of the emotional states and feelings that users experience before, during and between IVF treatment cycles: strong desire to have a baby; pressing uncertainty and puzzlement about why the "natural way" of conception (through sexual intercourse) isn't working; joyful confidence when doctors praise the "promising" follicle growth during hormonal stimulation of the ovaries; nagging envy of other people's having children "so easily", given the hard work and suffering they have already gone through; indignant deservingness of having a baby oneself; feelings of not being sufficiently supported or even betrayed by the partner who supposedly does not engage in the treatment process as whole hearted enough; devastating despair and self-doubt after a failed IVF cycle; relieved joy when a pregnancy is diagnosed; deep doubts when having to decide whether to continue ART treatment or not; panic and overwhelming fear of a (another) failure; and, not least and of paramount importance, probing hope that everything will turn out fine when finally holding one's own baby in one's hands.

Usually, both in clinical discourses and media accounts as well as in academic writing, such feelings are dealt with either as a matter of coping with the demands and suffering connected to IVF treatment, or as motivation for undergoing ART treatment, or as psychological factors which may hamper or support becoming pregnant. In any case, such feelings are seen as being external to the techno-medical procedures of IVF itself (e.g., Devonport and Lane 2013; Rockliff et al. 2013). From such perspectives, IVF and feelings are understood as quasi standing *vis-à-vis* each other. However, such conceptualizations fail to recognize the generative role that emotions and feelings have for technologies such as IVF in the first place.

To address this, I draw on Schatzki's work on social practices, in particular, what he calls the "teleoaffective structure." In his view, social practices, defined as "temporally unfolding and spatially dispersed nexus of doings and sayings" (Schatzki 1996: 89), are organized by various aspects. Among others, the doings and sayings of a social practice "hang together" through its teleoaffective structure. This is "[...] a range of normativized and hierarchically ordered ends, projects, and tasks, to varying degrees allied with normativized emotions and even moods" (Schatzki 2002: 80). These are normatively charged complexes of purposes and objectives (referring to the *telos*) and emotions, sentiments, and passions (the affective dimension) that govern which activities are regarded as "right" and/or "acceptable."

The teleoaffective structuring of IVF treatment as a social practice, I content, relies on and at the same time produces hope in important ways: hope aligns the doings and sayings of IVF treatment along its *telos*, having a hoped-for baby and becoming parents by both limiting and employing the multiple uncertainties involved in IVF treatment; hope is also nourished when one after another task necessary in IVF treatment is successfully worked off, enabling to proceed to the next.

At least two fundamental, interrelated characteristics of IVF are of central importance here: Firstly, IVF is a complex and uncertain technology that requires the concerted interplay of activities and capacities involving both technical procedures and (mostly female) bodies, yet—and depending on the individual situation—with more or less uncertain results. Both as a future possibility and as a past and current matter of fact, failure (of producing follicles, embryos, and ultimately pregnancy, to name but a few) is all too real, as IVF users painfully know after their first failed IVF cycle at the latest. When I asked Mrs Riedel (44 years-old, four unsuccessful IVF cycles) after she and her husband had stopped ART treatment, what had her impressed most during ART treatment, she replied:

> The first two attempts where the implantation [nidation] didn't work, the day when I got the menstruation, that's the thing that somehow stayed with me most. Because maybe beforehand the hope is pretty high that it [getting pregnant] could work, and then suddenly there is the bleeding. That is, that is a hammer. That was absolutely <Mrs Riedel laughs> a hammer. (Mrs Riedel)

The medico-technical IVF procedures, then, are to be understood as being necessary but not sufficient for pregnancy to occur: it also requires (female and, to a lesser extent, male) bodies to be successful. The biotechnological feasibility of IVF is giving nature a "helping hand" Strathern (1992); it can only enable pregnancy and make it more or less likely, but not directly cause it. The interplay of technology and biology remains unreliable and is often mysterious, which leads to multiple uncertainties. In our study (Hadolt and Lengauer 2003: 285ff) we identified three main types of uncertainty, which we called "uncertainty-of-occurring" ("Unsicherheit des Passierens")—Will there be enough good follicles? Will the retrieved eggs fertilize? Will implantation work? etc.—, "uncertainty-of-the-actual" ("Ungewißheit des Tatsächlichen")—What is really the reason that I cannot conceive a child? What exactly was the reason that the last IVF cycle didn't work? etc.—, and "uncertainty-of-the-best-possible" ("Ungewißheit des Bestmöglichen")—What should I do to make implantation as likely as possible? Should we change the clinic for our next IVF cycle? etc. Hope tackles—and relies on—such uncertainties by maintaining the potentiality of both a positive, albeit hidden reality in the past and present, and a positive outcome in the future. As a form of "embodied meaning-making" (Wetherell 2012: 4), hope does this by embodied feeling rather than cool, detached reasoning. Hope maintains movement towards a desired future in the face of hovering failure. Hope keeps the story/narrative of IVF going.

Secondly, IVF is a cumulative technology. Lasting between four to seven weeks, and IVF cycle consists of a series of phases or steps, including: ovarian hyperstimulation to produce up to 30 eggs capable of fertilisation; the "puncture" of the follicles that have developed in the ovaries to retrieve (or "harvest" as some doctors call it) the eggs; the fertilisation of the eggs with the sperm in the laboratory and the cultivation of the resulting embryos for up to seven days after fertilisation; the embryo transfer, in which one to three of the developed embryos are transferred back into the uterus; and the biological implantation of the embryo in the uterus (nidation), the success of which can only be checked by a pregnancy test after a further two-weeks of "waiting period" at the earliest. Every individual phase must be successfully completed to at least a satisfactory degree to maintain the possibility of becoming pregnant. If one phase fails, the entire IVF cycle has failed. With a highly cumulative trajectory IVF is like a "hurdle race" ("Hürdenlauf"), or "obstacle course" (Franklin 1997), in which all hurdles must be successfully overcome to emerge victorious.

Given this hurdle race structure, IVF treatment is firmly directed toward the future. In addition, after a failed cycle, IVF users are confronted with the decision whether they should try another cycle, and then probably another one. Structured by the interplay of failure and hope, a specific procedural pathway is laid out to be followed, both within and between IVF cycles. Junctures that afford alternative routes only exist at specific points of the process (e.g., when the number and quality of follicle during ovarian hyperstimulation is low), but most importantly in between IVF cycles.

IVF treatment, in its dramaturgy of hope and failure (or success), has at least a threefold temporal configuration: First, a step-by-step configuration that highlights the next task and the next milestone at hand and follows an individual IVF cycle's cumulative trajectory. The temporal horizon for action and hope is the next step/task. Second, the overall configuration of the individual IVF course has the successful IVF cycle as its hoped-for temporal horizon. Particularly in these two temporal configurations, hope is strongly framed by the threat of future failure. One way of dealing with this is to curb hope to a "proper" extent to avoid disappointment when the IVF cycle fails. Mrs Marek said about her hopes for a positive outcome when she started her first IVF cycle:

> No, I don't want to set my hopes too high, because otherwise I might be depressed afterwards, or I don't know. I'm the kind of person who can cope with something quickly or something. But I always lower my hopes. And if it does work out, I'm happy, but I don't have high hopes for the first time. (Mrs Marek)

Another reason for not committing oneself too strongly to a particular outcome of an IVF cycle is that failure is not pre-programmed by decrying it. E.g., during the waiting period during their first IVF cycle, 54 years-old Mr Riedel stated that he did not want to "talk about the bear's fur [getting pregnant] until the bear had been killed" ("über den Fell des Bären reden, bevor er erlegt ist"), because that would bring bad luck.

In the third temporal configuration, IVF, as part of the overarching project of having a child and becoming a parent, has its temporal horizon in having a child with or without ART treatment. IVF users emphasise this perspective before an IVF cycle starts or has ended, but much less so within an IVF cycle. Only after the failure of an IVF cycle do opportunities for strategic decisions arise: whether to attempt another IVF, when, in which clinic, under what circumstances, etc. Decisions must also be made during an IVF cycle, but these are largely left to the medical professionals or are based on the requirements of the next IVF step to be accomplished. Our informants experienced their decision-making options as very limited and tended to react to the medical instructions rather than actively acting; they practically never acted against the doctors' advice. In contrast, strategic planning became salient after the end of an IVF cycle, though even then people only cautiously considered plans beyond the next IVF cycle. Their considerations in this regard were not characterised by an if-then, but rather by a casual exploration of possible courses of action; "let's see" ("mal schauen"), as 38 years-old Mr Pichler often put it, when he talked about the future.

IVF users, therefore, tend to plan their quest for a child retrospectively about past events rather than prospectively. Such planning is used to lend a certain coherence to the quest of having a child and to evaluate past actions and events and give them meaning. So, while for IVF users planning that is focussed on the individual IVF cycle is prospectively limited by the possibility of failure, the experience of failure in their planning attitude in a broader sense is a kind of reflective pause to clarify the next steps and an essential element in the ways of how couples structure their stories of having a child and starting a family.

## Embryo transfer and waiting for pregnancy

On the biotechnical-assisted path to pregnancy, the embryo transfer, and the hoped-for implantation of the embryo in the uterus, also known as nidation, play a crucial role. Embryo transfer and implantation differ from the previous stages in several respects. Apart from the fact that implantation is the "decisive phase" in which it becomes clear "will it be something or will it be nothing," as Mrs Salzer put it, the result of the implantation phase not just concludes a stage, but the IVF cycle altogether. At the medico-technological level, the embryo transfer is the last medical act; from this point onwards, the conception process is considered as in any "normal" pregnancy, and implantation itself must be left to the "natural" processes of the female body; nothing more can be done to make pregnancy more likely. In addition, while the work and result in the stages of hormone stimulation, puncture, fertilization and, in the narrower sense, embryo transfer are characterized by their temporal proximity to each other, the result of the implantation phase, and by extension, the whole IVF cycle, only becomes apparent after a waiting period, which is about two weeks. Not least because of the high stakes, our informants experienced this waiting period, painfully characterized by inactivity and uncertainty, as particularly stressful and difficult to bear. E.g., Mrs Pichler, 32 years old, commented on the difficulties during this waiting period after her second unsuccessful IVF cycle:

> On the one hand, I'm happy, on the other hand I'm afraid. [...] of the result, of the urine test [pregnancy test]. Of that, yes. Otherwise, I don't mind. It's not so bad. But the fourteen days [of the waiting period], that's a disaster. (Mrs Pichler)

One might expect that implantation and, in consequence, pregnancy is a matter of either-or, either pregnant or not pregnant. This is indeed the case, but the temporal point of view from which implantation is evaluated is crucial here. Only from an *a posteriori* perspective, when a definite and unambiguous outcome of an IVF cycle is established, does the outcome take on the binary form of either-pregnant-or-not-pregnant. From an *a priori* position, however, before a definite outcome is reached, things often are not so clear; the bodily state of gestation is uncertain, and pregnancy is hopeful. This can lead to a situation in which pregnancy becomes gradable, a matter of more-or-less, and in which IFV users might feel "a little bit pregnant".

All our informants agree that a "real" pregnancy only exists when an embryo has been successfully implanted. However, since this event cannot be known when it takes place biologically, but only afterwards, by means of the pregnancy test, it is both uncertain if "it will happen" (a matter of "uncertainty-of-occurring") and if it perhaps has already happened (a matter of "uncertainty-of-the-actual"). Such uncertainty—which comes into being only through the knowledge about embryo transfer and implantation—opens a space of possibilities for understanding and experiencing pregnancy in novel ways. The embryo transfer is a central facilitator in this: having the embryo in the uterus after the embryo transfer—and being aware of it—creates an as-if pregnancy situation, because our everyday understanding of pregnancy is constituted by the idea of "baby in the womb." The fact that "having put the embryo into the uterus" is not the same as implantation becomes sublimated via qualitative induction (a method of inference in which one property of a phenomenon is used to infer the phenomenon as a whole): "having the embryo in the uterus" becomes quasi equated "baby in the womb", even though the process leading to a pregnancy is not yet completed.

But not completely so: In particular, during the waiting phase after the embryo transfer, our informants' attitude oscillated between knowing what it takes for a "real" pregnancy and hopeful feelings concerning the potential for pregnancy in the first two weeks after the embryo transfer, being cautious and hopeful at the same time. Many of them resolve the tension by feeling "a little bit pregnant", such as Mr Lang, who told us that his wife had a "feeling of being a little bit pregnant" when she waited for the pregnancy test after her second embryo transfer. Similarly, Mrs Koller, who repeatedly emphasised in our conversations how much she had learned about reproduction from a medical perspective since she started IVF, reflects on the time after the embryo transfer in her first IFV cycle, which was unsuccessful:

> Somehow you think, well, I mean that, somehow you think you're pregnant—a little bit. I don't mean that you feel it [...] as in stories about pregnancies, first when you feel sick. I mean, you don't really feel the pregnancy, [...] that you have a big belly, that you really experience—uh—[...] a physical experience of pregnancy, that's much later. But the thought, yes, this emotional feeling. [...] I mean, you kind of build up a little bit, that you say, [...] it's not certain yet. (Mrs Koller)

Mrs Marek also reported that she felt "somehow pregnant" during the time between embryo transfer and the onset of menstruation when she underwent her first (unsuccessful) IVF cycle. She said about her behaviour during this time:

> Well, when that [the embryo transfer] is over, you just walk like on raw eggs. <Mrs Marek laughs> You think: just don't move quickly! Yes, and then the waiting begins. That, the 14 days, that was somehow. Because you actually think about it every day. I think, one also feels somehow pregnant subconsciously, because you're totally careful and I hardly smoked anything. So that's already. Somehow, I mean, secretly you maybe DO hope that you're pregnant, but. Yes, it's just, after a day: do you feel anything yet? No, you don't feel anything. Yes, and then on the 15th day you take the [pregnancy] test. But I already knew one or two days before [that she was not pregnant], because that's when I started having cramps and light bleeding. (Mrs. Marek)

Mrs Salzer expressed the difference between feeling and knowing even more pointedly than Mrs Koller, quoted above, and said of herself that she had already had the feeling of being pregnant immediately after the embryo transfer, although she did not know this definitively:

> I mean, I already know that I'm NOT at that point, so [...] I mean, I already know that it's NOT necessarily [the case that she is pregnant], but from the FEELING? YES. From that moment on, I have the feeling [of being pregnant]. (Mrs Salzer)

Like most other IVF users in our study, Mrs Salzer was careful not to hope too much that she would actually be pregnant to avoid disappointment and despair if treatment proved to be a failure.

## Making pregnancy real

Remarkably, the possibility of being "a little bit pregnant" also exists from a medical point of view. Even after the two-week waiting period following embryo transfer has passed, it is not always possible to say with certainty "if it has worked out" ("ob es etwas geworden ist") or not, to use Mrs Salzer's expression. The onset of menstruation or a positive or negative pregnancy test is not necessarily the criterion by which such a clear result can be determined. If the pregnancy test is positive and no menstruation has occurred, doctors and the women concerned assume that there is a pregnancy. Such a "biochemical pregnancy" is then clinically confirmed a few weeks later by an ultrasound examination, making a pregnancy even more "real".

The situation is different, however, when no menstrual bleeding has occurred, but at the same time no clearly positive pregnancy can be determined due to ambiguous hCG levels on the pregnancy test.[3] Such a biochemical condition is sometimes referred to by some doctors in our study as "a little bit pregnant". In the case of the Mrs and Mr Lang, where this occurred during their first IVF cycle, blood was taken from Mrs Lang to determine the corresponding hormone status more precisely that by checking the hormone status in the urine. The couple was told in the clinic that the result should be available the same day in the afternoon. For Mrs and Mr Lang, 33 and 34 years old respectively, this increased their hope for pregnancy, but also prolonged the period of uncertainty. Their anger was correspondingly great when they only found out the result of the blood test the next day after several telephone calls. Mr Lang reported the negative result to us in an e-mail:

> Unfortunately, we were unable to find out yesterday whether we were allowed to celebrate or not. At 3 o'clock in the afternoon there was still no result. Today we tried again—8:40 a.m., still nothing, another hour's wait. We are not angry, but here too the procedure is incomprehensible: Ultrasound appointment,—no, but urine test,—but ultrasound—no, wait for urine test, – not clear, – so, blood test – result in the afternoon,—no, but not,—so tomorrow morning,—no, but not so

3 The pregnancy test works by measuring the amount of human chorionic gonadotropin (hCG), a hormone that only develops during pregnancy.

> early. Now, just after 10 a.m., finally the certainty. The waiting and hoping has come to an end. But unfortunately, the bad news. Not pregnant. That has to be digested in the first place. There were no tears, we are not upset. It's still too early. It wasn't meant to be yet [to become pregnant in the course of the first IVF cycle]. (Mr Lang)

Even if the pregnancy test is clearly negative, it can remain uncertain whether a pregnancy is present or not if there is no menstrual bleeding. This was the case for Mr and Mrs Pichler during their second IVF cycle and Mrs and Mr Salzer, also during their second IVF cycle. The following vignette describes the medical appointment to which I accompanied Mrs and Mr Salzer and at which the negative result of the pregnancy test, for which Mrs Salzer had previously given urine, was discussed:

> Dr Kramer greets us at the door of the consultation room and asks Mrs Salzer, who was the first to enter: "Are you bleeding?" Mrs Salzer denies this, shaking her head. Dr Kramer turns to Mr Salzer, who had entered immediately afterwards, and jokingly asks him too: "Are you bleeding?" Mr Salzer also, jokingly mocking his wife, says no. We all head to our seats as usual and before Mrs Salzer had even sat down, Dr Kramer announces that the pregnancy test unfortunately is negative: well, this would be just difficult now; if Mrs Salzer had already had her menstruation, it would be straightforward: pregnancy test negative plus menstruation; but it wasn't clear that way; it could just be the case that her menstruation would come later; but it could also mean that implantation had been delayed somewhat and that the hormone levels had therefore not yet built up.
>
> Mrs and Mr Salzer listen quietly with disappointed and annoyed facial expressions. Dr Kramer continues that unfortunately she could now only offer to do another blood test; but she would probably only have the results on Monday, because unfortunately it was already very late for today; in order to get the results today, the couple would have had to come in the morning.
>
> Mrs Salzer turns to her husband and says reproachfully: "I'll kill you!" [At Mr Salzer's suggestion, they had come to the clinic at 11 a.m., as Mr Salzer wanted to go to work for a few hours beforehand]. Mr Salzer defends himself, says it was not his fault. Mrs Salzer replies that it was certainly his fault, he had only wanted to come at 11 and now it was too late for the results of the blood test.
>
> Dr Kramer seem uncertain about what to do, first saying that it wasn't Mr Salzer's fault and then immediately agreeing with Mrs Salzer that it was too late and they should have come earlier.
>
> They then go on and on about whether Mrs Salzer could be pregnant or not and Dr Kramer keeps repeating that she was sorry that she cannot say anything today; everything is very complicated in early pregnancy and normally these steps that we observe go unnoticed.

At one occasion Dr Kramer asks Mrs Salzer if she feels pregnant. Mrs Salzer replies by asking how one feels being pregnant. Dr Kramer smiles and says that she could only tell from what others had told her, but if she simply feels different? Mrs Salzer: no, it is just like before the menstruation. Dr Kramer finally takes a blood sample from Mrs Salzer, whereupon a discussion ensues as to whether it might not still be possible to get a result today, which Dr Kramer again denies.
Dr Kramer leafs through the medical record again and says ponderingly that only three embryos had developed; but these would have been quite nice (she repeats this several times); but she had had a lot of eggs, a "huge pile of eggs" ("riesiger Eierhaufen"), but only three would have been fertilised. Mr Salzer admits: "Yes, that is also my poor [sperm] quality". Again, Dr Kramer says that if Mrs Salzer had got her menstrual bleeding, then one would know, but like this (?); there would just be pregnant or not pregnant. Dr Kramer then adds that there was also "a little bit pregnant", so the hormone levels had to be observed; but the pregnancy test was clearly negative. [...]
Finally, the meeting comes to an end and after arranging another appointment for the next week we say goodbye.
All the way to the exit, Mr Salzer talks to his wife and tries to convince her that they still had a chance for being pregnant. He calls Mrs Salzer (not very convincingly) a "slow breeder" ("langsame Brüterin") and that it could be the case that everything would just take longer. Mrs Salzer keeps repeating that she did not believe it, starting to cry. We stop and Mr Salzer hugs her for a few minutes, striking her head. Eventually we continue walking towards the exit.
Arriving in front of the hospital, Mr Salzer lights a cigarette—not two cigarettes, as he had done last time; Mrs Salzer had given up smoking in the meantime. Mrs Salzer says challengingly that she could now smoke again. Mr Salzer replies: no, she couldn't; it could still be that she was pregnant. And he finishes the cigarette on his own.
The following day Mrs Salzer calls me on the phone to tell me that her menstruation started, which unquestionably showed that this IVF cycle was again unsuccessful.

Apart from the social dynamics between Mr and Mrs Salzer and Dr Kramer respectively and the dramatic quality that medical appointments can have, especially at the very end of an IVF cycle when its ultimate result is not yet clear, this vignette also shows how hope and uncertainty are intertwined in the teleoaffectivities of IVF. Uncertainty, spanning what is actually the case now ("a little bit pregnant?") and how this will develop in the near future ("an established pregnancy?"), opens space for hope. Against the background of inconclusive test results, bodily states of feeling and organisational procedures, such hope is negotiated between the involved actors in terms of past events in the hurdle-race IVF, uncertain medical knowledge about reproduction, results of a urine test, ascribed personal qualifications and shared (or not shared) cigarettes. At times, hope is probing, taking on hopeful diagnostic possibilities again and again, then desperate or dwindling until it crumbles away and ends abruptly with the onset of menstruation—at least as far as this particular IVF cycle with its specific time horizon is concerned. After a break, Mrs and Mr Salzer will build up hope and try again and only stop ART treatment completely after a fourth unsuccessful IVF cycle.

If we look at it as a process, pregnancy may also be gradable rather than binary from a medical point of view. In any case, it needs to be made ever more "real", both physically and in terms of women's feelings, beginning with hormone stimulation and culminating in the pregnancy test. But even if a pregnancy is no longer questionable from a medical perspective because it has been "definitely" established through pregnancy tests and ultrasound scans, the making-real of pregnancy can continue. This takes two forms. The first concerns the feeling of being pregnant. Mrs Koller said in an interview one week after her pregnancy had been confirmed by the positive pregnancy test that she cognitively knew that she was pregnant, but that the corresponding bodily feeling had not yet set in:

> On the other hand, of course it was really nice when I heard [during the pregnancy test] that it was OK. And somehow it's also in my head: I mean, it's OK now and I'm now pregnant. But somehow, in terms of feeling it still needs time. [...] At the beginning [of a pregnancy] it's still most uncertain [that a pregnancy will last], or I mean, the danger of something happening is the greatest. (Frau Koller)

Although Mrs Koller already felt "a little bit pregnant" during the phase of implantation, her feeling after the positive pregnancy test was too little to "really" feel pregnant. What she missed in this context, as she explained elsewhere, were such typical signs of pregnancy as morning sickness and especially the baby's movements. As a contribution to making the pregnancy real, she also gave an important place to the ultrasound examination, which was scheduled for the week after the interview and which was intended to confirm the pregnancy clinically, because she hoped that this would make the pregnancy more visible. She said about the pregnancy test: "I mean, what's the big deal? I mean, something just changes colour."

In the above quote, Mrs Koller also refers to the second form of making the pregnancy real: the risk that "something will happen." Certainly, the positive pregnancy test is the first objective, albeit not always clear, sign of pregnancy and once this hurdle has been overcome, women no longer doubt that they *are* pregnant. What they do worry about is whether they will *stay* pregnant. Especially in the first twelve weeks of pregnancy, the threat of a miscarriage is experienced as a real possibility. Such a threat was perceived as even more serious if women and couples had already experienced a miscarriage, as was the case with the Durand couple.

To some extent, such a risk is certainly also perceived in the case of non-medically assisted pregnancies, although here, too, the first twelve weeks of pregnancy may be considered the "dangerous" ones even in this case. This is supported, for example, by the fact that the gynaecologist who cared for Mrs and Mr Durand during their pregnancy did not give Mrs Durand the *Mother and Baby Book* (*Mutter-Kind-Pass*)[4] until after the twelfth week of pregnancy. He explained several times that he would always do so in order to reduce disappointment in case of a miscarriage. However, IVF users seem to experience the risk of pregnancy as much more pronounced than with "normal" pregnancies due to the high stakes involved in ART treatment and the difficulties of getting pregnant in the first place. In addition, the way in which the early stage of pregnancy becomes "visible" in the context of IVF may also play a significant role.

## Precarious knowledge

In IVF treatment, precarious knowledge is everywhere—and so is certain knowledge in the very moment. To a certain extent, knowledge produces uncertainty, as this points to the parts that still are not yet known. In contrast to medically unassisted reproduction, where conception only comes conscious "after the fact" at a comparatively late state, medically assisted conception is characterized by its very early, conscious, and detailed perception. This also applies to the aspects that can "go wrong". As far as her theoretical knowledge of human reproduction was concerned, Mrs Koller emphasized that it was precisely the knowledge of the possible difficulties that was new to her:

> So to speak, how it works theoretically, uh—the fertilization and a pregnancy and so on, the development from the fertilized egg, that was COMPLETELY CLEAR to me. I mean, with all the stages, the biology of it. But what was, uh, very NEW for me was rather these things, that how REALLY possible it actually is that fertilization occurs. And that, first of all, it's not all that likely. And that if fertilization does occur, that even with NORMAL [pregnancies], as is often the case with one fertilized egg, but it aborts and you don't even NOTICE it and you just have your menstruation. [...] Somehow, I don't know, biologically speaking, OKAY: sperm cell, egg cell: kabong! <Mrs Koller and the interviewer laugh> It implants! But I mean, what kind of complications can there be UNTIL it implants! [...] So then, it's kind of like in the textbook: it works! But I know all the steps, where things may not work. This is what you do not know and this is what you realize then [when undergoing ART treatment]. (Mrs Koller)

4 In Austria, the *Mother and Baby Book* (*Mutter-Kind-Pass*) is a free of charge health prevention program for pregnant women and young children up to the age of five.

Mrs Koller's conviction that new knowledge is gained by going beyond textbook knowledge and by focussing on the potentially flawed parts of reproduction is striking. She focuses on what can "go wrong", which in turn is enabled by the fragmentation of the procreation process by undergoing the "hurdle race" of IVF with its various stages and cumulative outcomes. The complexity of the process turns much of the knowledge that she had known as unproblematic before her engagement with ART, precarious knowledge, knowledge until further notice. As a result, ART treatment also has the potential to make "natural" conception visible in a new way as an equally potentially ineffective endeavour. The need to make a pregnancy "real" after IVF treatment and the heightened awareness of how much can "go wrong" may extend to the post-IVF phases of pregnancy and further add stress to IVF users. In this sense, pregnancy after IVF may be by no means "completely normal", contrary to what medical professionals and the women and men concerned may believe.

## Concluding remarks

In this chapter, I have explored the entanglements of temporality, uncertainty, and hope as they become evident in the case of IVF treatment. I have argued that hope, in its relational and intentional mode, is intrinsic to IVF as social practice: as part of the teleoaffective structure of IVF treatment, hope holds together and organizes the doings and sayings of IVF, and by extension the human and non-human participants involved (Schatzki 1996; 2002). Against the backdrop of an often inconclusive past and present and potential failure in the future, hope both relies on and tackles uncertainty and—depending on where IVF users are in the process of IVF treatment and which temporal horizon is salient—maintains concerted movement towards a desired future; hope keeps the story/narrative of IVF going.

I followed IVF users in their dramatic quest for having a baby and becoming parents as they experience and deal with the necessities, predicaments and imponderability of IVF treatment. Focusing on the final phases of IVF treatment, I have shown their pragmatic stance by which they, being specifically situated, work through what needs to be done in the various stages of IVF treatment, make the best possible use of their resources at hand, imagine future possibilities, and try out new (and old) things to achieve pregnancy. In such a pragmatics of uncertainty (Whyte 1997), hope for a partially hidden favourable situation in the past and present and for positive outcomes in the future is carefully modulated, as their story unfolds: In order to make hope "bearing" ("tragfähig", in the words of Kinsky 2023: 34), IVF as social practice is organized in ways so that IVF users (and the doctors treating them) curb their hope to prevent too much disappointment, should an IVF cycle turn out to be unsuccessful, but nourish hope to the extent that necessary IVF work can continue and suffering be endured. In such a "paradox of hope" (Mattingly 2010), hope has intentionality; it is *hope for something*, thus bringing its referents (e.g., many eggs, embryos, and ultimately successful pregnancy and a baby) into play, charging them with embodied meaning and affective purpose, while simultaneously foregrounding potential failure.

Hope dwells in uncertainty about *what is*, *what will happen*, and *how best to deal with*. Knowledge brought into play as a means of dealing with uncertainty can also foster uncertainty, as detailed general medical knowledge about human reproduction makes visible the many aspects of conception that can go wrong, and tentative knowledge about the individual IVF cycle opens the space that makes gradable pregnancy in the form of "being a little bit pregnant" possible, both in the experience of IVF users and in biomedical discourse, and necessitates work to be done to make pregnancy "real."

I want to conclude by drawing attention to three implications that might prove useful for further research on uncertainty and hope beyond the case of IVF. The first concerns the central role that affects/emotions can play in social practices such as IVF. When taken seriously as relationally distributed among the (human and non-human) participants of social practices and not merely as momentary private states of feelings, hope can be probed for its function as an intrinsic constituent of social practices, furthering our comprehension of figurations that give rise to phenomena such as "being a little bit pregnant."

The second implication concerns the many forms and shades in which hope manifests itself in the stories of our informants, indicating complex feelings and functions: burgeoning hope, desperate hope, confident hope, reckless hope, comforting hope, etc. Academic literature lacks a sophisticated language of hope that could analytically capture this diversity. We could better grasp the significance of hope as a generative force in social practices by paying more analytical attention to such differences. Examining these across various socio-cultural settings might show that there are many more culturally marked idioms of hope than we can imagine.

Finally, the third implication relates to hope and uncertainty as they are temporally framed. Contrary to the taken for granted assumption that hope and uncertainty are always directed towards the future, our empirical material shows a much more complex situation, in which hope and uncertainty wander to the past and present and span to future events. By looking more closely at this temporality, we could gain a better understanding of how temporal figurations with their distinct temporal horizons are constituted and operate as social practices unfold.

## References

Ahmed, Sara. 2004. The Cultural Politics of Emotion. New York: Routledge.

Collu, Samuele. 2019. Refracting Affects: Affect, Psychotherapy, and Spirit Dis-Possession. Culture, Medicine, and Psychiatry 43: 290–314.

Devonport, Tracey J., and Andrew M. Lane. 2013. Emotions and Emotion Regulation in a Female Couple Undergoing In Vitro Fertilization Treatment. Psychology 4(6A1): 25–33.

Franklin, Sarah. 1997. Embodied Progress: A Cultural Account of Assisted Conception. London: Routledge.

Hadolt, Bernhard. 2005 [publ. in 2009]. Biotechnical Feasibility, User Agency and Patients' Strategies: How Unwanted Childless Women and Men Strategically Deal With the Uncertainties of In Vitro Fertilisation. AM. Rivista Della Società Italiana Di Antropologia Medica 19–20: 37–54.

Hadolt, Bernhard, and Monika Lengauer. 2003. Kinder-Machen: Eine ethnographische Untersuchung zur Handhabe von ungewollter Kinderlosigkeit und den Neuen Reproduktionstechnologien durch betroffene Frauen und Männer in Österreich. Vienna: PhD Thesis, Univ. of Vienna.

Kinsky, Esther. 2023. Gedankenspiele über die Hoffnung. Graz: Literaturverlag Droschl.

Mattingly, Cheryl. F. 2010. The Paradox of Hope: Journeys through a Clinical Borderland. Berkeley, CA: University of California Press.

Reckwitz, Andreas. 2016. Praktiken und ihre Affekte. *In* Praxistheorie: Ein soziologisches Forschungsprogramm. Hilmar Schäfer, ed. Pp. 163–180. Bielefeld: transcript.

Rockliff, Helen E., Stafford L. Lightman, Emily Rhidian, et al. 2014. A Systematic Review of Psychosocial Factors Associated with Emotional Adjustment in In Vitro Fertilization Patients. Human Reproduction Update 20(4): 594–613.

Schatzki, Theodore R. 1996. Social Practices: A Wittgensteinian Approach to Human Activity and the Social. Cambridge: Cambridge Univ. Press.

Schatzki, Theodore R. 2002. The Site of the Social: A Philosophical Account of the Constitution of Social Life and Change. University Park, Pa.: Pennsylvania State Univ. Press.

Strathern, Marilyn. 1992. After Nature: English Kinship in the Late Twentieth Century. Cambridge: Cambridge University Press.

Wetherell, Margaret. 2012. Affect and Emotion: A New Social Science Understanding. London: Sage.

Whyte, Susan Reynolds. 1997. Questioning Misfortune: The Pragmatics of Uncertainty in Eastern Uganda. Cambridge: Cambridge University Press.

# Part III: Health Management

# 7 Solo Living and Cancer in Denmark
## Understanding Care Politics as the Architect of Human Vulnerabilities

*Rikke Sand Andersen*

### Introduction

What insights can people who suffer from cancer and who live alone provide about relations between vulnerability and care politics? This is the question that underlines the discussions raised in this chapter, as I set out to understand ongoing shifts in care politics as they emerge and transform in the context of welfare. The empirical material is drawn from Denmark and from ethnographic work among people suffering from cancer, but it speaks to much broader changes in the distribution and definition of care, and the rise in solo living that are taking place across Scandinavia and elsewhere (Vaittinen 2015). Also, ethnographic engagements with people who suffer from cancer while sustaining life in the context of solo living, allows me to explore what it means when we say that vulnerability is—at the same time—both fundamental to human existence and political, such as noted by Judith Butler (2020: 20–22).

In Denmark and more broadly in Scandinavia, since the 1960s onwards, the distribution of care resources have been organized around the guiding principles of a care politics that emphasizes state-supported social security and individual independence from the family. Anthropological literature on Scandinavia often names this an egalitarian care politics, emphasizing how Scandinavian welfare politics aim to promote equal distribution of care both within the families and within society, and how this involved a substantial professionalization and institutionalization of care. Ideally, women should no longer rely on kinship or marriage for survival or for living socially acceptable or sustainable lives, and the elderly, disabled or sick should not rely on their families for care and survival (Gullestad and Segalen 1997; Bendixsen et al. 2017).

The aging of the Scandinavian populations means, however, that not only is there a dramatic growth in care needs, but also a diminishing professional workforce, and the family and people's private homes are increasingly reconsidered relevant contexts of care (Vaittinen 2015; Mattingly et al. 2011). Since 2006 one in five beds in Danish hospitals have been removed (Skovgaard et al. 2022), and "same-day-treatments" of cancer patients have gone up by 40 percent. Also, home care services are increasingly targeted at the neediest persons. Fewer older people receive municipality services (cleaning, shopping, care) from 18 percent in 2008 to the present 11 percent of persons 65+ in 2019 (Hjelmar and Rostgaard 2020). This mix of capacity reductions and political attempts to move care closer to the home of the patient mean that sick individuals must increasingly navigate treatment and care from a wide range of professionals, kin, and services concurrently (Skovgaard et al. 2022). Anthropologists have described how the transfer of care responsibilities to families may both heighten existing tensions and conflicts and promote experiences of belonging (Sparre and Rytter 2021; Grøn and Meinert 2017; Lamb 2014). But we only have sparse knowledge on how people who live alone experience and manage changing possibilities of care, or how shifts in the distribution of care resources reconfigure intergenerational responsibilities and vulnerabilities for individuals who live alone.

According to Eric Klinenberg, an American sociologist, the prevalence of solo living was minimal in societies worldwide prior to the 1960s (2013: 2–4). However, the number of individuals living alone has now reached nearly 30 percent of all households in the United States. Additionally, several major European cities have witnessed a surpassing of the 50 percent mark in terms of one-person households (Klinenberg 2013). In Denmark, four out of ten adults live alone, with the percentage of one-person households among the elderly exceeding fifty percent (Danmarks Statistik 2023). This chapter makes its initial contribution by highlighting the increasing number of individuals living alone, and I propose that examining how people suffering from cancer sustain life in the context of solo living provide a way to begin to understand and theorize emerging shifts in the distribution of care resources that are taking place in Denmark and across Scandinavia.

Introducing in detail the biographies and lived circumstances of Lise and Michael, two interlocutors that I worked with from April 2020 until August 2021, and drawing on the understanding of humans as embodied and vulnerable (Butler 2020; Guenther 2016) and upon critical feminist writings on care (Fischer and Tronto 1990; Buch 2018), this chapter makes its second contribution by pointing out that access to care is increasingly dependent upon social negotiation, and studying care in the context of solo living is a means of theorizing fundamental dependency and ethical responsibility in the context of welfare. With Elana Buch (2018: 12) I think of care as "the messy, disparate forms of practice through which people work to make life happen", and how these practices continually bring particular kinds of social relations, political economies, or vulnerabilities into being. Such a perspective on care reaches beyond the immediate, intimate context of care as practice, and it helps me acknowledge the polysemantic and shifting qualities of care and being that emerges when care politics change (cf. Meinert 2021; Fischer and Tronto 1990). I suggest that attending to the productive dimensions of care politics and care practices helps to direct attention to what care produces (Buch 2018: 18)—including new kinds of vulnerabilities that are historically and socio-politically distinct. Before I turn to Lise and Michal let me share some more reflections on what I mean when I talk about vulnerability.

## Vulnerability and care politics

Etymologically speaking, vulnerability means to be open to hurt. It comes from Latin *vulnerare*, to wound, hurt, injure, or maim. As a verb it specifies an action. That is probably why—in popular thinking and writing—vulnerability is often thought of as a state of being open to hurt from external risks (Vaittinen 2015: 104). A community can be susceptible to war, or a computer can be susceptible to damage. But as living, social organisms humans are also internally and persistently vulnerable to life itself; to the possibility of loss, destruction and to diseases such as cancer. There are no autonomous subjects without needs, "only degrees of embodied vulnerability" (Vaittinen 2015: 104) that elicits different care needs. In a similar fashion, Judith Butler (2020) says that vulnerability should not be understood as a static condition, but as a dynamic and relational process that unfolds in the context of social and historical relations. Humans are social bodies and therefore perpetually vulnerable to the loss of others, and to violence and disease. As humans we are "potentially undone by each-other" (Butler 2020: 23). Vulnerability, in this sense, is not a property of individual subjects, nor an external risk, but a product of social and political structures and processes. Vulnerability, Butler says, names "the porous and interdependent character of our bodily and social lives" (Butler and Yancy 2020: 483) and it invites discussions on how to live, how to face mortality and how best to make sense of the world (Butler and Worms 2023).

It is important to note that vulnerability to Butler, does not only gesture towards an existential condition. Instead, Butler advances vulnerability as an underlying aspect of human interdependence and coexistence, and one from which political principles emerge. Human vulnerability thus constitutes a repertoire of essentials that are subject to manipulation (for example through politics) and practice (such as care) for the purposes of producing what they call livable lives (Butler and Worms 2023: 27–28). Following this line of thought, I suggest that exploring solo living in the context of serious disease, testifies to the way in which care politics proposes itself as the architect of human vulnerabilities. I develop this argument by attending to what I consider to be emerging vulnerabilities in the context of solo living and changing care politics. The first being *relational vulnerabilities*, which refers to the increasing social and moral tensions that arise in negotiating access to care, and the second being *vulnerabilities to the self*, which I with reference to Lisa Guenther's notion of unhinged (2016), define as the loss of abilities to engage in world-making activities.

## Encounters with living alone

In this fieldwork, which I have done with my colleague Sara Marie Hebsgaard Offersen, we have worked with ten key interlocutors, all aged 54–84, who lived alone and suffered from cancer. To understand how people sustain life with cancer, we invited interlocutors who were in long-term care, and who, to some extent, were living with the prospects of "a life with cancer". Cancer is treacherous and unpredictable, though, and four of our interlocutors have passed away as I write.

The basic benefit of ethnographic fieldwork is its open-endedness (Rapp 1999). We conducted fieldwork from 2020–2021 (app. 14 months), but it did not work out as first planned. Our initial goal was to explore the social dynamics of care situations and to work with care workers and family caregivers as well as those in need of care. When the covid-19 pandemic broke out at the turn of the year 2019–20, enforced lockdowns challenged our presence at hospitals and other care institutions. Also, we were not able to visit with our interlocutors when home-care workers were present. We ended up spending many hours in the homes of our interlocutors, mostly being present when others were absent. Instead of witnessing the relational dynamics of care situations, we gained detailed insights into their life-histories, and through their experiences we learned about transformation in family- and gender values, intergenerational relations, and expectations to care; subjects of relevance to our understanding of care politics, and how it manifests in the minutiae of everyday life.

Some visits were structured around life-history interviews, or on mapping and narrating the web of social relations that made up their lives. Other visits were dominated by informal conversations on experiences and notions related to "family", "home" and "care". Sometimes we would go for a walk, act as chauffeurs to the hospital, or go for a drive and visit significant places such as former homes and communities where they had once lived. Also, we talked about experiences with living alone, and we shared quiet moments together. Due to the risk of covid-19, three out of ten interlocutors were only engaged with through online platforms. While the online meetings tended to be shorter, and made "hanging out" difficult, they allowed for regularity (we met often with these informants), and it was possible to both do semi-structured interviews and engage in informal conversations. We also interviewed three family members, one friend and one volunteer. In total we conducted about eighty interviews.

## Solo living in Denmark

Despite the moral dominance of the nuclear family and the detached house [parcelhuset] that developed during the 1960s and 1970s, the most dominant trend in living- and household arrangements in Denmark since the 1960s has been the rise in solo living (Klinenberg 2013). Today, there are 2.7 million homes in Denmark housing a population of 5.8 million people. In 1.3 million homes live only one adult (18+). People end up living alone for a variety of reasons and living alone is experienced and practiced differently. While research on Danish solo dwellers is very sparse Lynn Jamieson and Roona Simpson's research from Ireland (2013), as well as Eric Klinenberg's (2013) research from the US suggests that people who live on their own have different degrees of personal ties to kin, family, and friends. Some maintain relationships across households with partners, children, parents or friends, and others do not.

This diversity was also present in our material. Seven interlocutors lived alone because they had recently divorced, or their spouses had passed away, and three had lived alone most of their adult lives. Two of those had raised children on their own. None of them had actively chosen to live on their own, but that was "how life had turned out", as they would often say. There is thus an aspect of contingency and temporality to living alone. Some of our interlocutors had experienced it—at certain periods in their lives—as a source of freedom, while for others, and in other parts of life, it was associated with social isolation and hardship. None of our interlocutors, however, associated living alone with anything shameful, wrong, or dangerous (cf. Lamb 2022). Most of our interlocutors were middleclass, all lived in urban areas, and three, including Michael whom I will introduce in this chapter, lived lives that were burdened by poor economy and fragile relations.

In Denmark living alone is life-phase related and compared with other European societies such as France or Italy, inter-generational cohabitation is not very prevalent. Only three percent of all households in Denmark consists of three generations (Rytter et al. 2021). Living alone is considered part of conventional life-stages, and a source of "personal growth". Small children are trained to sleep on their own, to play in their own rooms, and young people are strongly encouraged to move out of their natal home to develop into a full person. Overall independency, which sometimes manifest as distance or self-reliance or living alone is considered a source of growth, and part of becoming a full person in Denmark.

In the 1970s one out of five elderly in Denmark, resided with the family of one of their children (Christoffersen 2004). Lise had, as the only one of the interlocutors that I worked with, lived with, and cared for her mother when her mother was aging. In 1972 Lise was in her mid-twenties, had a newborn daughter, and was going through a difficult divorce. She ended up moving in with her mother, who lived alone in a spacious flat. It was supposed to be a period of transition, but the three generations of women ended up enjoying the mutual care and support of sharing the same household right up until Lise's mother passed away. Lise is now in her seventies, and her daughter has established her own home and nuclear family, while Lise is living on her own in the flat that she used to share with her mother. I asked her if she had ever considered moving in with her daughter now that she has fallen ill. She responded laughingly and said: "I would never ask my daughter to do the same. I am not her responsibility. She has her own family now." Lise always refers to her relationship with her daughter as "very close" [meget tæt]. But establishing the kind of connectivity and relatedness that Lise treasures includes "not asking for too much help", even though she is dependent upon elaborate care and attention from friends and family to sustain a meaningful life with colon cancer.

I will return to Lise later, but for now, suffice it to say that her biography reflects historical shifts in care politics and cohabitation patterns in Denmark. The reflections she shares with me about her relationship with her daughter also reproduce taken-for-granted visions of old age and illness as a time for naturally needing and deserving care from professional care workers. Care politics are contingent in the sense that they have emerged through historical struggle (Tronto 2013), and through (inter)subjective, situated, motivated and creative questioning (Meinert 2021; Buch 2018). Following this I understand care politics in broad terms, as the distribution and definition of care resources and responsibilities; not in a static sense, but as the ongoing consolidation of sense-making, meanings- and practices that is contingently re-established, but which comes to function as a generative matrix for further practice[1]. We should, therefore, be careful to talk about care politics as something that axiomatically place care within the state or the family (Thelen and Alber 2018). But building upon Scandinavian care research, it is reasonable to say that care responsibilities within families have diminished due to the professionalization of care fostered within the context of the welfare state, and the structuring effects of an egalitarian care politics (Mikkelsen 2016; Ludvigsen 2017; Bendixsen et al. 2017: 5). As I will discuss further in the below, care, in the context of the family rather emerges into a relational ethics in the sense that it remains open to social and moral negotiation (cf. Andersen and Offersen 2022; Mikkelsen 2016). This perspective emphasizes the inherent vulnerabilities that are intertwined within the consolidating and generative effects of care politics, I suggest. In the following I introduce Michael and Lise, and I show how an increasing reliance on family and friends was—for some—a source of compromise and doubt, as well as of connectivity and relatedness; what I define as relational vulnerability. But for others, such as Michael, their homes were

1 I am inspired by Lisa Guenther's writings of quasi-transcendental structures in my definition of care politics. A full account of this concept and how it might relate to care politics is beyond the scope of this paper, but see Guenter (2021).

transformed into environments of unpredictability and instability. Difficulties in accessing care made Michael more vulnerable, and the enforced mobility between locations (in and out of hospital), imposed upon him a model of care, which he could not commit to and which—perhaps—ultimately contributed to his sense of abandonment and death; what I define as vulnerability of the self. Due to the complexity of Michael's case, I present his life and the conditions around his cancer care in greater length than Lise's.

## Relational tensions

Lise is a former manager in the public sector, and today a highly active pensioner. She has gone through surgery, and she is in chemo to "fight a cancer in her stomach", as she says. I visit her several times from spring 2020 until the early autumn 2021. I came to know her as a very warm and cheerful woman, with an extended and active network of friends and family. When I visit her in her large two-bedroom flat, we sit opposite each other in the large couches in her spacious living room. From where I sit, I can see her desk. It is loaded with papers signifying the mount of activities that Lise is engaged in as a volunteer in various associations [foreninger]. Her phone is always on the coffee-table that divides the space between us when we talk. The phone extends the sociality of the two of us to include her friends and the family-members that are calling to hear how she is. The text messages or the incoming calls function as invitations to share this and that story of a friend, or as a reminder for Lise to tell me who is acting as a chauffeur to the up-coming chemo-treatment. Lise's daughter, Ruth joins Lise for most hospital appointments, but chemo takes up a full day, and Lise's friend, Karen, whom she has recently met when she was volunteering in a local cancer support group, has "the chemo duty". Often Lise is very tired after chemo, and she cannot drive her own car. "Chemo-duty" therefore not only includes driving back and forth from Lise's home to the hospital, but also in assisting Lise climbing the stairs to the second floor and prepare some food in the kitchen while Lise gets undressed in the bedroom. Karen brings the food into the bedroom when Lise is comfortably placed underneath her blankets and sometimes, she keeps Lise company while Lise eats. Karen leaves when Lise is ready to sleep for a few hours.

Due to chemo-treatments Lise is often tired, and she needs help shopping for groceries and washing her clothes. Sometimes a neighbor stops by with a liter of milk and some bread, and Ruth and her granddaughter helps her bring her clothes down the basement, where the washing machine is placed. Also, she has had to adopt to a life with an ostomy-bag. Lise is a large woman, and she cannot clean the tubes and the bag herself. Every morning a home care nurse comes by and help Lise clean the tubes and get dressed. Also, every two weeks a care worker come by for 45 minutes and cleans her house. "It is not enough to keep the house clean", Lise says, and she often hesitantly accepts Ruth's offer to wash the floor in the kitchen when she visits. To withstand the loss of bodily integrity, her sense of control and familiarity with her own body, that cancer has brought onto her life, Lise must—daily—engage in care situations with a wide range of friends, family, and professional caregivers. When friends come over, do the grocery shopping, or drive her to the hospital, Lise is reminded of "all the love that she has in her life", as she says. Care in this sense, structurally supports her sense of self and her embodied capacities to engage in world-making activities (Buch 2018).

Shortly before the Christmas holidays, I call Lise to ask if I could come visit before the holidays begin, and she tells me—upset—that she has been through a very difficult period.

> Signe [granddaughter] was in here washing my clothes again. I was just so tired, exhausted... you know. I just lied there. I was like a whale in my bed. I couldn't do anything. I was so tired. Ruth was of course busy at work, but we had to call her. And she came as soon as she could. We were afraid that I would lie there and just die in their hands. It was terrible. I did not want Signe to see me like this. And I was so dependent upon them. You know they cocked and took me to the bathroom. Things I had otherwise denied that they should do.

Lise ends up spending two days at the hospital because her lung had collapsed. "But now I'm home again", she says. "It's lovely, and Mathilde [the care worker] now comes every morning and keeps an eye on me". Lise actively engages in many different relationships, but it is important to her to reciprocate the generosity of others, and she is most comfortable when she has the strength to co-define the terms of her relationships. After the situation with the collapsed lung, she offers her daughter to go shopping clothes for Signe, and she is planning how to "spoil Karen" with a nice dinner when she has regained her strength.

To Lise, as well as to our other interlocutors, the necessity of asking for help was both a source of relatedness and connectivity, but sometimes it was also uncomfortable fact of life, producing social and moral tensions, or what I call relational vulnerabilities. To the elderly in Denmark, it is considered normal to be cared for by professional care workers, and our interlocutors felt their life balancing precariously at a juncture between "doing for themselves"—which included "getting by" relying on what many of them considered to be sparse professionally provided care and asking for help from family and friends. Statements such as "I always try to even out my needs, so one week I ask my daughter, and the next, maybe a friend", or "I know my family would like to help me, but when? They have their own lives" were prevalent throughout our material. Lise's sense of self is inherently intertwined with her relationships and interactions with others, and care needs—in a sociopolitical context where care is often considered a condition of possibility (Guenter 2021) established by the state—often become a source of relational strains or disturbance. As noted in the above, Lise often felt defined by "the virtue of the address" (Butler 2020: 46), in the sense that her care needs sometimes compromised her sense of self as a capable person, and her notions of what constitutes "a good friend" or "a good grandmother".

In the context of solo living and cancer, embodied vulnerabilities are thus co-constituted by a repertoire of relational and meaning-making issues that must creatively be addressed to sustain life. Similar points have been raised by Buch (2018) and Grøn and Meinert (2017) in their work on care and relatedness, addressing the dark side of "kinship as a counterbalance to the recent illuminating preoccupation with kinship as belonging, relatedness and kinning" (Grøn and Meinert 2017: 583). Care is not only a "do-good-practice". When in need of care, the ties we have with others are delineated (Butler 2020: 22), and relational vulnerabilities emerge as part of a relational ethics that is contingent on the centrality of defining and negotiating care responsibilities. In the following I describe the case of Michael and how a comparable situation involving unresolved care needs unfolds in another combination of solo living, care, and vulnerability.

## A broken self

In early September 2020 Michael had a rectal cancer surgically removed. After a few days at the hospital, he was unwillingly returned to his home to recover. Every morning different home-care nurses visit him. They clean his surgical wounds, and the stoma-bag and tubes that has replaced parts of his intestines. But gradually Michael's wounds become infected, and he suffers from a pain that is brute and limiting, in the sense that he is confined to his bed, and it is difficult for him to move around in his home without assistance.

Michael is in his mid-fifties when I first meet him. We have talked on the phone a couple of times before I visit him one August-afternoon in the small, terraced house that he rents. Michael has worked on and off in casinos and had random chauffeur-jobs. For the past 15 years or so he has been "outside of the labour-market" [udenfor arbejdsmarkedet], living of social benefits. Before his life was interrupted by cancer and pains, he spent much time at the local library educating himself. Michael's curiosity and analytic interests in the world around him manifests in the ways in which he narrates and interweaves his own story with references to ongoing political debates on the state of the welfare society, lack of job-opportunities of political will to distribute resources more fairly. Michael is disappointed by the then sitting Sociodemocratic government, and he shares with me theories about the origins of what he calls "the flawed-well-fare-system" where well-educated managers and doctors [djøffere og læger] earn a prosperous living, while people like himself are abandoned to a life in poverty.

> When you are not working, you are not a real human-being in this system, and it is the managers and doctors who decide if you can ever become a human being again.

The only family he has left is his sister, Susan. Susan lives in the Northern part of Jutland, which is a two-hour drive from Michael's home. According to Michael it is a troubled relationship, and he has a two-year old niece whom he has never seen. Besides from two male friends, who occasionally drop by for a chat and a beer, Michael spends most of his time on his own in the company of his cat, Muffy. Despite the painful absence of company and intimate relations, Michael's home is organized in ways that reflect traditional values of sociality in Denmark. A large barbeque is standing in the front of his house, and he can pull up extra kitchen chairs to make room for four or five people to share a meal in his kitchen.

Perhaps to establish meaningful, temporal connections between his past and his present, Michael often repeats how his father, who had worked as a manual worker himself, never encouraged him to pursue any kind education. "A society is always in need of strong men, who are willing to work hard", his father had reasoned. This strategy had failed Michael and he blames the difficulties with building long-term-relations on his poor economy and failed social status.

> It is expensive to engage in friendships; to attend birthdays and eventually the birthdays of their children, participate in nights out—concerts and... so I guess that I gradually isolated myself.

Michael is eligible for public home care, which in Denmark is free of charge and provided by the municipalities. Every day he is brought a warm meal, and care workers clean his house every two weeks. Occasionally they will help him shower. Public care work is structured around tight work schedules, and care workers enter the homes of the elderly and sick with detailed, and temporally demarcated, task-lists. Elderly and sick people in need of home care on average receive 3.3 hours of care every week, and given the reduction in hospital-based care, they spend many hours on their own. Michael thinks "the homers" [hjemmerne] as he calls them—purposefully omitting "care"—are running in and out of his home, not really paying attention to him or his needs. Michael imagines that access to "proper care" [den rigtige hjælp] would repair the damage that cancer has done to his life, and that he, because he is living in a welfare society, is entitled to receive care from "the system" [systemet or det offentlige].

In Early December Michael estimates that he has lost 30 kg, and his skin is "hanging from his bones", as he phrases it. His surgical wounds are very sore, and he suspects that they are infectious. Most days he is too weak to leave his bed. Simple maneuverings such as brushing his teeth or going to the kitchen for a cup of coffee previously neutralized through embodied knowledge and strength are now impossible. Michael feels abandoned, and his capacities and desires to engage in meaningful relations are diminishing. I know from a care worker that visits him, that he has been offered support by the palliative care team at the local hospital, and a male care worker, whom Michael trusts and talks about with kindness, takes charge of the situation. In December and January 2021 Michael is in an out of the hospital a few times. It turns out that his wounds were infected, and the infections have turned into a blood poisoning affecting Michael's rectal areas as well as the rod of his penis. At the hospital he is constantly worried that they will send him home too soon, and he also worries about transport. He succeeds, however, in persuading a nurse to grant him a flex-taxi. Flex-taxies are paid for by the state and provide a means for people who are not able to drive themselves to get a ride home. "They keep asking if I do not have someone who can pick me up. God dam it, I have told them SO many times, that I live on my own".

From Christmas onwards I only talk to Michael on the phone. He calls me two to three times a week. Sometimes he is joyful and wittingly asks how my managerial-life [djøf-liv] is going. His voice gives away the ambivalence that is so characteristic of the way that he relates to me and the care workers that come to his house. He is both angry and warm. Both dignified and very vocal about the neglect he suffers. He is dependent upon care workers for care, and on me for having someone to talk to. I ask if I can visit him, but he says: "My house is dirty, I am dirty, it would not be a dignified visit". I bring him food a few times, but I am not invited in.

In early spring 2021 Michael learns that his cancer has recurred. He is offered more surgery, mostly to relief him of some of his pains. He refuses and tells me that he does not trust that they [the system] regard him "human enough" [de ser mig ikke som et menneske] to be granted the care that surgery requires. Michael eventually ends up at a hospice close to where his sister lives. He is there for a few weeks before he passes away. Eventually he is buried with his cat Muffy.

In the last months of his life, Michael is in despair, and his unmet care needs filters into a breakdown of himself as well as his domestic space. As his body and his home breaks down, Michael loses his abilities to engage in meaningful relations or other world-making activities (Buch 2018), which again adds to his isolation and maybe even to his death.

## Engaging accusations of abandonment

Michael—more so than any other interlocutor that we worked with—struggled to access the kind of care that was necessary for him to sustain life (Butler and Worms

2023), and in the end—abandoned by the system and his family—he gave up. In such complex stories, with accusations of neglect it is important to consider different and potentially conflicting perspectives (cf. Meinert 2021). I primarily had access to Michael's version, but I also talked to one of Michael's care workers and to his sister, Susan, with whom he eventually re-connected in early spring 2021, just before he came to the hospice. According to Susan, Michael did not find peace at the hospice, but he "was calmer than when he had been at home", and he had shared with her stories of gratitude about some of the latter encounters that he had had with the hospital. A few weeks before Michael ended up at the hospice Susan went to see him several times a week. At first, he had refused to accept her presence and help, but eventually he gave in. Susan tried to negotiate more public home care, cleaned up his home a bit, and sat with him throughout the afternoons when he was tired and in pain; making sure that his most basic needs of water and food were met. Eventually she was on sick leave from her job. She was exhausted and together with a care worker, she made plans for Michael to go to the hospice.

> I was constantly in a battle with myself. There was no way I could take care of Michael and my own family at the same time. Four hours in a car every time I went to see him. And feeling guilty, knowing that he was lying there, in pain all by himself when I left. What was I to do? I was glad when the hospice took him in, but also felt a bit guilty.

Michael and Susan's stories may be seen as everyday representations of an egalitarian care politics, as they both expect care responsibilities to primarily lie within the state. But their stories also exhibit the social negotiations and the porous connectivity that is fostered in the tension between Michael's care needs and Susan's insolvable situation, swaying between being able to help Michael, and being cut off, or not having the time and energy to care for him. The inevitability of Michaels care needs testifies to his basic, human vulnerabilities. The pain, his thirst, and immobility invite and demand resolution. Susan knew of this, and it haunted (Grøn and Meinert 2017: 582) her in profound ways. Like Michael she felt that they were let down "by the system", and she suffered from feelings of guilt and anger, because she was not able to support Michael in a way that she considered meaningful to him nor to herself.

I suggest that we see Susan's experiences with Michael as a testimony to the production of what I call vulnerabilities to the self. Lack of care made Michael's life and sense of self fall apart causing a profound unraveling of his life. He became unhinged (Guenther 2016) in the sense that he was unable to respond to any kinds of attention from professional care workers, from his sister and from me. He was increasingly disoriented and disconnected from the world, losing trust in the intentions of his sister and his other caregivers. Unhinged describes, according to Guenther, "what happens when the articulated joints of our embodied interrelational subjectivity are broken apart" (2016: 12). In her work on solitary confinement, Guenther shows how physical punishment, exhaustion and isolation put intense pressure on the capacity of American prisoners to relate to other people and to their selves. Prolonged isolation cuts prisoners off from their network of social, cognitive perceptual and affective support, and "structurally undermine their capacities for meaning making. They become unhinged. They lose their embodied orientation in the world and their sense of self" (2016: 154). I do not mean to indicate that Michael's life is comparable to the life of supermax prisoners, but I suggest that his lack of access to care and the immense pains and what he experiences as a social abandonment result in him falling apart. In this sense lack of care can be seen as a form of violence that erase a subject's connections to others, and reduce them to a bare, isolated self, which can no longer sustain life.

## The architect of human vulnerabilities

We are all given over to others and to life in ways that we cannot control (Butler 2020: 46). Cancer surely testifies to this. As attested by Lise and Michael, many embodied practices previously part of an everyday normal, such as taking a shower, cleaning the kitchen floor, or getting up and down stairs, are compromised, and in their attempts to sustain life they are forced to recognise and make visible to others "the basic vulnerable conditions of their embodiment" (Butler 2020: 26). For some, like Lise, asking for help, was a source of relatedness, but it was also a source of relational vulnerability, in the sense that access to care was contingent on inter-relational negotiations of care responsibilities. For Michael, social abandonment and lack of care transformed into a loss of self. He became unhinged (Guenther 2016) and lost his abilities to engage in meaningful world-making activities, suggesting that care resources may be distributed in ways that sustain or denies or erase certain forms of existence or subjectivity.

When care politics change, so does both the conditions and experiences of living, and more profoundly of living alone. Consequently, solo living may be seen as a way of life made possible by care, and a way of life which is lived and experienced in the tension between relationality and care politics. Care and the structuring effects of care politics are, in this sense, what makes life livable (Butler and Worms 2023: 15–18). Understanding relations between solo living, care politics and vulnerability thus also testifies to another anthropological testimony essential to the solo living research, namely that living alone is not merely a reflection of an inherent, human thrift for autonomy or freedom (cf. Coleman 2014). Vulnerability understood as a generalized fact of life in many ways marks the limits of individualism (Butler 2020; Meinert 2021), emphasizing that solo living is a political and social accomplishment sustained by care. This argument is important since it (once again) shakes the modern delusion of the human as potentially autonomous and independent, and it is consequential for our understanding of the role of care in society (cf. Tronto 2013). Exploring solo living in the context of serious disease, I suggest, testifies to the way in which care politics proposes itself as the architect of our human vulnerabilities, and it reminds us that vulnerability is not inherently individual, but distributed by structures of power, privilege, and oppression (Vaittinen 2015). When I say that care politics proposes itself as the architecture of our human vulnerabilities, I mean to emphasise that the ongoing, creative distribution and definition of care resources is a process that is intrinsically also shaping, designing, and producing human vulnerabilities. In this chapter I show how changing care politics produce both relational vulnerabilities and vulnerabilities to the self. Care is in essence both a treatment and an enabler of human vulnerabilities.

Attention to care as productive to relatedness (Carsten 2007) and social inequality or vulnerability (Buch 2018; Meinert 2021) is not new to anthropology. Recently, Sarah Lamb (2014) and others (Meinert 2021) have described ongoing shifts in care responsibilities between states and families that are taking place around the world. In India, Lamb says, rural-to-urban labour migration intersects with drops in intergenerational cohabitation and negotiations of care responsibilities of the sick and elderly, and a law from 2007 stipulates that children may be fined and jailed if found guilty of neglecting their aged parents (Lamb 2014: 50). This law brings to light the belief that the family, rather than the state, is the proper agent of care and, perhaps, the fear that this obligation will not be honored. It also, however, bears witness to the difficulties and often devastating care-caps that develop due to the speed of social change, and it affirms that creating a society that generates sustainable lives for people of every ability and background means recognizing the ways in which care is deeply entangled with household-structures and changes in co-habitation patterns (Lamb 2022; Klinenberg 2013), as well as notions of intimacy, belonging and relatedness.

Historically the welfare state has played a significant role in enabling the possibility of living alone, and the rise in solo living has been facilitated by those same supportive care infrastructures that are currently undergoing transformation (Klingenberg 2013). The figure of the elderly solo dweller—I believe—in many ways embodies a shared notion of what a successful welfare state looks like. It is important for me to stress that I do not wish to contribute popular or academic narratives that represent solo dwellers as *per se* vulnerable or lonely, or which equals solo living with social disintegration (cf. Grøn 2016; Lamb 2014). I would argue that we see solo living as an emergent sociality (see also Coleman 2009; Klingenberg 2013), partly made possible by an egalitarian care politics. Lise confirms this when she laughingly litters my inquiry about the possibility of her moving in with her daughter. "No, I am not Signe's responsibility", she says, reflecting, how an egalitarian care politics have historically normalized and supported the distribution of particular care responsibilities in Denmark. It is also important for me to emphasise that ongoing changes in the distribution of care, and the invention of private homes as contexts of care manifest in the everyday lives of sick people in a variety of ways (cf. Mikkelsen 2016; Andersen and Offersen 2023). But for all they set up the contours of a care politics in which the self, others and the home are brought into new forms of proximity, which may be a challenge for people who live alone. Solo living is, as noted in the above, regarded a normal way of life in Denmark. But it might in the future become a crucial site of political struggle and contestation, as current, intersecting conditions of care politics and embodied life are making solo living in Demark both possible, yet increasingly difficult.

## Acknowledgements

I would like to thank Lise and Michael, their families and the other interlocutors who worked with Sara Marie Hebsgaard Offersen and I, and who shared intimate details about their lives and relations with us. Without their generosity this chapter would not have been possible to write. I hope that the text reflects—to some extend—their experiences. Also, I would like to thank Maria Louw, Line Dalsgaard, and Sara Marie Hebsgaard Offersen for commenting on earlier drafts of the chapter. Also, thank you to Mette Terp Høybye and Maja Hojer Bruun for inspiring conversations on relations between solo living, health care and welfare. The chapter was presented in an early version at the XI MAAH Conference, 2021 hosted by Bernhard Hadolt and Andrea Stöckl in Austria, and I am grateful for the comments I received then and in their process of editing the book. The study was made possible by a grant from the Danish Cancer Society.

## References

Andersen, Rikke Sand, and Sara Marie Hebsgaard Offersen. 2022. Omsorgens Moralske Pionerer: Om at 'Bo Selv' og Forvalte Alenehed og Kræftsygdom. Tidsskrift for Forskning i Sygdom Og Samfund 19(37): 65–85.

Bendixsen, Synnøve, Mary Bente Bringslid, and Halvard Vike. 2017. Introduction: Egalitarianism in a Scandinavian Context. *In* Egalitarianism in Scandinavia: Historical and Contemporary Perspectives. Synnøve Bendixsen, Mary Bente Bringslid, and Halvard Vike, eds. Pp. 1–44. Cham: Palgrave Macmillan.

Buch, Elana D. 2018. Inequalities of Aging: Paradoxes of Independence in American Home Care. New York: New York University Press.

Butler, Judith. 2020. Precarious Life: The Powers of Mourning and Violence. London: Verso.

Butler, Judith, and Frédéric Worms. 2023. The Livable and the Unlivable. New York: Fordham University Press.
Butler, Judith, and George Yancy. 2020. Interview: Mourning Is a Political Act Amid the Pandemic and Its Disparities. Journal of Bioethical Inquiry 17(4): 483–87.
Carsten, Janet. 2007. After Kinship. Cambridge: Cambridge University Press.
Coleman, Leo. 2014. A View from Anthropology: Anomie and Urban Solitude. *In* The Handbook of Solitude: Psychological Perspectives on Social Isolation, Social Withdrawal and Being Alone. Robert J. Caplan and Julie C. Bowker, eds. Pp. 483–98. Hoboken, NJ: John Wiley & Sons.
Christoffersen, Mogens. 2004. Fra 1800-tals familie til moderne familie. Social Forskning (3): 10.
Danmarks Statistik. 2023. Husstande og familier. Statistics Denmark Report.
Fischer, Berenice, and Joan C Tronto. 1990. Toward a Feminist Theory of Care. *In* Circles of Care: Work and Identity in Women's Lives. Emily K. Abel and Margaret K. Nelson, eds. Pp.35-57. Albany NY: State University of New York Press.
Grøn, Lone. 2016. Old Age and Vulnerability between First, Second and Third Person Perspectives: Ethnographic Explorations of Aging in Contemporary Denmark. J Aging Stud. 39: 21–30.
Grøn, Lone, and Lotte Meinert. 2017. Social Contagion and Cultural Epidemics: Phenomenological and 'Experience-Near' Explorations. Ethos 45(2): 165–181.
Guenther, Lisa. 2016. Solitary Confinement: Social Death and Its Afterlives. Minneapolis: University of Minnesota Press.
Guenther, Lisa. 2021. Six Senses of Critique for Critical Phenomenology. Puncta 4 (2): 5–23.
Gullestad, Marianne and Martine Segalen, eds. 1997. Family and Kinship in Europe. London: Pinter.
Hjelmar, Ulf, and Tine Rostgaard. 2020. Supplemental Home Care and Topping-up: A Shift from Service Universalism towards a New and Privatised Public Service Model? International Journal of Social Welfare 29(2): 118–28.
Jamieson, Lynn, and Roona Simpson. 2013. Living Alone: Globalization, Identity and Belonging. London: Palgrave Macmillan UK.
Klinenberg, Eric. 2013. Going Solo: The Extraordinary Rise and Surprising Appeal of Living Alone. London: Duckworth.
Lamb, Sara. 2014. Permanent Personhood or Meaningful Decline? Toward a Critical Anthropology of Successful Aging. Journal of Aging Studies 29: 41–52.
Lamb, Sara. 2022. Being Single in India: Stories of Gender, Exclusion, and Possibility. Berkeley: University of California Press.
Ludvigsen, Bodil. 2017. Market Thinking and Home Nursing. *In* Emerging Socialities in 21st Century Health Care. Anita Hardon and Bernhard Hadolt, eds. Pp. 75–88. Amsterdam: Amsterdam University Press.

Mattingly, Cheryl, Lone Grøn, and Lotte Meinert. 2011. Chronic Homework in Emerging Borderlands of Healthcare. Culture, Medicine, and Psychiatry 35 (3): 347–75.

Meinert, Lotte. 2021. Vulnerability as Relational: Cash and Care for Elderly Ik in Uganda. *In* Vulnerability and the Politics of Care: Transdisciplinary Dialogues. Victoria Browne, Jason Danely, and Doerthe Rosenow, eds. Pp. 213–29. Oxford: Oxford University Press.

Mikkelsen, Henrik Hvenegaard. 2016. Unthinkable Solitude: Successful Aging in Denmark Through the Lacanian Real. Ethos 44(4): 448–63.

Rapp, Rayna. 1999. Testing Women, Testing the Fetus: The Social Impact of Amniocentesis in America. New York: Routledge.

Rostgaard, Tine, and Marta Szebehely. 2012. Changing Policies, Changing Patterns of Care: Danish and Swedish Home Care at the Crossroads. European Journal of Ageing 9(2): 101–9.

Skovgaard, Anna Louise, Marianne Jørgensen, Tine Tjørnhøj-Thomsen, and Mette Terp Høybye. 2022. Discharge Readiness as an Infrastructure: Negotiating the Transfer of Care for Elderly Patients in Medical Wards. Social Science and Medicine 312 (2022) 115388.

Rytter, Mikkel, Sara Lei Sparre, Abir Ismail, and Anika Liversage. 2021. Minoritet sældre og selvudpegede hjælpere: kommunal velfærd og omsorg i forandring. Aarhus: Aarhus Universitetsforlag.

Sparre, Sara Lei, and Mikkel Rytter. 2021. Between Care and Contract: Aging Muslim Immigrants, Self-Appointed Helpers and Ambiguous Belonging in the Danish Welfare State. Anthropology & Aging 42(1): 112–28.

Thelen, Tatjana, and Erdmute Alber. 2018. Reconnecting State and Kinship Temporalities, Scales, Classifications *in*. Reconnecting State and Kinship. Tatjana Thelen and Erdmute Alber, eds. Pp. 1–36. Philadelphia: University of Pennsylvania Press.

Tronto, Joan C. 2013. Caring Democracy: Markets, Equality, and Justice. New York: New York University Press.

Vaittinen, Tiina. 2015. The Power of the Vulnerable Body. International Feminist Journal of Politics 17(1): 100–18.

# 8 The Uncertain Future of Antibiotics
## Navigating Bacterial Presence in Hospitals amidst Antimicrobial Resistance

*Antonia Modelhart*

## Introduction

In recent years, antibiotics, one of the key pharmaceuticals of modern biomedicine, are increasingly a scarce good: rising resistances to the common substances and a dry antibiotic pipeline—a stalled development of new antibiotics—configure infrastructural uncertainties: the massive and far-reaching reliance on antibiotics for the function of not only modern biomedicine and but economies, security and modernity itself shape grim visions of a future without effective antibiotics (Landecker 2016; Chandler 2019).

In my research on antimicrobial resistance (AMR) in hospitals, I follow the uncertainties clinging to antibiotics and ask what this means for hospital staff in their everyday encounters with bacteria, infections, and growing resistances to antibiotics. Particularly, I look at hygiene practices as the old-fashioned and odd companion of the antibiotic era and argue that these practices play a central role in meeting and managing antibiotic uncertainties in times of AMR. Aligned with the volume's inquiry of how "hope and uncertainty take on particular meanings in the policing and managing of health, illness and wellbeing" I explore how hygiene practices shape the management of microbial encounters amidst antibiotic uncertainties. As part of AMR, these uncertainties are met with elaborate practices entailed in what is called hygiene management in German hospitals that give substance to microbiopolitics (Paxson 2008; 2012; 2014), where the governance of microbial presence is a key aspect of caring and managing individual and collective bodies. Approaching AMR through the meaning of uncertainty in the "policing and managing of health" opens a way to explore the multi-faceted nature of AMR: because AMR is a moving subject through scales, spaces and times, uncertainty figures on different layers, each layer telling us something about how we envision acting upon it as a health threat.

On a global scale, the uncertain future of antibiotics as effective substances against infections configures a looming global health issue that is both a present, but an even more pressing issue in bleak anticipations of a future without antibiotics. Relatedly, on a small-scale, health professionals in hospitals and especially hygiene professionals, build the awareness inside hospital walls that enacts this global health threat in daily practices and ways of doing medicine and healthcare. Here, hygienists embody the large-scale uncertainties of AMR put into practice in daily hospital flows, meeting hospital pragmatics infused by historical, political, economic, and material spheres. Further exemplified on a microscopic level, these uncertainties materialize themselves in the openness of bacterial compositions that can mean so many different things and must be managed accordingly to the hospital environment. Here, hygiene figures as the management of uncertain bacterial presence, or to be more precise, the uncertain processuality of bacterial compositions (which very well might be a deadly one for humans) linking back to the large-scale uncertainties clinging to antibiotics as an effective substance to control these presences.

I want to show how the emerging uncertainties because of resistant bacteria and ineffective antibiotics give rise to hygiene regimes where barriers, walls and borders play a crucial role: hygiene is an ongoing negotiation and oscillation between the inside of the hospital and the outside. I am particularly intrigued by how actors construe "the outside", i.e., the social being and living outside of hospital walls as relevant for hygiene matters inside the hospital, and ultimately, for managing AMR. While hygiene is often assumed to follow universal protocols for sterility and cleanliness, hygiene work encompasses intricate processes of considering various aspects and processes of the "outside" and thus configure and work along localized and local microbiologies (Koch 2011; Yates-Doerr 2017). In this regard, a patient's skin and the hospital's walls both present specific barriers that require complex considerations when enacting hygiene measures. The orchestration of hygiene is thus a delicate, nuanced practice for managing human life alongside microbial encounters.

In the first part of this paper I map the relation between the hygienic hospital and antimicrobial resistance. I follow the historical contextualisation of microbial encounters and shifting epistemologies mirrored in the transformations from Pasteurian and post-Pasteurian approaches to trace how hygiene practices historically engender different ways of approaching microbial life in relation to human life. In the second part, I explore how hospital staff and patients make sense of bacterial presence based on my empirical material. The procedure of risk-adapted screening of patients in hospitals serves as a case to analyse the rationale of hygiene. Along screening as one of the key hygienic measures in German hospitals, I question the large-scale, societal implications of such hygiene measures when viewed through a microbiopolitical lens.

The empirical illustration of the governing of microbes in the second part is structured along the process of admission and discharge. Both the situation of entering and exiting the hospital highlight how hygiene practices constitute a mediation between the inside and the outside of hospitals walls. Within the hospital, the mediation continuous as one between humans, microbes, and materials, where hygienic risk is allocated to specific bodies, patients, wards, and to spaces both inside and outside the hospital. Whereas inside the hospital, hygiene practices aim to exercise control and management over bacterial presence and compositions, this scenario changes abruptly once outside the hospital. These are the tensions I intend to follow in this chapter, as they present themselves in my material, being especially remarkable in the experiences of a patient, Nina. Illustrating the situatedness of hygienic risk, I will switch between Nina's perspective, a patient diagnosed with drug-resistant bacteria during a hospital stay, and excerpts from interviews conducted with the hygiene management professionals I name Paul, Elli and Carl as well as Dr Andress, a hygiene physician.

## Theoretical approach

The chapter's argument builds on recent theoretical approaches in thinking about microbes: a microbiopolitical lens (Paxson 2008, 2012, 2014) allows me to analyse hygiene practices in their relation to and their entanglement with large-scale politics, social practices, and biology while acknowledging the situatedness of bacterial materiality through borrowing from Landecker's (2016) *biology of history* and wider discussions of *local microbiologies* (Koch 2011; Brotherton and Nguyen 2013; Yates-Doerr 2017).

The addition of *micro* to Foucault's concept of *biopolitics* extends the analysis of how populations are governed to how populations are governed by and through their microbial encounters. Hygiene management, therefore, can be viewed as a microbiopolitical approach, following Paxson's understanding of "the creation of categories of microscopic biological agents; the anthropocentric evaluation of such agents; and the elaboration of appropriate human behaviors in relation to microorganisms involved in infection, inoculation, and digestion" (Paxson 2008: 17).

To account for the sociomateriality of resistant bacteria the concepts of *local microbiology* and the *biology of history* has proven fruitful. They both deal, in different registers, with the difficulty of accounting for the ever-changing material (*biology of history*) and the situational (*local microbiology*) nature of biological agents such as bacteria. Landecker's (2016) proposes *biology of history* to capture the enmeshment of bacterial evolution alongside the production of knowledge: As AMR illustrates, producing knowledge about bacteria and their evolution that resulted in the development and use of antibiotics, altered the materiality of bacteria themselves. The altered materiality of bacteria displays in acquired resistance mechanism that give rise to a biology of history, a materialized form of sociohistorical processes.

The concept of *local microbiologies* (Koch 2011; Brotherton and Nguyen 2013), a contribution to the concept of *local biologies* introduced by Lock (1994) in the 1990s, stresses the implicit co-productive processes of social and biological records in human–microbial relationships (Koch 2011: 84). Building on Lock's attempt to denaturalize the universal biological body with attending to *local biologies*, Yates-Doerr (2017: 382f.) further argues to denaturalize the *local* and specifically ask for the performativity of local biologies. In this vein, I look at the microagents of local biologies, bacteria, to explore what the localizing of biology means in the context of managing AMR in hospitals: what version of localities are actualized in bacteria's biology through hygiene staff?

This process of doing the local, I argue, is neither self-evident nor objectively innocent, no matter how geographically formalized the local microbiologies in the hospital are construed with the screening schemes (or in all the geographically distributed AMR-data). The microbiopolitics of hygiene work display the ever-changing ontological status of bacteria in everyday life. Hygiene practices epitomize the essence of locality, through its means and ends, and the way in which hygienists produce the hygienic hospital in a specific (microbiopolitical) way through localizing and historizing biology.

## Data collection and methods

At the core of this paper are questions about how living with—and being at odds with—bacteria give rise to practices around hygiene, health, and disease. What is done to act hygienic in view of the presence of bacteria? How is a hygienic hospital in times of AMR envisioned in Germany? These questions centre around a tension very central to my research on AMR in biomedicine: how hygienic risk in human-microbial encounters revolve around specific spaces, bodies, and materialities.

I conducted 13 semi-structured interviews in Germany that focused on either professional or personal experiences with diagnosed AMR. I visited four different hospitals in Hamburg, Germany's second largest city, and interviewed hygiene management teams, as well as physicians and nurses specifically trained in hospital hygiene who were responsible for hygiene issues across the entire hospital. In hospital A, I spoke with two hygiene specialist nurses (Elli and Carl); in hospital B, I interviewed one hygiene specialist nurse (Paul); in hospital C, I met with the hygiene physician (Dr Andress); and in hospital D, I conducted interviews with one infectiologist (Dr Krohn) and one microbiologist/infectiologist physician (Dr Spall), as well as a nurse from the intensive care unit.

In addition to the hygiene management teams, I interviewed professionals working outside the hospital, including a university scientist with a background in chemistry and microbiology who is conducting fundamental antibiotic research;

an expert at the municipal hygiene institute; two representatives of a company specializing in hygiene products; and three representatives of a city-wide network on multi-resistant bacteria, the Multiresistente Erreger (MRE) network. The MRE network essentially gathers participants in the health care sector, funded by the city's health departments, to discuss the issue of drug-resistant bacteria and its relevance to the working groups in hospitals, nursing homes, patient transport, and on an irregular basis, primary care. On the patient side, I interviewed one patient and one caregiver of an individual diagnosed with drug-resistant bacteria and was informally in contact with patients through online Facebook groups about drug-resistant bacteria, in addition to the methicillin-resistant Staphylococcus aureus (MRSA) patient organization in Germany. To guarantee anonymization, I use pseudonyms for the interviewees. There are 68 hospitals alone in Hamburg and I visited four of them. I only use interview excerpts that don't disclose any details about the specific hospital.

I analysed my material by applying *situational analysis* (Clarke et al. 2022) in conversations with constructivist *grounded theory* (Charmaz 2014). The *situational analysis* guided how I approached my data through mapping techniques, such as visualizing positions taken on hygiene, human–microbial relationships in hospitals, or risk-adapted screening. *Constructivist grounded theory* guided the coding of the data I analysed with MAXQDA, in which the core categories of human–bacteria relationships and hygiene management emerged along with the practice-oriented category of risk-adapted screening.

## The changing nature of infections: Hospitals in the antibiotic era

Following the widespread introduction of antibiotics in the middle of the 20th century, the hospital came to be seen as a healthy environment (Gradmann 2017): a clean place and the "best place to get better" (Condrau and Kirk 2011: 390). However, with AMR on the horizon the hospital's image changed, being again more a threat to health than a curative place as the German term for resistant bacteria *Krankenhauskeim* (hospital germ) aptly mirrors. Hospitals and AMR became deeply intertwined toward the end to the 20th century, which fundamentally changed the image of the hospital as a potentially dangerous, infectious "hothouse" (Gradmann 2017). Returning to the last century, Gradmann (2018) interrogates the shifting perceptions of hygiene and infectiology from the optimism of mastering microbial encounters to more dystopian visions of the future. The promise for both a cure and disease control, which was influential in the first part of the 20th century, changed the status of hospitals, which were viewed as places that were healthier and more hygienic than those outside the hospital walls (Gradmann 2018; Condrau and Kirk 2011). Despite changing disease dynamics in hospitals, however, including a reduction in cases of pneumonia or tuberculosis, an increase in other infections, particularly those acquired within the hospital setting, the promise of the hospital as a "beacon" of infection control vanished. Already during the 1950s, researchers complicated the promise of antibiotics for the elimination of infectious diseases with observations of how the widespread use of antibiotics drastically changed the nature of infections, including an increase in drug-resistant bacteria (Gradmann 2018: 107).

Landecker coins this changing nature of infections *the biology of history* because the materialization of socio-political processes of antibiotic use displays in the changing biology of bacteria as they develop resistances. Furthermore, the changing status of hospitals from "lighthouses to hothouses of infections" (Gradmann 2017) and inscribed visions of a controllable nature is paralleled by what Paxson (2008) elaborates on with her concept of microbiopolitics: the shift from Pasteurian to post-Pasteurian biopolitical versions of microbial encounters. While the Pasteurian approach to microbial encounters aimed at the elimination and eradication of pathogenic microbes, at controlling and mastering "nature", amid the buried dreams of a world without infectious diseases, a post-Pasteurian approach highlights the collaborative nature of human–microbial encounters and the situatedness of pathogenicity. As she notes, "post-Pasteurianism takes after Pasteurianism" in that it classifies microbes as good and bad, but the focus has shifted to make use of good microbes in dealing with the bad (2011: 118). Her examples of artisanal cheese making or the medical use of faecal microbiota transplantation (Lorimer 2020) illustrate this post-Pasteurian approach, as does the case of hygiene management in hospitals.

## Post-Pasteurian approaches in German hospitals: The work of hygiene teams

Today, in Germany, these epistemological shifts display in the ways that matters of infection, of microbial encounters, are enacted in hospitals. My analytic focus of hygiene management brings into focus the all-encompassing, infrastructural work enabling the curative and therapeutic logic of the hospital. Here, post-Pasteurianism articulates in the hygienic endeavours to weigh in on the uncertainties aligned to the issue of AMR: to manage bacterial compositions and avoid infection. This is the space where hygiene teams operate, between acknowledging bacterial presence and their potential to turn or be pathogenic: microbes are not understood as inherently pathogenic but might turn out as such. Thus, hygiene work revolves around evaluating and managing this post-Pasteurian spectrum of bacterial presence. And all this against a backdrop of complicated and far-reaching uncertainties attached to the use of antibiotics, both theoretically and practically: On a global level, AMR is discursively presented as a threat to global orders, and in daily personal encounters in hospitals, AMR materialises in patients who may already have resistance to substances and subsequently cannot be treated.

Every German hospital is required to have such a hygiene management team: a unit of their own that is concerned with all kinds of microbes and microbial encounters. Patients, materials, and health care professionals come with microbes, and it is the hygiene teams' tasks attend and make sense of them within the hospital setting. It is the hospital walls that give bacterial presence a specific relevance, and so does the entering body become something else: as Brown (2019) writes in reading Mary Douglas' *Purity and Danger* (1966), entering a building points to different entries, where "the bodies and buildings are awkwardly duplicated within one another, both symbolically and materially" (2019: 228). When entering the hospital, the patient's body mingles with the building, its logistics and flows, and its hygienic regime. This regime and its management entail a wide range of tasks and fields of activity. Paul, the hygienist, showed me how different the days might look like for hygiene teams: they document infections and antibiotic use on an Excel spreadsheet, adapt screening protocols or isolation plans, they carry out hygiene visits in different wards, train new staff, and advise colleagues on issues of hygiene, antibiotic use, and infection control. Every morning, Paul is responsible for scanning the data that the wards send to inform the teams' physician, who subsequently visits the wards and meets with the team there to coordinate and agree on appropriate antibiotic treatment, as well as the necessary hygiene measures. Hours later, Paul might need to monitor the flow and quality of water, the cleaning of technical equipment and the milk for new-born infants or might be called into meetings to discuss the planning and construction of a new ward.

The threads of these various hygiene practices all come together in the hygiene management team, but many other actors are also tasked with the day-to-day maintenance of hospital hygiene. Nurses screen newly admitted patients and perform smear tests. They also wash the patients in cases of unwanted bacteria or infection. Physicians and pharmacists adjust antibiotic therapy; cleaning personnel take care of professional cleaning; and the lab analysis team reports to the hygiene team. The hygiene teams' direct contact with patients is rare, but they typically make rounds through the hospital and are on hand to advise when needed or to observe during rounds.

Hygiene practices aim to understand microbial presence and prevent infection. Hence, in hygiene management workflows from different areas of the hospital, including wards, laboratories, pharmacies, clinical practice, and antibiotic surveillance converge. The screening practices clearly sanction this assemblage of microbiological and pharmacological knowledge with clinical practice and the hospital site. As one hygienist put it, a key task is to comprehend and record what they call the "microorganism clientele", moving through the hospital. This is done through screening, detecting, testing, documenting, quantifying, and reporting bacterial compositions.

In the next section, I will look at the ways of managing the "microorganism clientele" which revolves in a post-Pasteurian fashion primarily around managing bacterial presence to avoid people getting sick of it.

## "Preventing infection, accepting colonization"

In hospitals, hygiene is commonly perceived as a peripheral aspect to biomedical care, something that maintains the workings of the hospital, but that also interferes and disrupts the hospital's "real" medical work (Bose 2017: 49). Hygiene teams are often located in secluded areas in the hospital and both physically in their allocated space within hospital walls as well as from their social position within hospital hierarchies, they tend to act from the margins. As to not come off as the unpopular hospital police who just criticises ways of doing (like hand washing), besides the main task of negotiating human-bacteria relations a lot of effort goes into maintaining good relations to their colleagues.

It is often difficult for patients to grasp the processes of hygiene management and how it intertwines with care and therapy, as it is the task of physicians and nurses to consider the effects of biomedical interventions on microbial encounters. Thus, many interviewees working in hygiene shared a feeling for the specific responsibility of emotional labour as well. Thus, hygiene can be seen as a collective endeavour, where the care work encompasses relations to microbes as well as humans as patients and colleagues.

If a patient like Nina is admitted to the hospital, the medical staff must make sense of the patient in several ways. It may be important to know about any underlying medical conditions, the insurance number, or the weight of the patient, and in terms of hygiene, to evaluate the risks at stake: do they carry drug-resistant bacteria, which might lead to an infection? This evaluation is crucial and one of the first steps, because it specifies the flows, spaces, and practices a patient will find themselves in. As with Nina, the reasoning behind screening for drug resistant bacteria is two-fold: to secure the place and the patient.

In both admission and discharge, bacterial presence is crucial but with different implications: upon arrival, potential pathogenic and troublesome bacteria might enter with the patients, endangering the health of the patients and hospital flows. But not every patient's bacterial composition is relevant, and hygienic risk is distributed along specific criteria. These criteria play out in the decisions made about which patients are screened for drug-resistant bacteria and who is regarded as posing hygienic risk. These criteria also mirror a way of managing uncertainties about hygienic risk, of which bodies are risky at the same time (for other patients and the hospital), and are seen as at-risk because of their bacterial compositions.

## Admission: Situating human-bacteria relationships

> After weeks in a hospital abroad because of deteriorating health, Nina was transported back to Germany on a special flight organized by her insurance company. Her condition wasn't improving, and something had to be done. Admitted to a hospital in Germany with no diagnosis and vague symptoms, Nina was immediately isolated from other patients. Having returned from a non-European country, the reason for isolation stems from the concern that Nina might be carrying a contagious, "tropical" disease. The status of Nina as a patient and the reason for her ill health was yet unknown. Isolation was a means of practicing caution and providing safety not just for Nina, but for others as well, including other patients, the medical staff, and her family. A hospital is a densely populated place; thus, it was better to be "safe than sorry". Nina's isolation bought the physicians time to thoroughly investigate their microbial composition and the presence of possible pathogenic viruses, fungi, bacteria, or parasites without endangering other patients. (Field notes, Hamburg, 19.5.2020)

I analyse risk-adapted screening for drug-resistant bacteria as a standard hygiene procedure in German hospitals, using Nina's case. Screening, primarily done by nurses, serves to evaluate whether a patient should be tested for drug-resistant bacteria. Thus, upon arrival, the screening builds a basis for allocating hygienic risk. Although the screening protocols are provided by the hygiene management team, they are rarely executed by them. This screening process helps identify patients who might harbour resistant bacteria. If such a harbouring status is already known upon admission, if e.g., patient x was once discharged with a status of having resistant bacteria, the patient is immediately separated and isolated as hospital capacity allows. If the patient's bacterial composition is unknown, certain criteria point to the need of further clarification. It is exactly these criteria guideline that builds the risk-adapted screening protocol, which is practiced with a similar protocol across German hospitals. Ultimately, this evaluation aims to minimize two major risks: the ineffective use of antibiotics due to drug-resistant bacteria in patients and the potential risk that a colonized patient poses to other patients. Nurses decide based on a questionnaire defined by the Robert Koch Institute, the central administrative body of public health in Germany. In this process of risk-adapted screening, nurses working on the patient consider aspects of their medical but also non-medical biography and their reason for hospitalization: in some wards, such as the Intensive Care Unit, the screening criteria are broader, like wards with chronically ill or severely ill patients. In other cases, the specific bodily problem and the allocated ward determine who is screened for which bacteria: certain drug-resistant bacteria primarily pose a problem in gastroenterology wards; therefore, screening for specific drug-resistant bacteria is considered particularly important in these wards. Evaluating the patient's biography for making sense of bacterial compositions may include information from their medical history, traveling activities, geographical locations, or their occupation.

Nina's case was unambiguous: Having been transferred from a hospital outside of Germany, and even Europe, plus her unknown condition put her straight into isolation. Transfers from other hospitals always pose hygienic risks, so patients are automatically tested and, if possible, isolated. This routine serves also as a way for hospitals to demonstrate that the resistant bacteria was not acquired in-house but somewhere else. For Nina, screening for drug-resistant bacteria was just one part of the biomedical care she received and was not something she actively anticipated or was informed about.

This observation resonates with the situation of how hospitals deal with AMR in general and the often-drawn connection made by the interviewees between health status and drug-resistant bacteria. The situation where bacterial presence is regarded as relevant within hospital walls is build up through the patients, their whereabouts, their activities, and their wellbeing:

> What is inhaled outside, so to speak, is accumulated and amplified here [in the hospital]. Because this is where all the people come together. The big problem is that multi-resistant bacteria are above all a problem for people who are multimorbid. A healthy young person is usually not affected at all. (Interview Paul, hygiene specialist nurse: 479)

The hygiene specialist in the interview expresses a common argument, where resistant bacteria are problematic for specific bodies. The reasoning behind this framing is to grasp the complexities of the microbial spectrum, where the presence of drug-resistant bacteria does not necessarily indicate an infection. In healthy individuals, non-resistant bacteria usually out-compete or out-grow drug-resistant bacteria after a short time and are thus no longer detectable (though they may very well be there). For immunocompromised patients, however, the presence of drug-resistant bacteria might easily lead to an infection. Thus, an infection in such individuals can more quickly become a health threat. For patients, therefore, the hospital is potentially a threatening place, where care, therapy and recovery, the function of the place itself, might be endangered by the presence of drug-resistant bacteria.

Therefore, the exploration of bacterial presence in the hospital, relevant to certain patients in specific situations and within specific walls, allows for the detection of unwanted bacterial compositions in the first place (i.e., to identify a potential problematic bacterial presence). While usually the medical staff (e.g., nurses) carry out the practical steps involved in patient interactions, these are typically guided, supervised, observed, and sometimes controlled during so-called hygiene visits by the hygiene management team. Thus, a central task for the hygiene management team is to strike a balance between detecting certain bacterial presences and avoiding infection, as well as to pass on the necessary processes to the medical staff working with the patients. One hygienist told me how he himself experienced a moment of epiphany in terms of making sense of his profession and his daily practices:

> So that was a bit of an "aha moment" for me, that the focus is clearly on avoiding infection (...). The primary goal of hygiene measures ultimately is the prevention of infections. Not the prevention of colonization. And that is a very important point that we always have to remember. Because colonization itself is usually a temporary thing. As I said, these germs typically disappear again with sensible nutrition, normal diet, and normal personal hygiene. (Interview Elli and Carl, hygiene specialist nurses: 118)

In contrast to above statements about a healthy, young person being "fit" enough to deal with a certain bacterial presence, the temporality of this presence is brought up by the hygienist. The hygienist Carl employs practices like "diet" and "normal hygiene" as key, as technologies of the self to meet bacterial compositions, to build up the body capable of overgrowing resistant bacteria.

Therefore, of crucial importance is the evaluation of bacterial presence and their relation to the potential pathogenicity (infection) of their presence: hygiene is all about acknowledging bacterial presence while at the same time considering its temporality. And all this also to ultimately avoid unnecessary antibiotic use: as hygiene specialists point out, defining and diagnosing a patient's bacterial composition can only be considered a snapshot. Even in a case of certain stabilization after identifying the bacteria, it is only partial insofar as bacterial presence is understood as temporal. Nevertheless, once diagnosed, the bacterial status remains attached to the patient and defines their role during the hospital stay and far beyond. To rid themselves of the status of being colonized, a patient must prove with three tests over a certain period that the bacteria are no longer detectable. As Nina told me, once she was diagnosed with resistant bacteria and moved outside the hospital, she had to prove on three different occasions that the resistant bacteria were no longer detectable. Otherwise, entering the hospital with a known status of drug-resistant bacteria requires immediate isolation, which, as one of the interviewees pointed out, can be accompanied by stigmatization and neglect by the medical staff (Interview Dr Spall, infectiologist physician: 28).

Hygiene management is the solid ground upon which hospital business operates. Implementing risk-adapted screening, a rather complex process, as well as a dynamic field of developing knowledge, requires time and skilled personnel. However, at a time when care and hygiene practices are often outsourced or fragmented for economic reasons, practicing proper hygiene can easily become complex:

> The most common problem is actually the issues around screening. We have poured all this information into various standards and work instructions. But nevertheless, I can also understand that there are nurses on staff who are only here three or four times a month, because they have a part-time job, or only work in the middle of the night if there is an admission. They get this piece of paper, then they are supposed to interpret these crosses or checkmarks. And then they have to think about what do I do now? Do I have to swab the front, back, top, or bottom, perform a rapid test, PCR? And what do I actually need to do right now? It becomes more and more complicated over time. Because you simply learn more and more about these microorganisms. And it goes on and on: "Oh, we can make another special regulation." And that is also totally understandable and important from a technical point of view. But for the colleagues on the ward, exactly this kind of implementation can be super complicated, sometimes. (Interview Paul, hygiene specialist nurse: 371)

Standardized protocols and screening schemes cannot conceal the fact that hygiene is a complicated decision-making complex and involves an entanglement of practices of care based on attending to bacterial presence. Thus, hygiene management interferes with hospital architecture, everyday care, human-bacteria relations, systemic issues of organizational care, and patients' health conditions.

For example, a central aspect of hygiene management is concerned with the location inside the hospital where human-bacteria encounters unfold. The type of hygiene practiced depends on the vulnerability of the patients on the ward and the underlying causes for such vulnerability. In an intensive care unit or in transplantation wards, hygiene practices in general, and the bacterial threat in particular, are afforded more relevance than in other wards where less vulnerable patients are located. Hygiene management is a daily practice that involves negotiating multiple categories of relevance that are bound to hospital logistics and architecture, to the practices and resources of care and specialized wards, and to the bacteria and the patient. In addition, hygiene management depends on the patient's disease pattern, the type of ward, the bacteria in question, and which part of the body is the best location to swab for infection. This daily negotiation helps to configure the human-bacteria relation; the relation may become stabilized due to diagnosing a specific bacterial presence (as MRSA), but the diagnosis remains a temporal snapshot of a bacterial presence that is open to multiple outcomes, including infection, sepsis, death, disappearance, or overgrowth.

From the perspective of hygiene management, the evaluation of bacterial presence follows one important credo: accept colonization, prevent infection. As one hygienist emphasized, hygiene is not about preventing colonization and thus bacterial presence, rather it involves accepting bacterial compositions as a normal process and as part of the human condition. Hygiene practice includes the process of coming to terms with bacterial presence that informs the management of it. Risk-adapted screening is one example of how this management takes place in practice, approaching bacterial encounters on a spectrum (Huttunen et al. 2021) rather than by the dualistic classifications of good versus bad bacteria, which a screening questionnaire might suggest at first glance. This speaks to a post-Pasteurian microbiopolitical approach, where the bacterial composition is worked with and evaluated instead of just eliminated with antibiotics. While this certainly hints to a more generous encounter with microbial presence, it is also important to keep in mind that these elaborate practices of post-Pasteurian approaches are born out of a sense of necessity, of desperation and of the fear of a shortage in antibiotics.

## Discharge: Calibrating human-bacteria relationships

> After Nina had undergone countless tests, the period of isolation and hospitalization ended after a few days. Without a medical explanation for her illness, Nina was prepared for discharge from the hospital. Shortly before she left her room to exit the hospital, she was informed that resistant bacteria had been detected. This new information about her bacterial status, which Nina was told in passing, was unsettling: she was unsure if this is the diagnosis, the explanation for her ill health. On the way out, Nina was given some limited information about how to manage her drug-resistant bacteria and how to get rid of the status as a carrier. She should pay attention to her hand hygiene, and she should avoid contact with older or immunocompromised persons, as well as pregnant women and children. Nina could not make sense of this information if she is contagious and dangerous to others or herself. She was wondering why she is released despite this diagnosis. Already shaken by the experience of her illness and the lack of biomedical explanation for it, this new status of "being someone with something" in biomedical terms, further irritated Nina as she was released to the outside world. (Field notes Hamburg, 19.5.2020)

In Nina's case, a characteristic example of how hygiene proceeds, processes such as screening, testing, washing, or isolation are a peripheral aspect of care practices. The reasoning behind these practices is often unknown to the patients, as was the case with Nina. Swabs were taken from her skin, her nose, and the rectal area, but these appeared to be procedures like the others. Only upon leaving the hospital was she informed about her bacterial status, a diagnosis without a disease, an unstable bacterial condition:

> I remember, when I was discharged, that was also one of those moments; I was in an isolation room the whole time, you have a corridor, a showerhead for washing, a small room where the staff change clothes and disinfect everything, and I was just behind it. I am isolated and supposedly a danger emanates from me. The next day, when I was discharged, I was allowed to walk through the corridor without wearing a mask or gloves, which I found totally strange. Because a few hours before I was still in the isolation room, but now I was suddenly allowed to walk through the corridor, and touch the door handle, the light switch, the pen. (Interview Nina, patient: 9)

The immediacy and relevance for Nina of carrying drug-resistant bacteria was put into context and relativized by the medical stuff by associating it with her young age and overall health status. What was of utmost relevance inside the hospital was already changing as she left her room and headed for the exit. As the patient moves on to the outside, leaving the hospital walls behind, so does the bacterial composition: it becomes something else, and so do the hygiene practices. The practices of hygiene management are clearly bound to the hospital setting. For the patient this clear-cut division is often irritating and confusing. The professionals however argue for the temporal relevance of bacterial presence along giving a pragmatic picture of the patient concerning the overall health status and age:

> That is also the reason why in everyday life, where you don't have much contact with very sick people, you don't have to isolate yourself, for example. The need to be isolated is irritating for many patients here. They are isolated, almost like lepers, I would say, even though this is an exaggeration. Though you can only get into the isolation ward with a face mask and protective gown and everything. And then one day, the patient is discharged. They are put into the cab and take part in life again normally, just like that. Because the bacteria identified in their body are actually not dangerous for a healthy person. (Interview Paul, hygiene specialist nurse: 488)

This point is often exemplified in reference to people working with animals, whether in factory farming or as a horse trainer: Working alongside animals leaves an individual susceptible to drug-resistant bacteria, but at long as you are healthy or young or both, carrying drug-resistant bacteria is not likely to cause harm. Nina and other patients diagnosed with drug-resistant bacteria experience this situation as an ambivalent one. In the hospital, diagnosis with drug-resistant bacteria is considered highly relevant and is managed through various hygienic measures, such as screening, swabs, isolation, disinfections, and protective clothing. The way a patient is treated and cared for if diagnosed with drug-resistant bacteria differs materially, spatially, and therapeutically from other patients. With the departure from the hospital, this special role as a patient disappears, as does the relevance of the bacterial composition harboured by the patient, thus modifying the human-bacteria relationship.

## A diagnosis, but not a disease

Nina's confusion about harbouring drug-resistant bacteria—a diagnosis, but not a disease—points to the difficulty of integrating these hospital-bound practices, in conjunction with and against bacteria as contextual practices in an individual's everyday life and concerns about one's own health, body, fellow humans, and nonhumans (such as pets).

From the patients' perspective, hygiene practices often seem opaque. The patients may be screened, undergo smear tests, and are perhaps isolated and rigorously washed, but these are supplementary practices of the biomedical care that brought them to the hospital in the first place. They may receive an unlikely diagnosis: a diagnosis that not necessarily indicate a disease or pathology but nevertheless necessitates several hygiene measures. What follows is by no means simply "a fight against" bacteria. Hygiene management is a nuanced consideration of what might happen, and an anticipation of future harm caused by drug-resistant bacteria alongside local microbiologies.

By questioning, screening, and diagnosing, the vulnerability and ultimately uncertain meaning of being colonized by drug-resistant bacteria is evaluated and tried to be contained by isolation, protective clothing, hand washing, close monitoring, and sanitation. Isolation is a drastic intervention that cuts off the patient form physical contact and social closeness and ultimately covers the intricate processes at play to deal with bacteria. But in all that weighing of bacterial possibilities, the post-Pasteurian approach of exploring and managing instead of killing is strongly supported by the notion of healthy, adaptive bodies that are in a good position to fend off encounters with bacteria (Martin 1994; Brown 2019). One interviewee, a hospital-based physician for microbiology and hygiene, noted that the number one credo of hygiene in current practice is "to preserve the patient's own flora." Patients arrive at the hospital with their own bacterial diversity and this diversity, she emphasized, must be protected (Interview Dr Andress, hygiene physician). Hospital staff need to remain "neutral" in this regard, so as not to endanger the flora of the patients. And for this purpose, she argued, simply as it may sound, it is primarily about "hands, hands, hands, hands. Because the hand is the most important infection transmission site in medicine".

Hygiene practices like handwashing are necessary for the hospital to keep running smoothly, to allow for the flow of care, interventions, and therapy, in cases where AMR poses a major risk for this uninterrupted flow of care. The patient's body is biographized along their bacterial compositions and managed in its capability of position itself in microbial encounters and as microbial being.

Risk-adapted screening is one example of how hygiene management takes place in practice, approaching bacterial encounters on a spectrum (Huttunen et al. 2021) rather than by dualistic classifications of good versus bad bacteria, which a screening questionnaire might appear to suggest at first glance. This speaks to a post-Pasteurian microbiopolitical approach, where the bacterial presence is worked with and evaluated instead of just eliminated with antibiotics. While this certainly hints to a more generous encounter with microbial presence, it is also important to keep in mind that these elaborate practices of post-Pasteurian approaches are a necessity, configured through despair and fear of having no antibiotics, hence no thoroughly Pasteurian substance, at disposition.

The biology of history (Landecker 2016) is of large-scale induced bacterial evolutions—such as antimicrobial drug resistance—entangled with humans operating in the world as travellers, migrants (Kamenshchikova et al. 2018), farmers, and the chronically ill. These entanglements become meaningful in the hospital setting through localizing specific microbiologies such as bacteria. Locality here is done by mobilising specific types such as geographic, professional, or bodily locality that signify hygienic risk. The microbiopolitics at play rely heavily on the rationalities of creating an individual and collective body capable of embracing bacterial diversity. Hence, hygiene practices outside the hospital setting are far less rigid, in contrast to the potential menace of a healthy self and healthy environment. Health is not the absence of bacteria, but the equilibrium of the bacterial composition in and around the individual. Leaving behind the Pasteurian approach and a top-down *one-size fits all* concept in hygienic practices, the case of hygiene management demonstrates a post-Pasteurian microbiopolitical regime in the face of AMR, which emphasize bacterial diversity, the bacterial spectrum, locality, and situatedness over sterility and the killing of microbes as inherently pathogenic.

## Conclusion

Hygiene practices are an integral part of hospitals and multiple hospital workflows meet through the questions about care and therapy, of cleanliness and contamination, of design and architecture, of equipment and instruments, of construction, and of transportation or mobility. What does this specific mediation through hygiene work between the inside and the outside, spatially, and physically through walls, as well as bodies, tell us about the governance of microbes and bodies in general?

Returning to the eye-opening moment one hygienist shared about how hygiene management is not about having no bacterial compositions, but about avoiding infection: following Paxson's diagnosis, this approach marks a post-Pasteurian understanding in which good hygiene management is not a war against microbes but a balance act of making visible and thus managing bacterial presence. Still, there are such things as "bad" microbes, but only in relation to the humans: it is the human that needs to contextualize in face of bacterial presence. This in turn marks another remarkable observation: that post-Pasteurian approaches govern microbial encounters along with construing capable bodies: microbes are not necessarily bad; they are only bad if the human is ill-equipped to encounter them.

Like recent discourses about the danger of COVID-19 (for whom, or for which bodies?), a central category in situating microbial presence for anticipating their potential harm is that of healthy bodies. Certain bacterial composition remains a temporary status for the healthy body. "Healthy" in this case relates to the anticipated potential of the body's bacteria to out-compete drug-resistant bacteria, as the hygienist in the interview excerpt mentions, through "sensible nutrition, normal diet, and normal personal hygiene" (Interview Elli and Carl, hygiene specialist nurses: 118). The bodies in these narratives of drug-resistant bacteria are in Emily Martin's sense (Martin 1994; Brown 2019) pictured as "flexible", where the immune system works under the skin and inside the body to regulate bacterial balance and, therefore, good health. Martin's analysis of the ways in which metaphors and meanings of the body and the immune system have changed over time is helpful here because the "flexible body" of today is very much articulated in the foundation of hygiene management work: detecting bacterial presence and avoiding infection are key factors, as is mastering unstable and adaptable bacterial compositions created through the process of microbial balance.

I have shown how in Germany hospitals work alongside growing uncertainties about antibiotics and concern over AMR, hygiene staff enacts local microbiologies through the screening process. This can be understood as an effort to meet the growing uncertainties of antibiotics and the meaning of bacterial presence with partial control and manageability. These localizing practices and the construction of local microbiologies come with implications. Coming back to Yates-Doerr (2017) approach of denaturalizing the local the same ways anthropologists tend to do with the biological body, I want to conclude this chapter with following up on these implications. For example, situating the bacterial presence in medical staff is not considered necessary according to official guidelines. Moreover, medical staff may display their own local microbiology due to their workplace and daily work with patients with diverse bacterial compositions. But no one can manage these relationships. A diagnosis of an infection with drug-resistant bacteria is not considered an illness; however, it could endanger other patients, and medical staff with patient contact would have to stop working immediately without being able to take sick leave. Again, a diagnosis of harbouring drug-resistant bacteria stipulates a certain risk, but it is not a disease. This situation constitutes a legal grey area and exemplifies how bacterial presence is embedded in wider socio-political matrixes, and that human–microbial relationships are indeed a question of governance.

Research on AMR is often touted as a flagship effort for bringing together different disciplines in the fight against a global health threat, as expressed in a research program titled *One Health* (Hinchliffe 2015; Kahn 2017). Indeed, hygiene management practices typically incorporate multiple sites and localities, as the screening schemes show. However, this strategy carries the risk of naturalizing locality in local microbiologies and inscribing evaluation patterns in biological materiality. Thus, the locality in local microbiologies, as in certain bacteria, are handled not only as a matter of geography, but also as a matter of diseases and professions, or of all three taken together. While acknowledging the immensely important and delicate work hygiene management teams do on the frontlines of AMR, I also like to see this analysis as a point of departure for thinking critically about the underlying assumptions articulated in the localizing practices of hygiene work (and AMR practices more broadly).

Hygiene management is a microbiopolitical practice that connects the hospital arena to a broader vision of managing human life vis-à-vis microbial life. I have shown how the everyday negotiation of what hygienic action requires fits into the post-Pasteurian approaches to encountering microbes: the effort to identify risk in and for patients is focused on evaluating local microbiologies, how they are composed, and which locality needs to be actualized to be manageable. Thus, a local microbiology is a never-finished, partial, and temporary snapshot: Which local microbiology is actualized in any given moment depends on the hygiene regime established at a particular hospital.

Moreover, hygiene management also shows how so much of post-Pasteurian microbiopolitics rely on unhinged notions of the healthy body that is in itself capable of living the good life with microbes. But more often, it is not a choice, and humans are enmeshed in socio-political necessities that are neither microbe-free nor always healthy. It is these ramifications we should pay attention to in organising the healthcare system, in livestock farming, in our modes of production, and in the way we extract resources from humans and nonhumans alike.

## References

Bose, Käthe von. 2017. Klinisch rein: Zum Verhältnis von Sauberkeit, Macht und Arbeit im Krankenhaus. Bielefeld: transcript.

Brotherton, Sean P., and Vinh-Kim Nguyen. 2013. Revisiting Local Biology in the Era of Global Health. Medical Anthropology 32(4): 287–290.

Brown, Nik. 2019. Immunitary Life: A Biopolitics of Immunity. London: Springer.

Chandler, Clare. 2019. Current Accounts of Antimicrobial Resistance: Stabilisation, Individualisation and Antibiotics as Infrastructure. Palgrave Communications 5(1): 1–13.

Charmaz, Kathy. 2014. Constructing Grounded Theory. London: SAGE Publications.

Clarke, Adele E, Rachel Washburn, and Carrie Friese. 2022. Situational Analysis in Practice: Mapping Relationalities Across Disciplines. London: Routledge.

Condrau, Flurin, and Robert G. Kirk. 2011. Negotiating Hospital Infections: The Debate Between Ecological Balance and Eradication Strategies in British Hospitals, 1947–1969. Dynamis 31(2): 385–405.

Douglas, Mary. 1966. Purity and Danger: An Analysis of Concepts of Taboo and Pollution. New York: Praeger.

Gradmann, Christoph. 2017. From Lighthouse to Hothouse: Hospital Hygiene, Antibiotics and the Evolution of Infectious Disease, 1950–1990. History and Philosophy of the Life Sciences 40(1): 8.

Gradmann, Christoph. 2018. Natur, Technik, Zeit: Infektionskrankheiten und ihre Kontrolle im langen 20. Jahrhundert. *In* Medizin und öffentliche Gesundheit. H.-P. Schmiedebach, ed. Pp. 105–124. Berlin, Boston: De Gruyter Oldenbourg.

Hinchliffe, Steve. 2015. More Than One World, More Than One Health: Re-configuring Interspecies Health. Social Science & Medicine 129: 28–35.

Huttunen, Katriina, Elina Oinas, and Salla Sariola. 2021. When Cultures Meet: Microbes, Permeable Bodies, and the Environment. *In* With Microbes. C. Brives, M. Rest, and S. Sariola, eds. Pp. 121–142. Manchester: Mattering Press.

Kahn, Laura H. 2017. Antimicrobial Resistance: A One Health Perspective. Transactions of the Royal Society of Tropical Medicine and Hygiene 111(6): 255–260.

Koch, Erin. 2011. Local Microbiologies of Tuberculosis: Insights From the Republic of Georgia. Medical Anthropology 30(1): 81–101.

Landecker, Hannah. 2016. Antibiotic Resistance and the Biology of History. Body & Society 22(4): 19–52.

Lock, Margaret. 1994. Encounters With Aging: Mythologies of Menopause in Japan and North America. Berkeley: University of California Press.

Lorimer, Jamie. 2020. The Probiotic Planet: Using Life to Manage Life. Minneapolis: University of Minnesota Press.

Martin, Emily. 1994. Flexible Bodies: Tracking Immunity in American Culture From the Days of Polio to the Age of AIDS. Boston: Beacon Press.

Paxson, Heather. 2008 Post-Pasteurian Cultures: The Microbiopolitics of Raw-milk Cheese in the United States. Cultural anthropology 23(1): 15–47.

Paxson, Heather. 2012. The Life of Cheese: Crafting Food and Value in America. Berkeley: University of California Press.

Paxson, Heather. 2014. Microbiopolitics. *In* The Multispecies Salon. E. Kirksey, ed. Pp. 115–121. Durham, London: Duke University Press.

Yates-Doerr, Emily. 2017. Where is the Local? Partial Biologies, Ethnographic Sitings. HAU: Journal of Ethnographic Theory 7(2): 377–401.

# 9 Transfigurations of Lived Iatrogenic Risks in Switzerland

*Rachel Démolis, Thierry Buclin, and Rose-Anna Foley*

## Introduction

Polypharmacized[1] elderly individuals find themselves navigating uncharted territory. They must regularly consume multiple medications due to their chronic conditions while simultaneously remaining acutely aware of the potential adverse effects of such use on their body[2] and the lack of comprehensive evidence regarding the interactions between these numerous medications. This constant uncertainty surrounding their polypharmacy evolves over time, prompting them to develop strategies to manage these uncertainties. This raises the question: what transfigurative processes occur among polypharmacized individuals regarding their experiences of uncertainty related to iatrogenic risks?

The biomedical literature extensively documents the potential adverse effects that individuals living with polypharmacy may encounter. However, most of the existing literature approaches this issue from a medical, pharmaceutical, or public health perspective. In a recent work, Fainzang et al. (2019) dedicated a special issue to medication risks, addressing the topic from a socio-anthropological standpoint. However, to the best of our knowledge, there is limited literature that delves into the experiences and practices related to iatrogenic risks among polypharmacized individuals from a socio-anthropological perspective.

1 Polypharmacized individuals, also known as polymedicated individuals or individuals living with polypharmacy. In the context of this study, it characterizes individuals who have been consuming more than four medications per day for over three months.

2 According to Noaves et al. (2017: 878), "An estimated 5–78% of the elderly are subject to polypharmacy, 13–58% to drug–drug interactions." Long-term polypharmaceutical use is described in the medical literature as potentially inducing adverse effects. "In medicine, an adverse effect (AE) is a harmful and undesired effect resulting from a medication or intervention and procedures" (Rossini 2010: 89). According to Lalic et al. (2016), inappropriate medication prescription, distribution or use leads to higher hospitalization prevalence.

This paper is part of a broader socio-anthropological research project[3] focusing on elderly polypharmacized individuals' medication use and their interactions with their pharmacists in Western Switzerland. Using a critical interpretative approach, our investigation delves into the interpretations and meanings that individuals attribute to their illnesses, experiences, and health practices while considering the macro-social dynamics that influence these representations and practices.

In this text we argue that experiences of uncertainties associated with iatrogenic risks among polypharmacized individuals lead to the transfiguration of their medication use strategies. Specifically, individuals themselves are the principal actors in the transfiguration of their experiences, and pharmacists contribute to shaping and transforming these experiences. We also explore the transfigurative impact of their perception of time on their experiences of iatrogenic risks and, conversely, how polypharmacy-induced uncertainties affect individuals' relationships with time. To understand how these uncertainties are managed by both individuals living with polypharmacy and pharmacists, we approach the examination of medical uncertainties through the lens of two distinct analytical frameworks: the concepts of *transfiguration* and the temporal modalities of *kairos, chronos, and aevum*.

## Transfiguration

We draw upon Kehr et al.'s (2019) and Mattes et al.'s definition (2020) of *transfiguration*, which denotes the "continual, processual engagement and disengagement of humans with each other and their material and non-material worlds within and across particular figurations (i.e., relations of power and webs of social interdependences), each of which is imbued with its own specific logic that helps to hold the web together" (Mattes et al. 2020: 69). Kehr et al. recently used the concept of the *transfiguration* of health and the moral economies of medicine, describing "how pervasive and commanding many aspects of economics and finance – and the values and logics that the highly advanced capitalist world order is inflicting on all domains of human existence and wellbeing – have become over the last decades, not least with regard to the omnipresent politics and practice of neoliberal governance" (2019: 2). As such, medical products and health policies are *transfigured*, as they are "imbued with economic, ecological, scientific, political, cultural and moral values and norms that vary across place and time and are embedded in both local and global relations of (inter-)dependency and power."

3 Study financed by the Swiss National Scientific Foundation (SNSF), project n° 10001A 176336 by Foley, R.-A. entitled "Les personnes âgées face à leur polymédication: approche socio-anthropologique des usages des médicaments et relation au dispensateur" conducted between 2017 and 2022.

This conceptual lens is particularly compelling because it departs from conventional approaches that solely emphasize macro-social dimensions that shape meso- and micro-social dynamics. Instead, it offers a dynamic perspective through which to examine the reciprocal influence of structural figurations, health professionals, and health insurance policies, all of which are also transfigured as they interact with individuals' practices.

If Kehr et al. describe the economization of health as the primary transfigurative force affecting bodies and relationships, we contend that in the context of experiences related to iatrogenic risks, individuals themselves emerge as the primary transfigurative agents of uncertainties associated with medication consumption. We then show the roles of pharmacists in shaping and transforming these experiences. To comprehend uncertainty, we use the second analytical framework to delineate various perceptions of time and to understand how they influence the transfiguration of uncertainty. In this text, we refer to three temporal modalities.

## Kairos, chronos, and aevum

Trapani and Maldonado (2018: 279) emphasized the "new importance" given to *kairos* in the context of temporal modalities. Additionally, scholars such as Derbez et al., who refer to the work of Adam et al. (2004), have emphasized that "the notion of kairos has long been mobilized by sociologists of time, notably as being distinct from chronos" (2018: 14). Kairos denotes "the moments in which time is experienced as charged with significance," according to Svendsen et al. (2018: 23). *Chronos*, "in ancient Greek, refers to 'the mere passing of time'" (Svendsen et al. 2018: 23). It represents "linear, chronological, clock-time" (Wheater 2022: 12). Niles et al. highlight the interplay and sometimes the contradiction between these temporal modalities in their account of midwives' experiences, entitled "Kairos care in a Chronos System" (2021: 484). They discuss the challenges faced when striving to provide individualized care within a health system driven by imperatives oriented around efficiency and promptness. Another term used in the literature to describe different temporal modalities is *aevum*. As defined by Kermode et al. (2000: 461–72), "'aevum' in medieval Latin signifies a mode of existence situated between worldly time and eternity."

It is essential to distinguish between the perceptions of time held by individuals and pharmacists, as the perception of uncertainty is closely intertwined with one's personal view of time. Time exerts a transfigurative influence on experiences of iatrogenic risks, and the uncertainties resulting from polypharmacy significantly impact individuals' relationships with time. Using these analytical lenses, our inquiry revolves around several questions: What types of uncertainties do individuals encounter when faced with polypharmacy-associated iatrogenic risks? What strategies do they devise to navigate and cope with these uncertainties? Furthermore, what strategies do pharmacists adopt when addressing the uncertainties arising from polypharmacy? How do temporal modalities transfigure polypharmacized individuals' experiences and practices related to iatrogenic risks? Conversely, how do these uncertainties alter their perceptions of time?

We begin by uncovering the narratives surrounding iatrogenic polypharmaceutical risks in lay discourse. We then explore the strategies employed by our participants to navigate the uncertainties associated with iatrogenic risks. Next, we decipher how individuals experience various temporal modalities of iatrogenic risks and how living with polypharmacy transfigures an individual's relationship with time. Secondly, we examine how pharmacists develop strategies to navigate the uncertainties inherent in polypharmaceutical practices. These multifaceted dynamics also lead to variations in perceptions of temporalities among these health professionals, reflecting their unique economic temporalities. We finally discuss how the practices of both individuals and pharmacists contribute to the transformation of lived iatrogenic risks, and how this transfiguration extends to a global scale.

## Methods

The data for this study were collected as part of a socio-anthropological research project that focused on understanding the logics and practices of elderly polypharmacized individuals regarding their medication in Switzerland. We conducted 45 semi-structured home interviews with polypharmacized individuals aged 65 years and older. Additionally, we conducted focused observations of their household pharmacy supplies. The interviews lasted from fifty-five minutes to two hours. We also observed pharmacist-patient interactions during "polypharmacy interviews" or "polymedication checks" (PMC).[4] Furthermore, we conducted nine follow-up filmed interviews, which were specifically carried out for the purpose of creating a research film (Demolis et al. 2020).[5]

In addition to the interviews with individuals, we conducted interviews with four pharmacists who partnered with us in this research. Following the data collection, we fully transcribed all interviews and applied coding and crosschecking using MAXQDA software. Subsequently, we analyzed the subthemes using a content analysis method. The filmed interviews were integrated into the overall analysis and subjected to the same coding and sub-coding process.

4 "Since 2010, Swiss community pharmacies can offer a 'polymedication check' (PMC) to patients on ≥4 prescribed drugs taken over ≥3 months. The check is focused on adherence problems, drug-related problems, and the need for supply of prescribed drugs in a weekly pill organizer" (Messerli et al. 2016: 1071)

5 The film can be accessed at the following link: https://polymedication.hesav.ch/acces-film/

For this paper, we adopted a case study approach, wherein we thoroughly analyzed and synthesized all data relevant to our research question, yielding key results. We selected the most representative quotes from the narratives of the 45 participants whose data we analyzed; quotes from six protagonists were selected. Throughout the text, we provide information about the characteristics and contexts of these selected participants.

## Findings

### Individuals' various levels of uncertainties pertaining to their polypharmaceutical practices

Our participants shared their experiences and representations concerning iatrogenic risks associated with specific medications. They recounted risks such as dependency, undesirable side effects (e.g., dizziness, weight gain, drops in blood pressure, myalgia), and allergic reactions. Additionally, they expressed uncertainty related to iatrogenic risks when using several medications simultaneously, including concerns about overconsumption, drug interactions, and the consequences of long-term daily exposure to pharmaceutical chemicals. However, for some participants, mandatory polypharmacy was non-negotiable due to their medical conditions, resulting in heightened levels of uncertainty. We will describe these various types of uncertainties.

First, when faced with the combination of several medications, which some participants referred to as their "medication cocktail," they grappled with uncertainties regarding its potential outcomes.

> Monsieur Boichat is an 80-year-old retired cook who lives in the countryside with his wife. He trained as a cook and travelled internationally during the first part of his career before settling down as a hospital cook. His father was a farmer. He has two sons, one of whom works as a state worker and the other as a lorry driver. He has kidney failure and has a knee prosthesis and currently lives with diabetes and high cholesterol.[6] He takes seven medications per day on a chronic basis.

Monsieur Boichat stated the following:

> The cocktail [...] may well lead to something not good [...] Nobody knows what happens with several medicines [...]. The medication cocktail [...] when you make

6 Participants' pathologies are indicated the first time they are referred to.

cocktails with liquors and things like that, it can bring about things that are not good. (Monsieur Boichat, July 13, 2018[7])

Some participants expressed uncertainty regarding which specific medicine among the cocktail may be responsible for potential harm.

Monsieur Courvoisier is an 85-year-old retired train conductor. He received professional training in mechanics and electronics. His father was a mechanic who became a market gardener in his later life. He has two children, one of whom works as a pharmacy laboratory technician. He lives with his wife in one the main towns of western Switzerland. He has a mechanical aortic valve and suffers from lower gastrointestinal bleeding, obstructive voiding dysfunction, and hypertension. He takes five medications per day and takes three more occasionally.
Because I took medication for a long time...I think the one harmful to the kidneys is... Aldalat, I don't remember which one. (Monsieur Courvoisier, October 8, 2018)

Additionally, the form of harm that may be caused is uncertain, as illustrated by Monsieur Courvoisier: "If we took it for a long time, it may have an effect on the kidneys, or I don't know what."

Another cause for uncertainty was the perception that high medication use may at some point become harmful; however, they were uncertain when or if this situation would arise.

Madame Rosselat is a 66-year-old retired trade union secretary. She also used to work as a social educator. She trained in sales and then completed her education to become a social educator. Her illnesses drove her to be medically discharged five years before her retirement. She lives by herself in one the main cities of western Switzerland. She is from the Swiss Jura. She is divorced and has one daughter, who is a psychologist. She lives with rheumatoid arthritis, clogged coronary arteries, asthma, hypertension, cholesterol, and osteoarthritis, and she currently takes 10 medications per day.
You have to get check-ups on your liver; you have to get check-ups on your kidney: I wouldn't be surprised if one day I had either a kidney or a liver problem. (Madame Rosselat, July 27, 2018)

This uncertainty stems from the awareness among most respondents that despite significant scientific and technological advancements, the intrinsic unpredictability related to their polypharmaceutical consumption remains. This uncertainty persists because not all medication combinations have been scientifically documented for

7 The day on which the interview was conducted is indicated at the first mention of each participant.

elderly patients. However, they cannot discontinue their medication, leaving them with no viable solution. Madame Rosselat expressed the following: "I would like to stop but I can't!"

## Relying on and constructing medical common-sense discourses

Faced with these uncertainties, study participants created a series of common-sense medical discourses for themselves; they often referred to them as belonging to the realm of common knowledge:

> Madame Bovet is a 67-year-old retired psychologist. She has four children and began her studies after raising her children. She lives with her husband, an engineer, in one of the main towns in Switzerland. She currently lives with refractory chronic low back pain, hypotension, *age-related macular degeneration* (ARMD), and urinary and fecal incontinence, and she takes nine medications per day and takes another 10 medications occasionally.

She stated the following: "Everybody knows these side effects." (Madame Bovet, September 20, 2019)

The primary cornerstone of this medical common-sense knowledge is the recognition of hazards associated with high medication consumption.

> Monsieur Griset, a 90-year-old former army instructor, is a widower living in the periphery of a major town with his grandson, who attends a university nearby. He has three children. Since retiring, he has become very involved in charity work, providing school and medical supplies to low-income countries. He lives with postural back pain and sciatica, lumbar spinal stenosis, acute hearing loss in one ear, and insomnia, and he currently takes nine medications on a regular basis and four medications occasionally.

He stated the following: "We well know we shouldn't consume too much, that if we consume too much, there is the negative side." (Monsieur Griset, May 17, 2019)

Secondly, the consequences of iatrogenic polypharmacy are frequently described in relation to specific bodily functions. Most participants highlight the impact of polypharmacy on organs such as the kidney, stomach, and liver, as exemplified by Monsieur Courvoisier, who stated the following: "Maybe not all of them but some of this medication surely harms the stomach." (Monsieur Courvoisier, October 8, 2018)

Thirdly, the vocabulary commonly used to describe polypharmacy frequently includes terms like saturation, exaggeration, and accumulation of medicines within the body. Monsieur Griset expressed the following: "There is such a huge panoply of medication!"

Massé (1995) invoked the concept of idiosyncratic knowledge, referring to an individual's beliefs derived from their own observations, reinterpretations of information in their environment, and corporal personal experience. In our study, we propose the term "medical common-sense," drawing from C. Geertz's conception of common sense, which encompasses an assembled and reassembled, evolving, and constructed "interpretation of the immediacies of experience" (1975: 2).

## Individual strategies for navigating uncertainties associated with lived iatrogenic risks

While facing the uncertainties described above, our participants have developed strategies to navigate the challenges associated with iatrogenic risks.

### Medication moderation, avoidance, and compensatory strategies

The primary strategy involves moderation and avoidance.

> Madame Duret is an 82-year-old former commercial employee who lives in a small town with her husband. She received a secondary school education. Her husband, a retired carpenter, used to own a carpentry business and then worked as an employee. She has three children. She currently lives with chronic refractory pain, fibromyalgia, rheumatism, osteoarthritis, hypertension, and thyroid disorders, and she takes six medications per day and another one occasionally. She also uses alternative and complementary medicine.

She indicated that despite her chronic pain, she limits her use of paracetamol: "One must not do too much [i.e., take too much medication]" [...] "I am allowed to use it, but I avoid it because we know that these products are not good for the liver and all that."

Madame Bovet states that they are consequently abiding by the rule of exception: "Sometimes, we really need it. I want to avoid taking anything and everything." Monsieur Courvoisier describes himself as avoiding resorting to statins at all costs, as he views this as a step towards "sparing his stomach." Madame Bovet is wary of succumbing to a medication "spiral": "Sometimes you would have to take a pill to treat the secondary effects of another medication; in this case I would rather not take it than get into the spiral."

Similarly, Madame Duret avoids resorting to sleeping pills and anxiolytics. Despite her severe sleep disorder, she refuses to take sleeping pills: "...if I can manage like that...when you have not slept for three or four nights, the fourth night you sleep better." This strategy is intended to limit the potential negative secondary effects. Several respondents therefore refrained from using antalgic medication. Monsieur

Griset stated the following: "...it helps a little bit ...but I don't feel like taking it all day though. Because the truth is, when you take it, it knocks you out afterwards."

In these circumstances, caution and abstinence sometimes also extend to refraining from experimenting with "natural products," as emphasized by Madame Duret, who expressed the following: "As far as natural products go, I do not try any medication that would be inappropriate."

Consequently, patients frequently turn to compensatory strategies to reduce their reliance on conventional medications. Several participants describe resorting to dietary measures as a means of protection against the adverse effects of medications. For example, Madame Duret opts to eat yogurt as a stomach protection mechanism rather than using proton-pump inhibitors. Similarly, some participants avoid taking certain medications, such as anti-inflammatory drugs, on an empty stomach, as mentioned by Madame Bovet. Monsieur Courvoisier, on the other hand, eats apples rather than taking statins. Similarly, some participants have explored non-medication-based strategies. Madame Duret, for instance, opted for an intrathecal pump delivering morphine derivatives to reduce her medication consumption: "In order to have less medication [...] in order to limit the use of the Oxynorm, which did not suit me."

In some instances, participants decide to use non-medication therapies or turn to "natural" treatments. We observed two primary approaches to natural treatments. In some cases, participants avoid adding natural or homeopathic treatments to their allopathic treatment, while in others, they use natural treatments to achieve medication sobriety.

## Developing experiential expertise

A core strategy developed by elderly individuals resides in developing experiential lay expertise (Epstein 1995). Madame Bovet illustrated how she mitigates underlying uncertainties by leveraging her own knowledge regarding iatrogenic risks: "I know side effects, I am careful [...] I know what substance is adequate for each thing. I have integrated it well. I know. It prevents me from taking anything and everything, which I don't feel like doing."

Other participants documented their medication use meticulously over time in notebooks. Several study participants incorporated the reading of medication information leaflets into their self-examination process, to determine if a negative feeling may be assessed as a side effect of the introduction of a new molecule in their cocktail. Monsieur Griset states the following: "I take the medication, and then, if I notice I don't feel good, I look at the information leaflets."

Developing and exercising this experiential knowledge is pivotal to circumventing these uncertainties. As Fainzang has noted, we observe in this case the development of a "lay pharmacovigilance" (Fainzang 2014: 334); individuals develop strategies not only to maximize efficiency, but also to minimize risks. We shall use the term “lay pharmaceutical vigilance” to distinguish it from “pharmacovigilance” as a formal system. This differentiation is crucial because it distinguishes the systematic approach from individual observations of medication's effects on oneself.

To consolidate their experiential expertise, participants also rely on technologies that enable them to assess treatments' effectiveness. Monsieur Boichat monitors his insulin level as part of this process. Participants may also depend on laboratory analyses ordered by their physicians to evaluate the suitability of consuming new molecules, thereby strengthening their expertise. Monsieur Courvoisier, for example, conducts such controls to identify “which medication causes greater harm than gain.” Similarly, using blood tests, Madame Duret regarded positive results as evidence that she has not exaggerated her medication use. This prompts us to question the notion of iatrogenic risks as developed in public health policies. These actors develop individual lay expertise and, in some cases, challenge existing figurations. For instance, while researching information about her thyroid therapy, Madame Duret collected data that she provided to her general practitioner and her pharmacist. She also shared experiential data with her migraine specialist who then used it in treating other patients.

Madame Rosselat, on the other hand, suffered severe adverse reactions while using Chinese herbal medicine recommended by a Chinese medicine practitioner. She reported this incident to her health insurance company, which reimbursed her for the treatments. In these cases, it is evident how experiential pharmaceutical knowledge is employed by study participants to both inform and challenge current medical practices concerning iatrogenic risks.

## Living with iatrogenic risks in chronos, kairos and aevum temporalities

Our participants navigate different temporal modalities. They live within a “chronos system” where the clock relentlessly ticks, age advances and, for most, the burden of managing pathologies and the associated medications accumulates. Despite witnessing the “mere passing of time” (Svendsen et al. 2018: 23), their perception of time is marked by inexorability. Regarding their medication regimen, it is unlikely that their prescriptions will become less complex. Thus, the passage of time frequently translates into heightened medication-associated risks. As discussed previously, Madame Rosselat anticipates the time when she will encounter liver or kidney problems due to her polypharmacy. This mirrors another Greek mythical reference to living under the Sword of Damocles, a sentiment shared by many participants:

> Because it's true that it does improve health. But I think that on the other hand, it must alter certain things. If one day someone says to me: ‘you have a sick liver,’ I won't be surprised. Or the kidneys, that's it. That's why we check twice a year. (Madame Rosselat)

In certain circumstances, one might argue that polypharmacized individuals live in a state akin to "aevum," especially when they undergo altered states of consciousness. For instance, two participants have described feeling "out of it" during extended uses of morphine. However, all participants reject this altered perception of time and choose to discontinue opioid use when the dosage is too high or when it induces a distorted perception of reality. Madame Rosselat, for example, stated the following: "TARGIN is a morphine derivative—I don't take it more than three days in a row because after that I can't remember my name... my memory isn't as good, my head is fuzzy, it's no fun."

The lives of polypharmacized individuals are also characterized by kairotic moments. Drawing on Taylor's interpretation of kairos (2007), these are instances when "extraordinary things occur that break everyday life routines" (Derbez 2018: 14). Several experiences within the realm of polypharmacy can be described as kairotic times. To illustrate this, medication-related accidents constitute a departure from the ordinary routine of daily life. For example, Monsieur Griset recounts an incident of accidental overmedication that resulted in hospitalization.

> So, they told me: "You did well to come because... it could have been... something serious. And if it happens again, you come straight away. And then they changed the medicine.

As cited earlier, Madame Rosselat also recalls her intense experience, as the Chinese herbs she was counseled to use triggered adverse reactions. Some medical appointments may become life-altering consultations; receiving laboratory or tests results may be of immense significance, as they indicate positive or negative news. Similarly, medical consultations are in some cases moments of revelation that may have major significance for the future.

> Monsieur Treboux is an 80-year-old retired sales representative living with his wife in the countryside. He suffers from diabetes and non-alcoholic liver cirrhosis and currently takes seven medications per day.

He expressed that learning about his liver cirrhosis diagnosis was a life-altering moment for him: "Around three years ago, I said, ""Now I have for how long?" And then the... the diabetologist he said to me, 'don't make any... any big commitment to more than a year and a half.' So, it's up to me to make an interpretation."

Conversely, some consultations and encounters can be deemed auspicious. These are the moments when participants discover solutions that enable them to reduce their medication intake or acquire new insights into appropriate medication usage. In this regard, polypharmaceutical interviews led by pharmacists can be viewed as transformative and positively life-altering.

Additionally, these uncertainties significantly influence how individuals' perceptions of time become intertwined with their daily experiences of chronic illnesses and polypharmacy. Many participants in our study have multiple health conditions, necessitating several medical appointments per month and, in some cases, daily or weekly visits from healthcare professionals. Their lives are frequently punctuated by these medical appointments and check-ups. Living with several pathologies and with polypharmacy transfigures their relationship with time. It becomes marked by their medication routines throughout the day and the medical appointments they attend over the course of months. These uncertainties regarding their health and medication usage serve as the foundation for the strategies that participants develop to address doubts associated with high medication consumption.

## Strategies employed by pharmacists to address uncertainties associated with iatrogenic risks

These dynamics are intricately interwoven with other social domains that influence individuals' practices in relation to iatrogenic risks. Pharmacists play an essential role in the transformation of individuals' experiences of iatrogenic risks.

We conducted interviews with four pharmacists who collaborated with us in the study. They facilitated participant recruitment within their pharmacies (in situ) and allowed us to observe the polymedication checks (PMCs) they conducted with study participants. Two of the pharmacists were managers in a large pharmacy chain, with one located in the city center of a major city (pharmacist 1) and the other on the outskirts of a large city in Switzerland (pharmacist 2). Another pharmacist worked in an independent pharmacy in a very small town in Switzerland, primarily serving patients from rural areas (pharmacist 3). The last pharmacist was the owner of an independent pharmacy in a small town in Switzerland (pharmacist 4).

We uncovered three practices employed by pharmacists to address the challenges associated with iatrogenic risks arising from polypharmacy. These practices include a) pharmacists making calls to physicians to seek prescription clarifications or to notify them of potential inconsistencies or incompatibilities, b) the utilization of clinical decision support software, and c) the conduction of polypharmacy interviews.

### Calling the physician to obtain prescription clarifications

To manage the risks associated with polypharmacy, pharmacists must perform several verifications. One interviewee described her role as the "patient's last safety net" because she is the final health professional responsible for verifying prescriptions, dosages, and the medications that her patients consume before delivering them (Pharmacist 2, February 27, 2020). Pharmacists do not have access to a complete patient file containing all medical information regarding the patient, as the

"Dossier Électronique du Patient (DEP)," housing comprehensive medical records, is still in the process of implementation and has not been universally activated by all patients (Bünzli et al. 2023). In Switzerland, health insurance is not free. It is provided by private companies and is mandatory for all residents. Patients can choose their health insurance provider among approximately 60 insurers. The pharmacists we interviewed in 2020 did not have access to patients' electronic files, and physicians do not transfer any medical information to them. A pharmacist we interviewed described operating "blindly," "guessing" the patient's diagnosis, and "reconstituting" the consultation and being relegated to the role of "drug merchant", who "doesn't need to know" (Pharmacist 2). In such cases, pharmacists frequently need to call physicians to obtain clarifications regarding prescriptions, a process that requires diplomatic skills and is embedded in the power dynamics between physicians and pharmacists. In a context where physicians can recommend different pharmacies, maintaining a positive relationship with the provider is of critical economic importance for pharmacists. Trust in one's physician is frequently regarded as a cornerstone of a patient's treatment 'adherence' or appropriation. The pharmacists we interviewed also emphasized that trust between the pharmacist and the physician is a crucial element in resolving prescription clarification issues.

### Using clinical decision support systems

Furthermore, to mitigate polypharmaceutical uncertainties, clinical decision support systems have become ubiquitous in pharmacies. These systems flag potential drug–drug interactions and provide information about their severity. Pharmacists may use their judgment to interpret this information considering whether the patient has previously experienced these medication combinations. However, these systems, while considered indispensable, can be problematic, as they "always pop up," potentially creating a "false sense of security" (pharmacist 2).

The temptation to rely solely on the tool's output underscores the importance of maintaining a dialogue between the pharmacist and the patient to assess the potential severity of the risk and its detectability. Consequently, this dialogue must remain linked to the traditional role of pharmacists in discussing the patient's experience with these medication associations.

### Performing polymedication checks

Polymedication checks (PMCs) offer a glimpse into how issues involving polypharmaceutical iatrogenic risks are intertwined with more global economic and political concerns, shedding light on ongoing power dynamics. PMCs, a service offered in Switzerland, enabled polymedicated patients to engage in 20-minute discussions with their pharmacist to address medication-related issues, including interactions, understanding the purpose of education, and increasing medication confidence and adherence (Krähenbühl et al. 2008; Messerli et al. 2018). These PMCs represented a major advancement in defining the pharmacists' role in Switzerland by emphasizing their specific training and dispelling the perception of their "drug merchant" role. It also underscored the pharmacists' qualifications as healthcare professionals capable of providing recommendations. Notably, this service was reimbursed by insurance companies and did not require a physician's prescription. One of the pharmacists we interviewed revealed that the pharmacy chain he worked for placed particular emphasis on polypharmacy interviews, accounting for approximately half of the PMCs conducted nationwide. Employees were encouraged to conduct these interviews, with PMCs listed as part of their annual corporate objectives (Pharmacist 1, February 3, 2020). Interestingly, representatives from this chain described the service as non-commercial and viewed it as a public health commitment. The incentive was not primarily commercial but to enhance the public image of pharmacies as providers of patient-centred care and to elevate the profession's profile as service providers. Identifying the profession as service providers was regarded as vital by this pharmacy chain. However, reimbursement for these interviews was rescinded after a six-year trial period. Another pharmacist, well-versed in local financial dynamics within the pharmaceutical and insurance sectors, stated the following: "insurance companies are not willing to reimburse simply for the sake of patients' trust in their treatment. Proof of safety, efficiency, and cost effectiveness" was not established (Pharmacist 4, March 7, 2020). Most pharmacists were unwilling to advocate for the ongoing reimbursement of this service, as they perceived it as not being cost-effective. This perspective was described by a pharmacist working for an independent pharmacy in a small town in Switzerland (Pharmacist 3, February 26, 2020).

## Discussion

### Medication users as key actors of the transfiguration of their lived iatrogenic risks

In response to the uncertainties related to iatrogenic risks, individuals employ various strategies. Participants in our study drew upon experiential pharmaceutical knowledge to confront these uncertainties. They actively informed and challenged prevailing medical practices concerning iatrogenic risks. However, these efforts were undertaken individually within the context of their interactions with healthcare practitioners, operating in parallel rather than in coordination. We observed incremental parallel transfigurations of practices for assessing iatrogenic risks.

Although these learning processes and challenges are typically experienced by individuals separately, it is important to recognize that information circulates among patients and caregivers (Fainzang 2001), particularly among patients who suffer from chronic illnesses. Over the course of their medical trajectories, patients' representations are likely to be largely influenced not only by medical discourses but also by natural therapists and pharmacists. Individuals frequently discuss their personal medical concerns with friends and family, and some may join patient associations dedicated to scrutinizing the iatrogenic effects of medications. Furthermore, we consider that medical professionals play a crucial role in facilitating the dissemination of these individual medical experiences, thereby transfiguring individual separate experiences of polypharmacy-induced risks.

Individuals also cultivate experiential expertise and develop lay pharmaceutical vigilance practices and discourses, adopting precautionary strategies. These strategies are often intertwined with broader medication-related concerns that surface among our study participants' discourses. There is a prevalent skepticism directed towards pharmaceutical companies, which participants frequently describe as prioritizing corporate and financial interests over individual access to health. These pharmacovigilant practices are closely connected to a more general aversion to "chemical" products with a preference for natural alternatives. In some instances, they align with global ecological concerns, reflecting a desire to detoxify both the planet and our bodies.

The presence of this "ecological discourse" among the elderly has been documented for some time (Collin 2001). However, our findings suggest that it has gained greater prominence on a global scale, influenced by policies and advertising campaigns aimed at addressing climate change. Additionally, local political and cultural imperatives in Switzerland, exemplified by referendums regarding synthetic pesticide use in agriculture and waste management policies, have contributed to the amplification of these concerns.

Medication moderation dynamics are exhibited by our study participants and are also co-constructed and interwoven with more global, institutional dynamics. This is evident in the implementation of deprescribing policies in hospitals and nursing homes (Cateau et al. 2020) that are co-constructed with evolving institutional, and hospital offers. For instance, advancements in pain treatment technologies, observed in the pain clinic we studied, contribute to reducing medication usage or dosages, in alignment with the global deprescribing movement. It is noteworthy that moderation practices among poly-medicated elderly individuals extend to the use of "natural" products, thereby deconstructing the preconception that simply switching from chemical to natural products is a magical solution that addresses iatrogenic risks. This observation lays the foundation for further research into the perceptions of polyherbacy-associated iatrogenic risks among the elderly and the wider population.

In this sense, the transfiguration of iatrogenic risks precipitated by individuals' own vigilance is intertwined with global criticism directed at pharmaceutical companies, the growing international preference for "natural" and local products, and decisions made at the local political level. Individual transfigurative actions related to perceptions of uncertainty regarding iatrogenic risks intersect with global and local dynamics.

## Lived iatrogenic risks across kairos, chronos, and aevum temporalities

Individuals living with polypharmacy experience uncertainties within various temporal frameworks. To better interpret these notions, we will examine more closely the literature describing these concepts. Wheater describes *kairos* as "a favorable moment, an opportunity, what one would call today the 'appointed time,' the 'crucial moments,' or the 'best times'" (Wheater 2022: 12). Lanz notes that Ramo's description of kairos (1999) was "originally named from the Greek god of the favorable moment" (Lanz 2021: 2). For Trapani and Maldonado (2018: 271), "it has enabled granular distinctions between closely related notions like the 'opportune,' the 'appropriate,' and the 'possible'". "Kairos can be considered in itself as an event. Indeed, the specificity of kairotic time appears especially when extraordinary things occur that break everyday life routines" (Taylor 2007; Derbez 2018: 14). Kairos has been described as "one of the deities of 'magical moments'" (Adam 2004: 8) and as the "God of lucky coincidence and the right moment for favorable action" (Derbez 2018: 14). Regarding action and its effectivity, every moment is not equal. There are "good" and "bad" moments.

Chronological time (chronos) is the conception of time that holds great significance in our secular modern era (Taylor 2007). It refers to uniform, repetitive time composed of hours, minutes, and seconds that can be measured, "what is commonly called the clock-time" (Derbez 2018: 14).

Within the chronos temporality, individuals' polypharmacy becomes integrated into their daily routines, and they address it by incorporating it into their temporality. As the number of their pathologies and medication regimens increases, individuals' perception of time becomes transfigured. Their lives become punctuated by their medication use and medical appointments.

When viewed through the lens of aevum, the lived experience of iatrogenic risks is one that participants reject when they cannot actively participate in the transfiguration of their experiences of uncertainties. This is an indication that individuals are not passive observers of various temporalities. They actively incorporate their medication routines into their chronological time, which they embrace. However, they reject medication that induces an altered state of consciousness—an 'aevum' state—where their agency is diminished.

Experiences of iatrogenic risks are prevalent within kairotic time, which occurs during life-altering events, such as medication accidents or when patients discover medication-induced complications. Kairotic time is also at hand during polymedication checks (PMCs) when patients learn more about their own treatment. During these kairotic moments, actors from various social domains converge. Particularly during emergencies, all actors cooperate to transfigure iatrogenic risks, such as when a medication accident occurs.

## Pharmacists' practices that transfigure individuals' experiences of iatrogenic risks and their perception of time

Uncertainties are undergoing transfigurations due to technological advancements over time. The use of computer-assisted analysis and various forms of software by physicians and pharmacies has exerted a profound impact on the provision of instantaneous answers related to polypharmaceutical risks. Similarly, the development of DEP is expected to accelerate access to information for both individuals and health professionals. This technological development is progressively transfiguring perceptions and practices related to polypharmaceutical uncertainty. It is also reshaping the power dynamics among health professionals and changing the nature of relationships between patients, physicians, and pharmacists. The computerization of pharmacists' practices and the DEP will contribute to merging various temporalities experienced in parallel by patients, physicians, and pharmacists.

The strategies developed by pharmacists to address polypharmacy-induced risks underscore the fact that patients, physicians, and pharmacists operate within a similar clock time, but their temporalities diverge. Pharmacists, who bear responsibility for ensuring the safety and suitability of treatments and their delivery, operate within a distinct temporal framework compared to primary care physicians. They receive the prescription after the doctor–patient consultation and engage in a distinct interaction with the patient.

This discrepancy also underscores the fact that various interconnected social domains evolve within different economic temporalities. Economic considerations play a pivotal role in mitigating polypharmacy-induced uncertainties. PMCs, for instance, could empower patients to better comprehend and manage their treatment. However, the sustainability of such services is subject to national economic and legal rationales, frequently determined by national pharmacist organizations (Swissmedic) assessing the safety of therapeutic products and the economic feasibility of these interventions. For patients, their economic temporality revolves around their monthly health insurance payments and other healthcare-related expenses, which are intertwined with their broader financial circumstances. Pharmacists find themselves navigating multiple temporalities, including those of patients, physicians, insurance companies, and the legal bodies that dictate the duration of PMCs and whether they will continue to be reimbursed.

## Global transfigurations of lived iatrogenic risks

The issues surrounding iatrogenic risks among polypharmacized elderly individuals are of global concern, generating scientific research across various domains, including pharmaceutical research, health economics, computer sciences, medical sciences, and chemistry. Software developed to facilitate medical decision-making, for instance, might be created in Canada[8] and subsequently be sold and utilized in locations as distant as Madagascar or New Zealand. The collective efforts to mitigate uncertainties related to polypharmaceutical iatrogenic risks are, indeed, global in nature.

Furthermore, certain historical and global pharmaceutical events can be considered pivotal and transformative, contributing to shifts in how the pharmaceutical industry is portrayed in the media and perceived by individuals. For example, the Vioxx scandal in the USA in 2004 left consumers skeptical of the pharmaceutical industry's vested interests. A similar event occurred in France when the Mediator treatment was trialed. More recently, the pharmaceutical company Purdue Pharma, known for producing opioids, has faced numerous legal charges. Their marketing strategies have been criticized for inducing opioid dependency among the patients they were serving. These events have further intensified the critical attitudes held by the media and the public toward pharmaceutical companies. These incidents resulted in a long-lasting paradigm shift, eroding people's trust in the pharmaceutical industry. These paradigm shifting events may be interpreted as kairotic times, crucial moments, which played a pivotal role in a global transfiguration in the perception of the pharmaceutical industry. Patients became more critical toward them and more cautious in their medication use. These historical events induced institutionalized doubt and precipitated the emergence of deprescribing movements, such as the "less is more" movement in the USA, the "overdiagnosis" movement in the United Kingdom and Australia, and the "Smarter Medicine" movement in Switzerland (Angel 2004; Goldacre 2012). Transfiguration, in this context, should therefore be understood as a dynamic process of evolving social representations.

## Conclusion

Elderly individuals living with polypharmacy in Switzerland encounter a multitude of uncertainties linked to their high medication intake. These uncertainties encompass questions regarding the potential outcomes of their medication cocktails, including which specific medications might pose risks and the nature of harm that

8 Canadian software used globally which helps professionals and patients to reduce their medication use.

could result. They are aware that not every medication combination used by elderly persons can be subject to scientific study. These uncertainties find expression in common-sense medical discourses.

In response to these uncertainties, individuals develop various mitigation strategies. These strategies encompass medication sobriety, avoidance, and compensatory measures. Additionally, individuals cultivate lay pharmaceutical vigilance practices. They often express concerns about the perceived "unnaturality" of pharmaceuticals, the inherent toxicity of "chemical products," and the influence of consumerist society and profit-driven pharmaceutical corporations. In their quest to navigate uncertainty, they construct a "medical common sense" to interpret and cope with the uncertainties associated with polypharmacy-induced risks.

While public health policies typically frame these risks as adverse events that are "combated by both the health insurance system and health professionals" and that "affect mostly the elderly "[authors' translation]"[9] our findings suggest that individuals themselves also play an active role in combating iatrogenic risks, thus transfiguring their own experiences. They are not merely passive recipients of protective measures provided by the healthcare system; they are also proactive agents in evaluating and exercising vigilance over their own polypharmaceutical regimens.

The research conducted by Kehr et al. (2019) highlights the intricate interplay between the practices of individuals and healthcare professionals, situated within economic and power dynamics operating at both local and global levels. Our study revealed that these practices are embedded in complex economic and power dynamics, which operate on an individual level and on a meso-social level. Representations of iatrogenic risks have become deeply ingrained within evolving local institutional and hospital policies, in alignment with the emerging global trends that prioritize medication sobriety and deprescription practices.

The use of the transfiguration concept allows us to delve deeper. The transfiguration of uncertainties in polypharmaceutical practices may be understood in various ways. For individuals living with polypharmacy, their perception of time is transfigured. Their perception of chronos, or "clock-time," becomes increasingly intertwined with the timing of medication intake throughout the day and their adherence to medical appointments over the course of the year. They also encounter kairotic times, wherein medication accidents or medical appointments take on life-altering significance.

The transfigurative role of time in the lives of individuals living with polypharmacy operates at the individual level. Individuals' lay vigilance practices also transfigure several figurations. When narrating their firsthand experiences of iatrogenic

9 https://www.ameli.fr/assure/sante/medicaments/medicaments-et-situation-de-vie/iatrogenie-medicamenteuse; last accessed on 24.11.2023

risks, they have the potential to influence the practices of healthcare professionals and, in some instances, to impact the policies of health insurance providers.

Pharmacists' temporalities also differ from those of physicians and patients. Their capacity to mitigate polypharmaceutical uncertainty hinges on their ability to navigate the power dynamics between physicians and pharmacists. Additionally, they are subject to various economic temporalities, including decisions made at the national level, deeming polymedication checks (PMCs) non-cost effective. The evolution of information technologies, such as the use of DEP and software supporting clinical decision-making, also results in the transfiguration of pharmacists' processes and temporalities involved in solving polypharmacy-associated uncertainties. Consequently, interactions between different social domains are also transfigured.

On a global level, some pharmaceutical "scandals" have unleashed transformative effects by eroding public confidence in the pharmaceutical industry. These events have contributed to the transfiguration of uncertainty in pharmaceutical use.

In summary, elderly individuals and pharmacists are essential actors in the transfiguration of iatrogenic risks. They are entangled in broader dynamics, including reimbursement policies, pharmaceutical controversies generating media attention and growing skepticism toward the pharmaceutical industry. This entanglement is also rooted in global and local shifts in attitudes toward chemical and imported products. Polypharmacized individuals reject medications that cause unwanted side effects. They avoid medications that would confine them to an 'aevum temporality', which would make them passive participants. It is crucial for them to exercise lay vigilance over their polypharmacy. This underscores the vital role polypharmacized individuals play in reshaping their experiences of iatrogenic risks. Their control over the temporality in which they live is a critical factor in this process. Individuals and pharmacists often operate under distinct temporal frameworks. For pharmacists, chronos time revolves around selling merchandise and preventing medication accidents, while individuals' chronos time involves incorporating medication consumption into their daily lives. However, their temporalities intersect during kairotic moments, particularly in emergencies when the risk ceases to be a mere possibility and becomes a reality, as in the case of medication accidents. In such situations, both parties strive to draw upon their accumulated experiences during their separate chronos time. They can then integrate the new knowledge acquired in this kairotic time to enhance their understanding and practices of polypharmacy in their chronos time. Ultimately, kairotic time enables them to jointly transfigure the experiences of iatrogenic risks.

## Acknowledgements

We would like to express our heartfelt gratitude to all the members of the MAAH conference for their feedback on the initial draft of this document, with special thanks to Sangeeta Chattoo. We are also deeply appreciative of the input of the book's coordinators and Raphaël Hammer for their revisions in the later stages.

## References

Adam, Barbara. 2004. Time. Cambridge and Malden, MA: Polity Press.

Angell, Marcia. 2004. The Truth About the Drug Companies: How They Deceive Us and What To Do About It. New York: Random House Trade Paperbacks.

Buclin, Thierry, Rose-Anna Foley, and Francoise Livio. 2019. Pharmacovigilance, Hémovigilance, Vaccinovigilance, Tératovigilance...: Quelles Retombées Imprévues pour les Patients, Les Intervenants De Santé Et Les Systèmes De Soins? Anthropologie & Santé 19. https://doi.org/10.4000/anthropologiesante.4937.

Bünzli, Dominique, Sylviane Boissard, Philippe Eggimann, and Vladimir Mayor. 2023. Dossier électronique du patient: les médecins dans l'expectative. Revue Médicale Suisse 19(828): 1055–1057.

Cateau, Damien, Piertluigi Ballabeni, Stéphanie Mena, Olivier Bugnon, and Anne Niquille. 2020. Deprescribing In Nursing Homes: Protocol for Nested, Randomised Controlled Hybrid Trials of Deprescribing Interventions. Research in Social and Administrative Pharmacy 17(4): 786–794.

Collin, Johanne. 2002. Observance et Fonctions Symboliques Du Médicament. Gérontologie Et Société 25/ N103(4): 141–159.

Démolis, Rachel, and Fazia Benhadj. 2020. Le Film De Recherche Comme Modalité De Production d'un Discours Scientifique En Anthropologie De La Santé. Anthropologie & Santé 21. https://doi.org/10.4000/anthropologiesante.8141.

Derbez, Benjamin. 2018. Is There A "Right Time" For Bad News? Kairos In Familial Communication on Hereditary Breast and Ovarian Cancer Risk. Social Science & Medicine (202): 13–19.

Epstein, Steven. 1995. The Construction of Lay Expertise: Aids Activism and The Forging of Credibility in The Reform of Clinical Trials. Science, Technology & Human Values. 20(4): 408–437.

Fainzang, Sylvie. 2001. Médicaments Et Société: le Patient, le Médecin et l'Ordonnance. Paris: Presses Universitaires De France.

Fainzang, Sylvie. 2014. Managing Medicinal Risks in Self-Medication. Drug Safety 37(5): 333–342.

Fainzang, Sylvie, and Ashley Ouvrier. 2019. Face aux risques médicamenteux. Dossier Thématique. Anthropologie & Santé 19. https://doi.org/10.4000/anthropologiesante.5261.

Geertz, Clifford. 1975. Common Sense as A Cultural System. The Antioch Review 33 (1): 5–26.

Goldacre, Ben. 2012. Bad Pharma: How Drug Companies Mislead Doctors and Harm Patients. London: Fourth Estate.

Kermode, Frank. 2000 [1967]. The Sense of An Ending: Studies in The Theory of Fiction. Oxford: Oxford University Press.

Kehr, Janina, Hansjörg Dilger, and Peter van Eeuwijk. 2019. Transfigurations of Health and the Moral Economy of Medicine: Subjectivities, Materialities, Values. Zeitschrift Für Ethnologie 143 (1): 1–20.

Krähenbühl, Jean-Marc, Anne Decollogny, and Olivier Bugnon. 2008. Using the Costs of Drug Therapy To Screen Patients For A Community Pharmacy-Based Medication Review Program. Pharmacy World & Science 30(6): 816–822.

Lalic, Samanta, Janet Sluggett, Jenny Ilomäki, Barbara Wimmer, Edwin Tan, Leonie Robson, Tina Emery, and Simon Bell. 2016. Polypharmacy and Medication Regimen Complexity as Risk Factors for Hospitalization Among Residents of Long-Term Care Facilities: A Prospective Cohort Study. Journal of the American Medical Directors Association 17(11): 1067.e1–1067.e6.

Massé, Raymond. 1986. Culture et Santé Publique: Les Contributions de L'anthropologie à la Prévention et à la Promotion De La Santé. Montréal, Paris, Casablanca: Gaëtan Morin.

Mattes, Dominik, Bernhard Hadolt, and Brigit Obrist. 2020. Introduction: Rethinking Sociality and Health through Transfiguration. MAT-Medical Anthropology Theory 7(1): 66–86.

Messerli, Markus, Noortje Vriends, and Kurt Hersberger. 2018. Humanistic Outcomes and Patient Acceptance of The Pharmacist-Led Medication Review "Polymedication Check" In Primary Care in Switzerland: A Prospective Randomized Controlled Trial. Patient Prefer Adherence (12): 1071–1078.

Niles, Paulomi Mimi, Saraswathi Vedam, Amy Witkoski Stimpfel, and Allison Squires. 2021. Kairos Care in A Chronos World: Midwifery Care as Model of Resistance and Accountability In Public Health Settings. Birth 48(4): 480–492.

Taylor, Janelle. 2008. On Recognition, Caring, And Dementia. Medical Anthropology Quarterly 22(4): 313–35.

Trapani, William, and Chandra Maldonado. 2018. *Kairos*: On the Limits to Our (Rhetorical) Situation. Rhetoric Society Quarterly 48(3): 278–286.

Wheater, Kitty. 2022. No Time Like the Present: Mindfulness, Temporality and the Therapeutics of Kairos. Anthropology Today 38(2): 9–12.

# 10 "Skyped, Zoomed and WhatsApped"

## Practicing Psychotherapy in Pandemic Times

*Andrea Stöckl*

### Introduction

In this paper, I will reflect on my experiences as a practicing psychotherapist in Austria from an auto-ethnographic point of view. Having worked as a medical anthropologist in a medical school in the United Kingdom for nearly 17 years made me all too aware of the regulations of medical and allied health professional training. Being a student again at 40, when I started psychotherapy training, gave me another perspective together again. At 53 I was finally equipped to leave the academic world behind and start the adventure of opening my private practice, when all of a sudden, a pandemic was announced by the WHO. I was suddenly confronted with using Zoom, Skype, and the Smartphone as allies in the healing process. This brought more uncertainty and insecurities to my life as I was unsure how my professional life and practice would change.

In this chapter, I reflect on the changes in interactions and treatment in my psychotherapeutic practice from 2020 to 2023, when I suddenly had to switch from seeing clients in the privacy of the consulting room to seeing them as "talking heads" on Zoom. The COVID-19 pandemic was declared shortly after I had set up my private practice in Innsbruck, Austria, in January 2020. Apart from familiarizing myself with the complexity of diagnosing mental health disorders and finding dysfunctional patterns that caused my clients problems in everyday life, I had also finally mastered the problematic tasks of noticing, naming, and communicating what in psychotherapy is called "transference" and "countertransference" in the sessions in real-time. Transference occurs when a patient, based on their experiences and neurotic or dysfunctional interpretations of these experiences, casts other people as actors in their inner world and sees their actions and ways of being only through the lens of their dysfunction, leading most often to a repetition of the original trauma. In any therapeutic relationship, psychotherapists will also be given a role in this "play"; the therapist is more or less aware of the role they have been given in the client's world, and the reaction to this role is called countertransference, which any good therapist will be able to recognize and use in the consultation room to make the implicit and unconscious "game" that the client is playing explicit. Learning to deal with this countertransference and its manifestations in the psyche and body of the therapist is one of the most challenging skills to master on the journey to practicing the "impossible profession." For this chapter, it is essential to conceptualize transference and countertransference because it helps us understand which challenges psychotherapy must face using video telephony.

Every school of psychotherapy has a model of transference and countertransference (Levy and Scala 2012). In my experience, I knew I had started to master this skill when I noticed that the sensation of my bodily affects had changed. Suddenly, I felt nervous on the way to my consulting room and didn't quite know why, or I made sure that I would wear more expensive items of clothing on a day I knew a specific client would be coming to see me or that I would worry about the quality and brand of the tea and water I would sometimes offer my clients. Reflecting on these "worries" in areas of my life in which I felt comfortable made me aware that a difficult client with severe narcissistic traits would wait for me, traits that I had not yet consciously made sense of in terms of diagnosis. Similarly, I started to notice very unusual exhaustion in the evenings on days in which depressed clients had come to see me, yet grieving clients did not have the same effect: I knew that despite the same symptoms they presented with as depressed clients, theirs was not a far less hopeless struggle. Likewise, I had started to use forms of somatic attention (see also Csordas 1993) with my clients: could they sense trust and certainty in their embodied feelings rather than in their thoughts? Could they move from cognitively analyzing whether they could trust someone, which often leads to obsessive thought patterns, to an intuitive sensation of trust in themselves, their partners, and their therapist? Could they distinguish a sensation of anxiety from the nervous tingling that hope engenders? Could they move from overthinking to focusing on these somatic modes of interpreting emotions and the world around them?

Just about when I noticed that I could use these newly honed skills of somatic attention to my feelings in the consulting room, everything changed: the pandemic COVID-19 hit us, and consultation in person was, in most cases, not possible anymore. I had to adapt to new versions of treatment quickly. While the professional body of psychotherapists in Austria, the Österreichischer Bundesverband für Psychotherapie (ÖBVP), viewed the delivery of mental health care via technology with a lot of scepticism because of a lack of evidence-based research (Finger-Ossinger 2021) my clients welcomed the integration of tools such as Skype, Zoom and WhatsApp in their search for an answer to their ailments.

After initial confusion about data protection and "safe" delivery of the consultation online on Zoom video-telephony, my clients and I settled into the new routine of "being" with each on Zoom. Not only would we now see each other only as "talking heads," i.e., the face and upper torso rather than the whole body, but in addition, we would also see our own faces talking in the more minor pop-up of the Zoom interface mirror. We would no longer share a bodily presence in the same room. How could we carry on working on embodied emotions? How could I use my skills of noticing transference and countertransference in the virtual world? These were the questions that I started to ask myself increasingly. Furthermore, I was concerned about my private space and the framework in which therapy should and could be delivered. The correct setting is a significant factor in psychotherapy. It is not an accident that we refer to therapy as "going to therapy" and "coming out of a depression". The consulting room provides the client with a setting and a framework for feeling safe and thus being able to trust. Words that cannot be spoken anywhere else can be uttered there and nobody would or should ever hear them again. Walking or driving back home gave the client with enough time to process what happened in the session so that everyday life could be lived without intruding on therapy. All this would change by using online tools to deliver therapy directly to the client's room and to their psyche.

It is also a truism that psychotherapy is an "impossible profession" because similar to social anthropology, it deals with a person's ideas of the past, the present and the future; sometimes it deals with waiting for the right moment to put into action what had been imagined and desired for a long time. One becomes all too aware of the passage of time when the past, present and future are condensed into a 50-minute session. The past and what we remember of it shape our present and influence what we fear or wish for the future.

Psychotherapy is an impossible profession because one can never know if the therapeutic relationship works, if there is an outcome and if there is an outcome, whether this outcome is what the client wanted or, rather, what he or she feared the most. Therapists work with aspects of the unconscious, with the numinous, with aspects of a person's life that are sometimes not known and sometimes not felt, yet these aspects are there and manifest in symptoms such as anxiety disorders or depression. If therapy is successful, these aspects of a client's personality are unearthed and made conscious. Happiness is not always achieved, but the client sometimes leads a more fulfilling life, and, in the best case, is equipped with the ability to make decisions when it is the right time or has the skills to wait until it is the right time. Holding the space of indecision is a critical element of good mental health. Hope is what brings people into therapy, a hope that the future will be less burdensome than the present, and fear or desire makes an uncertain future often hard to imagine. I was presented with these challenges at the beginning of my new career and had to navigate these by using newly developed technology such as Zoom and WhatsApp.

Having outlined all the above, let us now have a look at how health authorities in Austria dealt with these challenges. Then I will discuss the impact of using Zoom in my own private practice.

## Regulating the impossible profession: Governance of online therapy in Austria

Practicing counseling and psychotherapy has changed over the last 30 years ever since the advent of personal computers and, more recently smartphones. Before 1991, practicing psychotherapy was not regulated by the Austrian government. The Psychotherapy Act (Psychotherapiegesetz), introduced in 1991, has provided a legislative framework for the profession. This framework governs training, practice, and the recommendations concerning professional development. Austria, the country where psychoanalysis and psychotherapy were developed at the beginning of the 20th century by Sigmund Freud and his circle, has chosen a unique path to train prospective psychotherapists: people of all professions can take up psychotherapy training. This means that anybody with an interest in psychotherapy who has a "sense of calling" can apply to a commission within the Ministry of Health to pursue professional training. This application must be argued for by the applicant and granted on a case-by-case decision. Once this has been granted, the applicant can go on to study the principles and basics of psychotherapy (Propädeutikum) at either a university or at a private institution with university status. The degree obtained falls short of one semester's duration and thus does not align with the Bologna legislation. Consequently, upon completion, graduates cannot carry any title such as Bachelor of Arts or Bachelor of Science but can only use this degree to gain access to one of the 40 training institutions in Austria. These institutions offer psychotherapy training in one of the 23 recognized psychotherapy forms, such as cognitive behavioral therapy, psychoanalysis, or humanistic psychotherapy. Teaching and training based on the Psychotherapy Act does not equip the student psychotherapist; however, with knowledge of the code of ethics surrounding online psychotherapy or data protection, two significant developments in social aspects of providing healthcare that have changed since 1991.

Austria has stringent laws on confidentiality obligations (see Rechtsinformation des Bundes). It ensures that the relationship between therapist and client is legally regulated. Clients must feel safe, knowing and trusting that their secrets remain with the therapist. A usual setting is when a client visits a therapist's treatment room. The therapist must ensure that the room is soundproof. With the rise of online therapy, all these issues of assuring that trust can be maintained have been challenged because of the vulnerability to security breaches of electronic communication and the setting of the client's location at the time of consultation. Can clients arrange a space where they are free to talk without being listened to?

In Austria, psychotherapy is regulated alongside the medical ethics principles of the Hippocratic Oath which is based on confidentiality and non-maleficence. Furthermore, similar to other countries, the Declaration of Geneva, formulated by the World Medical Association in 1948, states that patients' rights need to be respected regardless of age, disease or disability, creed, ethnic origin, gender, nationality, political affiliation, race, sexual orientation, social standing, or any other faction to intervene between duty and patient. The duty of confidentiality is part of the respect that a medical professional has toward his patients. In the case of psychotherapy, it does not even end with death, but secrets told in the sessions must be maintained even if the patient dies. Confidentiality must also be maintained towards relatives, the police (with a few exceptions), other therapists, and medical doctors. Even the fact that someone is in treatment is a secret and must be treated as such. Information that can lead to a patient's change in economic or social standing must be treated as secret. There is, however, an exception, which is when the clients are planning to harm someone else or when they are planning to harm themselves and when children or adolescents are in danger of domestic violence.

As mentioned above, clients and therapists have requested videotelephony because of the ever-growing demand for psychological help in what is perceived as an era of increasing uncertainty. As such, online therapy can be placed under the umbrella of the newly emerging field of telemedicine (TM). In principle, telemedicine means that medicine is delivered and practiced from afar, using a digital device. In recent years, it has not only been used to diagnose conditions but also to instruct patients on how to treat themselves (Waller and Stotler 2018). Functionality, application, and technology have been defined as the taxonomy of TM (Bashshur 2011). These include consultation, diagnosis, monitoring, and mentoring (Waller and Stotler 2018). In terms of time, telemedicine can be asynchronous, which means that diagnostic images, exams, and other medical interventions could be delivered at different times, whereas a synchronous event is interactive and occurs at the same time (ibid.).Telemedicine can be delivered via mobile phones on apps, Zoom, or Skype. These applications proved to be increasingly difficult because they could no longer guarantee that meta-data would be protected from commercial interests. Zoom nevertheless became the market leader for the delivery of online therapy in Austria because the company behind Zoom could guarantee that meta-data were not shared with other cyber-companies. Yet it came with a caveat: after 40 Minutes, the free trial version of Zoom would cut conversations short, and one would have to restart the conversation. Therapy sessions usually last 50 Minutes. Normalization and professionalization thus meant purchasing the anual subscription to Zoom so that the 50-minute session could be guaranteed without interrution.

Ever since 2020, 30 percent of consultations in total are allowed using video-based consultations in Germany, but the first point of contact must be made in person. In Austria, a new legislation coming into force in 2024 will probably allow for video-based psychotherapy, especially ever since the COVID-19 pandemic in 2020 to 2021. This legislation will consider what has already happened, namely that "cybertherapy", or the "virtual couch", is here to stay. The new legislation will have to consider that therapists are aware of the pitfalls of data protection when they use online tools such as Skype (which is not officially recommended) or Zoom. They must use a certified video service provider, guaranteeing that data is encrypted and no contact sharing happens. They also need to ensure that the client has privacy in their personal space to guarantee privacy. The therapist must be in his consultation room and not in his own home. Yet, WhatsApp—which clients frequently used to communicate with me, shares data with its mother company, Facebook or indeed Meta Platforms, Inc.

Zoom, Skype, and WhatsApp thus confronted me with several ethical questions: how would I respond if a client sent me a WhatsApp messages, which happened frequently? Should I buy a second phone and get a new phone number? Suddenly, patients appearing on my Facebook feed became a common occurrence. Would I also appear on their Facebook feed? Was it time to make my profile completely private? Would I be sued for being negligent? Could I be sued for breaching the confidentiality contract? These are issues that the incoming legislation will have to regulate.

Let us go back to the argument about the importance of somatic attention in psychotherapy that I mentioned above. Let us consider taking somatic modes of attention into account to understand why these changes need more debates rather than only legal regulation.

## What is psychotherapy? A moment in time in which past, present, and future collide in sensations and interpretations?

The characteristic of psychotherapy is that a spoken word is a tool; that is why psychotherapy is also called a "talking cure." But the spoken word is not the only tool that therapists use. Increasingly, psychotherapists have become aware that body language and the transmission of affect in corporeal sessions are as influential as the spoken word in the session. When a problematic topic is discussed, the atmosphere in the room often says more about what is happening than the spoken word. Psychotherapy is much more than traditional medicine but also a corporal relationship; as such, it has much in common with the other allied health professions, such as physiotherapy or osteopathy, that treat the muscles and bones of a "touchable" body. In Austria, these somatic modes of experience can be studied as continuous professional development after therapy training. They are seen as an addition to the talking cures.

This paradigm shift to relational psychotherapy had already begun with the development of object relations theory in the 1950s, e.g., with Melanie Klein's discussion on object relations (see Mitchell 1987). This laid the ground for relational concepts, which focus on intersubjective views and embodied knowledge of both the client and the therapist. From this perspective, a therapist combining both the psychodynamic perspective and embodied, implicit, intuitive knowledge would also consider the experience of the lived body of the client. The therapist would also be aware of their countertransference, manifested as lived-body sensation. Psychotherapists working from this perspective would be trained to notice any slight change in the atmosphere in a room which would indicate the mood surrounding the client. The client is "in a mood" to speak from a phenomenological perspective, and the psychotherapist also enters this mood.

Even more so, a therapist considering embodiment would notice how their body is tuned with the body of the client in countertransference, caused by affects that are primarily implicit in the body but cannot yet be voiced or made explicit in words and language; words which signify emotions but are not yet found. The German psychiatrist Thomas Fuchs, who also works from this interrelation embodied stance, distinguishes between "the phenomena of bodily expression, bodily presence, intercorporeal resonance and synchronicity as well as intercorporeal proximity" (Broschmann and Fuchs 2020: 460).

These new approaches in psychotherapy thus do not only deliver us a new perspective on the somatic expression of psychological pain, commonly referred to as psychosomatic medicine or psychotherapy, but they also allow us to understand bodily processes in the therapist during and after the consultation and thus to understand psychological phenomena such as grief, depression, and anxiety disorders from an entirely new perspective. A therapist trained in this tradition often experiences on a somatic level the pain which the client feels but cannot yet allow surfacing from their unconscious, due to the hypothesis that on a neurotic level, human beings all function similarly, otherwise the act of mentalisation (Fonagy 2008), i.e., implicitly and in anticipation knowing or feeling what another person is going through, which makes human interaction possible, could not take place. This phenomenon is increasingly incorporated into psychotherapeutic theory and practice, again basing this on what developmental psychologists call implicit relational knowing (Lyons-Ruth et al. 1999).

These developmental psychologists propose that in addition to being able to learn to verbalize knowledge as children, we human beings are already born with the knowledge of how to do things with intimate others, which they would refer to as "implicit relational knowing" of client and therapist that "intersect to create an intersubjective field that includes reasonably accurate sensing of each person's way of being with others, sensings we call the 'real relationship'" (Lyons-Ruth et al. 1999: 282).

A predecessor to these debates was the philosopher and psychotherapist Eugene Gendlin, who already in the 1960s, started to combine the philosophy of implicit experience with a new form of psychotherapy based on making the implicit explicit by guiding the client to feel what he referred to as the "felt sense." A felt sense is a bodily sensation that is an intuitive body feel for unresolved issues. This philosophy of the felt sense gave rise to the development of what is now referred to as "focusing," a psychotherapeutic technique that allows the client to "focus" on this implicit bodily sensation to make it explicit cognitive knowledge (Gendlin 1996). Gendlin might be seen as a philosopher who anticipated more recent debates on the role of the microbiome of the gut in producing moods, which can then, in turn, lead to mood disorders such as major depressive disorder (Borkent et al. 2022). Suppose we take this type of research seriously: in that case, sensations and moods are "produced" or "created" in the abdomen before traveling upwards to the brain, where they are processed and turned into cognitive knowledge.

## Mental health in modern times

Feeling uncertain about where things are going in your life, fearing the worst, feeling depressed, unhappiness, impatience, just wanting to cry, to run away, wishing you were someone else, in some other place, or in with someone else, losing all hope that your life and your work in this world make any sense at all—these are all states of being that every human is familiar with. When these states of being become permanent and won't dissolve, when we cannot control them any longer by sheer willpower, when we have lost hope that things will change, we speak of poor mental health. We find ways of naming these states which then manifest in diagnosis so that we can treat these manifestations.

We create metaphors to speak about these manifestations (see Kirmayer 2004) and we nominate and train people to treat these manifestations. In some cultures, these people are called shamans; in Western societies, caring for ailments of the soul has been institutionalized as counseling and psychotherapy (Kirmayer 2004). The healer restores the faith of the afflicted in the world and makes sure that the uncertainty of living and being is transformed into trust and the capability to rely on oneself and on others. In the best case, a sense of awe and beauty of life itself and the world around us is restored. In the best-case scenario, a sense of self and belonging in the bigger scheme of life is found (Frankl 2006[1959]). The person is capable again of leaving his or her inner shell and going out into the world to transcend himself and contribute to what anthropologists refer to as "dwelling" (Ingold 2011).

A healthy person can resonate within any given lifeworld (Rosa 2019) so that inner and outer needs are found and fulfilled. As such, everyone contributes to the best of all worlds. This is how sociality functions in the best of cases. Of course, this best-case-scenario is most of the time only held together by the worst-case scenario: people increasingly live on their own and only communicate via premeditated technology, which does not allow them to create inner spaces of being with their own self, what psychoanalysts call the "inner garden" (Kristeva 1982). Climate change and new global-scale diseases remind us every day that certainty in necessary security to lead our lives is only a dream, a long-lost hallucination. Beauty is increasingly only found in protected areas of the world where human beings are not allowed to dwell as they like. Increasingly, people lead lives online rather than in the real world. Sociologist Christopher Lasch (1991) has already 1991 pointed out that narcissistic traits such as taking the self as a reference point rather than adhering to the values of a wider community have become mainstream in the contemporary USA. The need for permanent self-improvement and the need to compare oneself to others in a competitive spirit fosters depression and anxiety and a sense of weariness, as described by sociologist Alain Ehrenberg (2010). This is not the place to discuss the complexities of the contemporary state of mind, so to speak, but the cultural diagnosis of these two sociologists should remind us of the tasks of contemporary psychotherapy as a type of social work. The need for constant self-improvement, alienation, and isolation all contribute to a diminished sense of social coherence and social resonance, as described by Hartmut Rosa (2019). Would telemedicine and cyber-psychotherapy contribute to this trend of increasing isolation and alienation?

Let us have a look at how I experienced the change from delivering health care in the consultation room to having to use digital media.

## Auto-ethnographic observations: The transfiguration of the therapeutic relationship

As I have already mentioned above, virtual communication tools such as Skype, Zoom, and WhatsApp replaced face-to-face meetings and the intimacy of the space in the consulting room. When I first started using these tools, the clients seemed to adapt to these new technologies much better than I did: they cherished the convenience that they no longer had to leave the house for an appointment. They could see me, come rain or sunshine, early in the morning or late at night. They often needed to find a space in their home where they felt safe and protected to speak to me and tell me about their lives, but once they had arranged this, they were fine. With some of them, the change to using Skype or Zoom—we had moved to Zoom after initially using Skype but stopped it because it did not provide the safe digital space that I was required to use—even provided them with a much more intimate space than the consulting room.

I noticed that they started to talk about issues that had been difficult to talk about in my consultation room; once they had gotten over the uncanny feeling of seeing themselves and me on the same screen, they started talking about topics that in other settings are much more difficult to talk about, such as e.g., body dysmorphia, issues with substance misuse, and difficulties with their partners. Sometimes they stepped away from their screens, seeking retreat in the areas of their rooms that I could not see. This seemed to give them more freedom to control their own space, especially their own private space. It felt as if they were more in charge of regulating their free associations, a technique pioneered by Sigmund Freud. Freud asked his patients to lie on the sofa and he would sit behind them so that the patients could just say what came to their minds rather than having to have a conversation with the therapist. They could freely speak without censoring what they would say to me so that they would not have to feel a sense of shame. Sometimes they sat at their desks, having become part of the home office movement, and showed me their favorite books; sometimes, they would arrange their books so that I could appreciate their intellectual curiosity. My younger patients were already equipped with the professional tools of the YouTuber generation and were proud to show me their equipment such as vintage-style microphones.

For me, it was a much more difficult move. I often found that having to keep up with the rapid changes in how to use online video telephony is stressful. At first, I was also concerned about seeing myself in the little pop-up window that comes up when the Zoom sessions start. Was this what I looked like? Was this the expression I unconsciously made when someone told me about stressful events or difficult emotions? I wanted to minimize this pop-up window even more, but I soon learned to cherish it: at least I could now study myself and observe my own unconscious reactions and mimics.

I could learn from this, knowing that patients very much try to "read" the facial expressions of their therapists. Already established trust can be ruined within one mini-second of a therapist's raised eyebrow. Seeing and being seen becomes part of the therapeutic process. I needed to learn to own my face and my expressions. I needed to learn to take care of my expressions. Mental health and psychological well-being are tied to seeing and being seen. The image I want to present to others, the (imagined) need to invent a respectable persona that hides my true inner self, the fear I have of being judged on my looks, the terror of seeing myself reflected in the mirror after a sleepless night: who is not familiar with these feelings?

Eating disorders and body dysmorphia are some of the most common psychological disorders that people present in the consulting room and that are a direct result of not being seen from a kind and favorable perspective. Thus, suddenly, here we were, having to look each other in the eye on Skype or Zoom, but not only that, but we also had to face our own faces, so to speak. Suddenly, I saw my own twitches of the eyelid in close-up, and I became aware of the micro-expressions of my own mimic. I became painfully aware of how often I waved my hands around while speaking, trying to emphasize my point. Had I always been like that? How could I look others in the eye while trying frantically to ignore my own reflection in the Zoom mirror? I suddenly not only had to be aware of and process the micro-expressions of my clients, but also those of myself. Did the horror of seeing myself reflected whilst thinking and speaking signal that I was suffering from body dysmorphia myself or was that just a normal reaction to a new phenomenon? Was this even a phenomenon I could use and discuss with my patients, thus sharing the common experience? Suddenly, we no longer had to painfully go through the exercises of getting to know—and hopefully like—our own reflections in the mirror, which is a much-used tool in the treatment of body dysmorphia. Suddenly, I and the client had both arrived in the desert of the real, to quote Slavoj Žižek (2002).

Yes, that was us, talking to each other as we really were, not our imagined persona. As Freud observed, when two people make love, there are always at least three people present because one of the parties involved in physical contact would dream of an imagined perfect erotic partner whilst pretending to be in touch with the present partner. Current relational psychoanalysis knows that this is true: when we communicate, we always communicate with an imagined other who then, in turn, communicates with us as the imagined other. What we refer to as our "real selves" is often painful and shameful to experienc, and often, we do our utmost to hide it and invent personas. Yet, in the Zoom meeting, even though it was a virtual space, it was a space that was more "real" than the real space. Yes, this was us: unkempt, crying, in need of coffee, in pajamas, and without make-up. With a twitching eye (my own neurobiology of stress expressed itself) and red cheeks (the neurobiology of the client's shame). One more phenomenon often jokingly referred to as the "séance-quality" of online meetings had to be dealt with. "Are you there?", "I cannot hear you," "Are you still with me?", "I can only see your frozen image, but I hear your voice!", became standard sentences in the Zoom consulting room. How would these disturbances interfere with the intense process of the emotions that we were just discussing and trying to understand? And strangely enough, yes, we could. Sometimes, these disturbances even became jokes, which lightened up an already emotionally laden session.

As I already discussed above, recent developments in psychotherapy made us aware that bodily presence is as significant in the consulting room as the narrative that is being constructed in mutual talking engagements. Co-regulation of breathing is as important a factor in establishing a trusting relationship as is nodding and making reassuring sounds and noises. The sense of sharing a bodily space of being together, of sharing a place and feeling safe, is as important in counseling as is the clever interpretation of a dream and the wise insights of shared experiences. Was this possible on Zoom? Was it possible to feel connected and yet be in two different rooms? A strange phenomenon occurred: yes, it was possible. Sometimes the shared virtual space was even more intimate than the shared physical space could ever be. Suddenly some strange form of democracy started to take shape: the client no longer came to my room only. I no longer had the privilege of "being at home" while the clients had to create a place for themselves in my space.

Suddenly, we both shared only the online space. Often, this led to some interesting exchange: Me: "What lovely curtains you have, and I really like your sofa!" or "I had not realized you were on a beach in Brazil?", until I noticed that one could "fake" the environment on Zoom. Interestingly, after approximately 5 minutes these environments were forgotten: oftentimes, a much more intense space between the client and me developed in these virtual spaces. Yet, the need for "faking" the background of the Zoom meeting also allowed me to understand more aspects of client's needs: the need to conceal parts of the self and the home environment often disclosed more about them than they wanted to let on. And yet, the phenomenon remained that there was a felt-sense of greater shared space on Zoom. This continued to amaze me when, after we were allowed again to meet in person and my clients returned to my consulting room, there was a strangeness in the air, as if we had come too close online and now had to re-establish corporeal boundaries.

The last aspect of telemedicine I wanted to discuss is the impact of mobile phones on the communication between therapists and clients. As I mentioned above, WhatsApp also became a lifeline for some of my clients. In some treatment contracts, I allow suicidal clients to add me to their list of people to be contacted if a crisis occurs, and for some of them, this became a lifeline. We later also switched to SMS or iPhone messenger again because of data protection and WhatsApp becoming part of the Meta-group to which Facebook also belongs. One of the aspects that WhatsApp also "allowed" or indeed "afforded" me to do was to notice when clients were last online, which sometimes meant that they were online all night when they could not sleep. Despite warning them about this feature, some clients found it comforting that I would know that they were still alive. This feature entered my everyday life. I could hear the "ping" when a new message arrived. I also wondered what it would mean when they switched off the function that I could see when they had read my message. What did it mean when I noticed that someone had sent me a message but then deleted it again? These functions of technology and the mobile phone became part of the consultation outside of the consultation room. Going back to where I started this discussion, I had to learn not to always be in "somatic modes of attention" and to consciously switch off the hard-learned bodily sensation of transference and countertransference. For my clients, mobile phones and messenger services such as WhatsApp became a lifeline in their search for hope and certainty.

## Conclusion

I have described above how cultural commentators such as Julia Kristeva, Christopher Lasch and Alain Ehrenberg have tried to construe the contemporary self. They diagnose a lack of inner mental space, increased traits of narcissism, and, following on from that, weariness. Hartmut Rosa reminds us to resonate with our environment to stay sane. At the same time, communication between human beings, which helps to regulate emotions, fosters empathy, connections, is increasingly aided by technological devices. This is also the case in psychotherapy. My question thus was whether the use of telecommunication tools in psychotherapy would contribute to the trend of alienation and isolation.

The usage of Zoom, Skype, and WhatsApp has entered the therapeutic space between psychotherapists and clients and, in all likelihood, is here to stay. Even though clients are again allowed to leave their houses and see the therapist in private practice in their consulting rooms, the Austrian government has not yet decided to regulate the usage of the communication tools as was the case before the pandemic. We can thus assume that they will become part of the therapeutic alliance between clients and therapists. The fact that these technologies allow us to create a different, sometimes more intimate, relationship with the clients should let us embrace these technologies rather than legislate against their use. Cyber-psychotherapy will become part of telemedicine in the near future, and this will be a good thing because it allows clients to stay in their own familiar environment, in case they cannot reach a psychotherapist. Legislation will come in that will regulate the governance and ethics aspect of this kind of telemedicine, such as which software is safe to use and how often therapists and clients will have to meet up in person. However, some other aspects of the therapeutic alliance will have to be redefined if we take video telephony as a unique tool seriously.

My research sample has only been I, so it is hardly representative, but I would like to propose a few aspects that might shape future discussions. First, I think that the online relationship does not impact transference and countertransference. We human beings seem to be able to relate on a somatic level, even mediated by a computer or by a mobile phone. Discussions on the alienating characteristics of these technologies will have to be reimagined because, from my limited experience, these technologies sometimes even allow us to build deeper connections and relationships. Thus, rather than contributing to more alienation, they allow us to relate on different levels of intimacy and privacy. Some aspects of our somatic experience will have to be adapted, e.g., the phenomenon that for some clients, corporeality in the consulting room can be intimidating and hindering their willingness to discuss certain aspectst of their lives, e.g., shame and guilt. The notion of being able to control the environment, crucial for patients with anxiety disorders, might be helpful for them. In conclusion, I would like to suggest that a lot of research is needed to understand the impact of these new technologies on the therapeutic relationship so that they can be used to their full potential.

## References

Bashshur Rashid, Elizabeth Krupinski, and Jim Grigsby. 2011. The Taxonomy of Telemedicine. Telemedicine and e-Health 17(6): 484–494.

Borkent, Jenny, Magdalini Ioannou, Jon D. Laman, et al. 2022. Role of the Gut Microbiome in Three Major Psychiatric Disorders. Psychological Medicine 52(7): 1222–1242.

Broschmann, Daniel, and Thomas Fuchs. 2020. Zwischenleiblichkeit in der psychodynamischen Psychotherapie: Ansatz zu einem verkörperten Verständnis von Intersubjektivität. Forum Psychoanalyse 36: 459–475.

Csordas, Thomas. 1993. Somatic Modes of Attention. Cultural Anthropology 8(2): 135–156.

Ehrenberg, Alain. 2010. The Weariness of the Self: Diagnosing the History or Depression in the Contemporary Age. Montreal: McGill University Press.

Finger-Ossinger, Margarete. 2021. Internetberatung und Psychotherapie: Reflektierte Erfahrungen von Psychotherapeuten_innen und Klient_innen. Psychotherapeutisches Forum 25(3-4): 115–123.

Fonagy, Peter. 2008. The Mentalization-Focused Approach to Social Development. London: Routledge.

Frankl, Viktor. 2006 [1959]. Man's Search for Meaning. Boston: Beacon Press.

Gendlin, Eugene. 1996. Focusing-Oriented Psychotherapy. A Manual of the Experiential Method. New York: The Guildford Press.

Ingold, Tim. 2011. Being Alive: Essays on Movement, Knowledge and Description. London: Routledge.

Kirmayer, Laurence. J. 2004. The Cultural Diversity of Healing: Meaning, Metaphor and Mechanism. British Medical Bulletin 69: 33–48.

Kristeva, Julia. 1982. Powers of Horror: An Essay on Abjection. New York: Columbia University Press.

Lasch, Christopher. 1991. The Culture of Narcissism: American Life in an Era of Diminishing Expectations. New York: W.W. Norton and Company.

Levy, Kenneth, and Wesley J. Scala. 2012. Transference, Transference Interpretations, and Transference-Focused Psychotherapies. Psychotherapy 49(3): 391–403.

Lyons-Ruth, Karlen, Nadia Bruschweiler-Stern, Alexandra M. Harrison, et al. 1999. Implicit Relational Knowing: Its Role in Development and Psychoanalytic Treatment. Infant Mental Health Journal 19(3): 282–289.

Mitchell, Juliet, ed. 1987. The Selected Melanie Klein. New York: Free Press.

Rosa, Hartmut. 2019. Resonanz: Eine Soziologie der Weltbeziehung. Frankfurt/Main: Suhrkamp.

Rechtsinformation des Bundes. 2023. Bundesrecht Konsolidiert: Gesamte Rechtsvorschrift für Psychotherapiegesetz. Fassung vom 22.11.2023. https://www.ris.bka.gv.at. Accessed on 22.11.2023.

Waller, Morgan, and Chad Stotler. 2018. Telemedicine: A Primer. Current Allergy and Asthma Reports 18(54): https://doi.org/10.1007/s11882-018-0808-4.

Žižek, Slavoj. 2002. Welcome to the Desert of the Real. London: Verso.

# Part IV: Individual and Socially Distributed Emotions

# 11 Affective Processes and the Diagnosing of Chronic Fatigue

*Mette Bech Risør and Nina Nissen*

> … I have always felt strong, and suddenly I do not have it in me, and cannot plan. I try to keep up just to do something, this is what I need somehow. I need to find a way to cope with this, acceptance. I cannot find the balance between [doing] too much and [doing] too little… I blame myself. I am angry with myself, but I also tell myself that others are in worse trouble… I think that sometimes I can… I am terrified to become too passive, I feel trapped …
> *(Trond)*

Imagine a life dominated by a constant sense of tiredness, feeling exhausted and overwhelmed; trying to make sense of an unpredictable and fluctuating, intense bodily sensation, while simultaneously experiencing how fatigue impacts your cognitive and physical capacities and your identity as well as depriving you of social and intellectual functions. Imagine further that the causes of this sensation of tiredness are not identified despite multiple medical examinations, tests and assessments.

Based on a study of people suffering from fatigue and hoping for help by taking part in a diagnostic assessment for conditions of chronic fatigue, we argue that the diagnostic process is enacted as a shared affective effort and that this effort is constituted and materialized in the relationality of the clinical encounter. With Manning we ask: "What if, instead of placing self-self interaction at the center of development, we were to posit relation as key to experience?" (Manning 2013: 2).

Several sociological and anthropological studies have scrutinized and elaborated the enactment of diagnoses and temporality in clinical settings and encounters (e.g., Büscher et al. 2010; Chew-Graham et al. 2010; Gardner et al. 2011; Gardner and Williams 2015; Mol 2002; Moser 2010; Smith-Morris 2015). These studies explore the making of a diagnosis in collaborative, relational practices of assessment as a material-semiotics approach to the assemblage of diagnostic processes. By contrast, Tessier (2018) presents an analysis of diagnosing dementia by drawing on early theories in psychiatry, particularly *Gefühlsdiagnose*. Tessier demonstrates how health professionals used their own feelings and reactions towards a patient as an instrumental effort to enable contact with the patient, making diagnostic work an assemblage of stabilized concepts built on sensory experiences of "affordances." Tessier concludes: "Medical expertise is still bound to a sensible experience of the world that is never given *a priori*" (Tessier 2018: 125). That is, stabilized biomedical knowledge and reasoning are combined with or perhaps guided by "feeling", by "our own affectivity" (cf. Minkowski, in Tessier 2018: 124) in a concrete and affective meeting with the patient.

This focus on affect is also taken up by Hadolt (2018) in a study of genetic counseling. He examines how a counseling situation is organized, stressing a specific style of affectivity that influences rationale, client-centeredness, and professional compassion. Hadolt argues that the counselor and counselee "connect and resonate with each other as experiencing and receptive bodies" (Hadolt 2018: 136). He employs the concept of "affective coordination" to analyze a process of shared and mutual attunement, whereby affect brings about affordances to which each person must respond. Collu (2019) likewise explores affect in psychotherapy sessions with a couple. Especially attentive to a crisis unfolding during a specific session, he elaborates how its affective moments move things (Stewart 2007), while "possessing" the couple and the therapists involved. He suggests that "we cannot understand therapeutic efficacy if we focus only on language and discourse" (Collu 2019: 290). Accordingly, we may benefit by asking what the impersonal and evanescent qualities of affect may offer to the analysis of therapeutic sessions or, in our case, diagnostic processes during the assessment of chronic fatigue (cf. Swallow and Hillman 2019).

The sparse anthropological literature which explores fatigue or tiredness does so through studies of chronic fatigue syndrome (CFS), cancer, or fibromyalgia (Hay 2010; Risør and Lillevoll 2021; Seppola-Edvardsen and Risør 2017) and tends to position the tired body in relation to, for example, illness narratives and diagnostic negotiations (Sachs 2016). Further, Ware's work on CFS (Ware 1992, 1999) demonstrates how life is lived in the context of specific cultural expectations that prompt a social course dominated by marginalization and social distance, while other scholars emphasize the embodiment of suffering (Addison 2013) and the legitimacy of a diagnosis and its medicalizing effects for possible CFS patients (Sachs 2001, 2016). Limited research has inquired how a diagnosis of CFS or related disorders such as medically unexplained symptoms (MUS) materializes (Chew-Graham et al. 2010; Hydén and Sachs 1998; Rasmussen 2017).

CFS is a debilitating multifaceted disorder, characterized by fatigue, muscular and joint pain, extreme exhaustion after exercise and long recovery time, sore throat, flu-like symptoms, unrefreshing sleep, cognitive impairments, and sensitivity to sound, smell, and taste, however, not all patients experience all symptoms. CFS constitutes a profound challenge for those affected and for health professionals. Patients are often offered a variety of assessments, sometimes based on interdisciplinary, biopsychosocial approaches, followed by advice on activity regulation, psycho-education, and classes teaching coping and daily management strategies.

The diagnostic processes are, however, often surrounded by uncertainty, despite a presumed "aura of factuality" (Geertz 1993) of biomedical knowledge. Epistemic uncertainty becomes especially prominent when the classification of diseases is contested due to a misalignment between symptoms and established disease models; in other words, when the indexical aspect of the biomedical sign is denied (Staiano-Ross 2012). This is precisely the case for patients suffering from chronic fatigue where diagnostic assessment rests on a disorder with no clear etiology in the borderlands of disease classification.

In this study, we explore how the interplay between a patient, health professionals, diagnostic criteria, advice on regulated activity, emotion and affective interaction shape and enact the diagnostic assessment. In our analysis, we integrate how organizational routines, neoliberal health ideologies, gender and social circumstances work as a wider context for such an assessment, inducing an ambiguous complexity of concerns and matters-at-stake involving all parties.

## Affect, affective atmosphere, and attunement

Anthropologists have increasingly attended to affect and affectivity which encompass ordinary activities (Stewart 2007). This affective turn reacts to textualism and cultural theory (Stewart 2007; White 2017). It emphasizes what slips and evades, what is maybe ineffable (Brown and Tucker 2010) or non-representational (Thrift 2008) but nevertheless significant because it moves and drives processes forward. Particularly related to a critique of dyadic encounters, this affective turn posits that intensities and potentialities emanate from atmospheres and non-individualized relationality rather than from subjective agency (Anderson 2009; Massumi 2002). Accordingly, affect is embodied and instills agency not in individuals but rather in and through relational experiences.

Attending to affect has helped anthropologists to examine the senses and sensations and the materialities of lives that are lived through body and mind (Stewart 2017). This focus rests on an ontology that, as Manning (2013) argues, is based not on a fixed notion of self, subject, or agency, but rather on the relation as the prominent analytical unit. Thus, the clinical encounter can be understood as a performance of mutual responses and resonances in the actual moment of a clinical process, accounting for emotions, sensing, adapting, mirroring, and sharing of knowledge as well as intersubjective experience. The social also encompasses moods, atmospheres, and rhythms that come from places where language stops or is insufficient (Knudsen and Stage 2016). Overall, bodies have the capacity to affect other bodies and to be affected by them (Anderson 2006). Attention to affect and its potentiality may illuminate change and movement in specific encounters.

Differences between affect and emotion are often debated (e.g. Swallow and Hillman 2019) and may be difficult to distinguish. However, following Massumi (2002), different logics and orders pertain to emotion and affect. An emotion holds subjective content, a qualified, owned, and recognized intensity. Affect is not part of a determined regime; it is not prescribed; it is prior to but potentially able to become something. Other researchers link affect and emotion (e.g. Ahmed 2004; Wetherell 2012), arguing that affective practices entangle emotional, bodily, social, and material figurations, and combine affect with meaning-making and the discursive. We acknowledge this understanding; however, we wish to remain close to the notion of affect as a felt intensity that is primarily experienced bodily. The intensities noted in this study were embodied and shared and also affected the first author and prompted her to try to understand their potentiality and their movement. Without abandoning discursive matters, cultural mechanisms, and templates that mediate clinical encounters and which are part of the assemblage of a diagnostic process, we attempt to choose another—bodily—scale of attention (Hastrup 2013) in order to grasp intensity and affective moments.

To concretize affectivity, we draw on the notions of affective atmosphere and affective attunement. Anderson states that perhaps "the use of atmosphere in everyday speech and aesthetic discourse provides the best approximation of the concept of affect" (Anderson 2009: 78). Like affect, atmosphere denotes an intensity, but it draws attention to something shared, something overflowing in space and time, without belonging to a specific body but still being embodied. The atmosphere of a situation is undetermined because it is not fixed, yet it is there and affects the situation.

Further, by drawing on affective attunement, we may understand how bodies react to cues or atmospheres, either creating sameness or distinction depending on the bodies' dispositions (Knudsen and Stage 2016). Manning, paraphrasing Stern (1985), notes: "Affective attunement is key to interpersonal becoming. Affective attunement is another mode of immanent relation where the relation radically precedes the purported unity of the self. Attunement is a merging-with of vitality affects across experiences toward emergent events" (Manning 2013: 7). We aim to show how patients and health professionals attune to each other in this way, resonate and create or transform emerging affordances or matters, giving way to potentiality and movement.

Lastly, hope anticipates the indeterminate that has not-yet-become and dispositions of hopefulness may move suffering bodies (Anderson 2006), creating specific hopes. Hence, potential is central (Massumi 2002) and speaks to the intensity of hope. Taussig et al. (2013) explore potentiality as something that can be imagined and talked about but does not (yet and never may) exist. It may denote something about to manifest itself when comparing what "is not and what might never be" (Mattingly 2010: 3). In this sense, there is a close affinity between affect, hope, and potentiality; i.e. hope as an ability to affect and be affected by the world (Anderson 2006: 747).

## The study

This study is based on fieldwork in a Norwegian university hospital clinic specialized in diagnosing chronic fatigue. Participants in the study were patients who had been referred from primary care to a specialist fatigue clinic for CFS assessment. All the patients had a long-standing history of fatigue as a dominant health complaint, and all had experienced several examinations and tests in primary care as well as in hospital departments in order to ascertain mechanisms or reasons for their symptoms. On being referred to the specialist clinic, the patients primarily expressed nervousness ("How would it go?") but they were also relieved, hopeful, and excited to possibly be at an endpoint of their diagnostic trajectory, being seen by CFS specialists. Their long history of complaints and various symptoms had severely impacted their professional life, their social life, and personal identity. Some expressed a desire for a CFS diagnosis, others merely clarification and support. Personal endeavors, ambitions, hopes, and concerns were at stake and patients sought support to enable a more manageable life. This was the case for both Anna and Trond whose clinical encounters we analyze below.

To carry out the study, the first author collaborated with a specialist team at a university hospital, consisting of a physician, a psychologist, and an occupational therapist, occasionally substituted by a physiotherapist. By coincidence, all the professionals on the team were women. During spring 2017, the first author conducted fieldwork at the clinic where the team is based and followed twelve patients during three consultations, one with each health professional. The team assessed two or three patients each week, and patients spent an hour, sometimes longer, with each health professional, depending on the conversation and the problems discussed. Consultations were spread over two days and would eventually result in a diagnostic decision—a CFS diagnosis, an alternative fatigue diagnosis, or no diagnosis at all. Further, the final fourth session with all health professionals was also observed. Here, the professionals first discussed their individual conclusions and arrived at a joint diagnostic decision and then summoned the patient to explain their decision and offer advice. The verb "to summon" is deliberately chosen to describe the tension, nervousness, and atmosphere of anticipation associated with a verdict. Patient participants, waiting for this consultation had, for example, slept badly the night before, were exhausted, sweating and finally bursting into tears as both Anna and Trond did. The following analysis draws predominantly, but not exclusively, on this final session.

Fieldwork with the intention of analyzing a relational setting and grasping how patients and health professionals sense each other, and how they adapt, mirror, resonate, and respond to each other is not a straightforward task. A methodology that seeks to identify affective processes requires an understanding of what affect is and how it might be traced (Knudsen and Stage 2015; Staunæs and Pors 2021). Affect may be best studied if linked to a specific situation and to the bodies involved in that situation, including the researcher-body. To this end, the first author—by using her own body—noted the intensities of statements, reactions to these, responses in words and body, non-verbal language and expressions, moods, the intensity of voices or lack thereof, and the affects which were expressed verbally. Even though we allow for affect to be expressed through articulations of meaning (Wetherell 2012), in the following we primarily trace affective attunement and atmosphere through embodied fieldwork, for example by attending to more-than-representational layers of experience, sensory work, and bodily sensations, and how these intertwine with biomedical agendas, the materiality of the setting and resulting atmospheres (Knudsen and Stage 2015: 16).

## The CFS landscape in Norway

CFS is a disorder that has increasingly been diagnosed in Norway during the last few years. How many people are diagnosed is uncertain since registration is unreliable and contradictory. An estimated 10.000-20.000 individuals currently have this diagnosis and the media mention a five-fold increase between 2008 and 2015, especially among young people and adult women. The increasing number instigates debates about the impact of societal strains on people. It also spurs academic and clinical debates about diagnostic borderlands. On the one hand, the expansion of disease boundaries increasingly specifies more and more bodily states as diseases and, on the other hand, this introduces continuous contestation and ambiguity related to illness experiences, exposing what is outside the borders of disease (Rosenberg 2006). Several patient associations, medical societies, and lay media vigorously take part in debates about both diagnostics and recovery strategies.

To meet the growing demand for assessment and treatment of possible CFS, specialist teams were established in several Norwegian hospitals from 2013 onwards. The national guideline on assessment, diagnostics, and care (Helsedirektoratet 2015) constitutes the backbone of the work of these teams. Assessment includes physical and psychological examination, history taking, and differential diagnoses (based on, for example, blood tests, diagnostic imaging, and the use of depression and anxiety scales). The Norwegian guidelines base the diagnosis of CFS on the Canada consensus criteria (Carruthers et al. 2003; Helsedirektoratet 2015), which are considered to be conclusive for a diagnostic decision. These criteria measure and operationalize levels of fatigue by assessing whether a patient has a 50 percent reduced activity level, compared to self-reported previous activity levels. This supposedly objective measurement is decisive for a diagnosis, being the principal criterion to sustain or dismiss the overall symptom presentation.

Norwegian guidelines further provide advice to patients on how to regulate their everyday activities, for example, through adjusting and balancing activity according to individual capacity. Accordingly, talk about activity was the most important focal point of the observed consultations, defining the agenda of the encounter, i.e., talking about activity levels "before" and "after" in order to determine reduced capacity and establish details on general activity to advise on regimens suitable to a patient's situation. The term "activity" thus references a specific assessment criterion integral to "activity levels", but also everyday activities, and care, revealing tensions and discrepancies in perspectives.

Being active is a cultural and social norm for all patients. Due to physical constraints and fatigue activity, "doing" is connected to what has been and what is longed for. For the patient, activity is embodied, practically embedded, and inscribed with despair, anticipation, and hope (Adams et al. 2009). All participants deeply regret what they no longer can do, while also trying to explain that they are still active, in their own way and on their own terms, thus embracing hopefulness as well as a prevailing notion of agency (Laidlaw 2010). In the medical context, the notion of activity is closely related to productivity, agency, and competence, and activity levels constitute a biomedical diagnostic criterion. This transformation of activity into a supposedly objective measure of activity level detaches activity from its subjective meaning. Thus, the perceptions of activity generate moments of hope and intensity for all parties, however in different ways.

## The case of Anna: Resonance through hope, fear and passion

Anna, in her mid-thirties, is a single mother of two children. The first author meets Anna in the waiting room at the university clinic, where other patients wait too. We sit next to each other while Anna awaits her first consultation with the occupational therapist (OT). The first author asks her some questions about her situation, how long she has waited to be referred, where she lives, whether she has children, and related questions about these kinds of topics. Anna makes the first author feel a bit hesitant about asking, not inviting much to the conversation, just answering politely. But when talking about her children, Anna happily shows pictures of them playing football. We continue talking more about them and my children as well. While waiting, Anna wears her overcoat—dark, somewhat out of shape—which she also keeps on during consultations.

During the consultation with the OT, Anna is met with eager questions about her everyday activities, her daily rhythms, and her resources; all very concrete, routine questions for the OT. Anna answers quite briefly, giving the impression of being very exhausted, sad, and dejected. She remains wrapped in her thick coat, sits with her hands clenched and hardly moves when talking. When answering there is a tone of sorrow and a heaviness to her voice and bodily presence—at least this is how she affects the first author and how she interprets the mood of the scene. Anna adds information about her lived life, past and present troubles and efforts, feelings of regret and grief because she was unable to keep the job she enjoyed, can no longer undertake outdoor activities with her children, and no longer has any social life. Anna emphasizes that her main concern is to be a good mother to her children.

The OT seems affected by Anna's narrative and the emergent mood. She tunes into Anna's history, makes eye contact with her, nods, and shows openness in her body language by leaning towards her. Eventually, the OT moves on to her routine advice about activity regulation for managing daily tasks, while also trying to inspire Anna to be in charge of her life. Talking about the need for and control of activity highlights a paradox in the affective atmosphere—the co-existence of tragedy and exhaustion with clinical empowerment. Anna's response to this atmosphere is to keep emphasizing what she manages to do despite debilitating pain and fatigue in addition to managing the effects of domestic violence. This paradoxical pattern repeats itself during Anna's later consultations with the other health professionals. All the health professionals are moved by her; they have, we would say, empathetically attuned to her hardship which fills the room with both words and sensations.

Before Anna meets the three professionals in the final consultation, the professionals discuss their assessment, their clinical as well as person-oriented impressions and conclusions, and how they may help her:

*Psychologist:* She pushes herself, pulls herself together. She wants them [her children] to feel good, it is as if she needs to perform, and it is probably an important priority in many ways, pushes herself when they are at home, and thinks that they should notice as little as possible that she is ill, does not want to pull them into her illness.

> *OT:* She pushes herself and I get the impression that it's not because she suddenly has a lot of energy, but she says anyway that she functions better when she has the kids. Since when she does not have them, she just lies down. I think that is

perhaps not typically CFS, but I don't know really, because you can mobilize a lot if something is important enough.

*Physician:* But she is maybe not that good at doing things for herself then ...

*OT:* No, there are few things like that ...

*Psychologist:* She also does not do anything with the kids that she used to do. Her life was about hiking, trips, and out-door life for a large part and she does not do that now.

This conversation jumps from summing up Anna's history with violent or game-addicted husbands to emphasizing how she has tried to cope amidst periods of depression and making ends meet to give her children the best conditions, even attempting to arrange for them to see their father. While talking, the professionals are clearly touched and moved by Anna's history, but they also assess her hardship professionally to reach a conclusion—is it CFS or not according to the criteria?

When the health professionals summon Anna to present their conclusion, they explain their rationale about a possible diagnosis, while acknowledging and feeling sympathetic about her struggles and efforts. Anna seems quite tense. In the waiting room, she confided her fear that the health professionals might report her to the child welfare authorities. At the start of this final consultation, she answers very briefly and while she does receive a CFS diagnosis, she hardly reacts. The OT asks: "What do you think about that?" Anna answers: "I don't know, I .... what is the prognosis from now on? Is there anything that will make me well?"

This brief exchange provides the cue for the rest of the consultation. The OT, physician, and psychologist grasp the opportunity to passionately offer Anna different types of help which Anna responds to positively but also hesitantly, because she might not have the energy, as she says. Importantly, Anna's cue contains hope, for herself and her children; a hope projected into the future imagining recovery. The resulting hopeful atmosphere in the room seems to affect everybody. The health professionals talk energetically, they perceive a chance to help and make a difference; they bodily show relief. A "collective condition" of hope and future seems to be established (Anderson 2006). Especially the OT shines when there is an opening to give detailed advice on energy management, which Anna promises to think about. Anna herself appears increasingly comfortable, relaxes bodily, and slightly laughs for the first time when she says to the OT, in response to very detailed activity advice: "One would think you were in my head!" This makes everybody laugh. The intensity in the room is characterized by a shared optimistic tone: advice is given, courses on coping are recommended and Anna accepts and nods. Eventually, the psychologist says: "[...] I have been surprised many times by how big constraints people have in their lives and what people experience, but also [...] how capable and coping people are, and how much they manage to become good parents anyway, yes, I have to say this, and I just want to say to you ... much suffering and much coping [...]."

Anna reacts with humility expressing that "one has to learn", and right after as a final outburst, she vehemently says while crying: "Thanks for the help, you don't know how grateful I am ... you will get paid in heaven [all health professionals start laughing]."

Anna came to the clinic with hope and fear. She hoped for help, not necessarily a CFS diagnosis, but help to be able to live a life with her children the way she feels they deserve. She also feared that coming would have consequences for her role as mother, and this fear, the first author realized just before the last consultation, was perhaps just as intense as her hope. Fear might have made her extra conscious about stressing her competencies. However, she also needed to balance her fear by staying with her main issue: hope to receive help. Before Anna was summoned for the final consultation, the health professionals did discuss the children's welfare but decided that they did not see reasons for making a report. Overall, the consultations built up an atmosphere of mutual resonance, where the health professionals met Anna's concerns and hope, where they were led by feelings of empathy for a struggling mother, and possibly shared life experiences, just as much as by diagnostic criteria. Affected and gendered bodies moved the diagnostic process, making it fluid and contingent.

## The case of Trond: Transformation of hope

Trond, in his mid-40s, is a man who likes to talk, also with the first author in the waiting room, apparently unconcerned about other patients overhearing the conversation. A big, bearded man, he resembled a bear who is down on his knees because of his many health complaints. He eagerly expresses his hope for help to be able to recover to some extent, not only hoping for a CFS diagnosis.

Trond's story as told to the first author and the health professionals, one by one, centers on several issues: being tormented by poor concentration, poor memory, and exhaustion while also trying to recover mentally and physically from the effects of malpractice when having had cancer. He tells his story in quite an overwhelming way, taking up more time in each consultation than the other patients. Also, Trond actively engages in weekly support groups for cancer patients and exercises twice a week. He says he gains a lot from helping others, but he is tormented by the things he no longer can accomplish, having been used to a very active life. He experiences his lost abilities as a personal failure.

In the final session during which the health professionals discuss Trond's case, the first author sits as usual next to the table where the professionals have assembled. Trond has not yet been summoned. Everyone hesitates, fiddles with their papers, and chats with each other, waiting for the physician to give her assessment first, as usual. The physician has the role of the medical expert who can make the authoritative distinction of whether a patient meets the diagnostic criteria or not. She is also the one who tends to bring up activity levels as the decisive criterion in accordance with the Canada criteria. Anticipation affects us all: What will happen? What does each person bring to the final session on this patient, who—everyone had expressed previously, judging from their individual consultations with him—was rather perplexing and overbearing?

The physician eventually begins, noting first that Trond's poor experience of cancer treatment dominated her consultation with him: "It's not a case that's quite closed, so it's kind of still lying there, that's how I see him. It's like it's still lying there muttering, everything about it, so it's like he doesn't really move on, sort of." Responding to the physician's introduction, the OT and the psychologist modify this and emphasize that having experienced cancer malpractice is not an exclusion criterion *per se*. The physician agrees but also repeats her statement, then notes that the blood test results "looked nice." She then quickly begins to talk about activity levels. She finds that Trond has less than a 50 percent reduction in activity level, so the criteria are not met. The psychologist is surprised and disagrees. All three discuss back and forth how they may interpret what Trond has told them about his activities, i.e., how many percentage reductions may be assigned. There is suspense in the room. Particularly the psychologist becomes insecure, hesitates, tries to find her notes, and initially defends Trond—until her voice loses power.

The physician continues to argue that Trond presents with less than 50 percent activity reduction. By listing his many different current activities and his varying exhaustion levels after each effort, she reiterates that these do not fulfill the Canada criteria. The OT declares that Trond is not a classical CFS patient and somewhat supports the physician, while the psychologist still contests this. Though the OT initially mediates, she then argues with the physician that Trond's previous cancer and his long history of poor treatment may explain his fatigue. The psychologist then turns to Trond's very high score on the self-reported anxiety scale and while all three agree that he does not appear to display clinical anxiety, they consider possible trauma or a diagnosis of posttraumatic stress disorder (PTSD). This turn from activity levels to a topic that allows the psychologist to show her expertise seems to lower the intensity of disagreement and the clinicians now seem united, eager to reach a consensus. The physician summarizes their views:

> I think that his fatigue may be excluded by the cancer. You may think that his great strain is due to this, in relation to his maltreatment, and that he has huge exhaustion, and then, in a way, as we discussed yesterday, he does not, in a way, fulfill the Canada criteria concerning loss of function. But he does have a considerable loss of function anyway, so …

No one objects now; tensions seem resolved and positions renegotiated. All are now very empathetic towards Trond and his constraints and the discussion moves on to how his functional level may be improved and how to help him, for example, through regulating activity. Trond has "regulation potential", they all agree.

Trond is then asked to join the session. Before the physician starts explaining their conclusion to him, he tries to sum up, quite despairingly, how he has tried to address his exhaustion and cognitive problems:

> I don't remember everything, so that's what ... forget quickly and then I try to remember what we've talked about and then, I probably would have remembered more I wanted to bring up, but, but I feel, you know that [sighs deeply] the things you showed me, I've tried in a way to do those things, you know, those things, sort of that I try to make something robust, that it will work somehow, and then in a way, I'm so afraid that then it'll be too much and I get worse; as I mentioned, I've really pushed myself, because it got a bit too much, right, and then you don't feel well [...] I feel I cannot get out of this by myself.

Trond refers to mental and physical challenges, particularly his efforts to try to follow earlier advice. He is active but also desperately wants help. The health professionals, however, are eager to convey their diagnostic conclusion and actively discourage any further elaborations. When learning that he does not receive a CFS diagnosis, Trond neither objects nor comments directly; instead, he reiterates his long and complex story about his complaints while trying to justify his recovery efforts. When he mentions his previous assessment for trauma, everyone grasps the opportunity to discuss this. Eventually, the health professionals suggest a new referral for anxiety and PTSD assessment. Trond responds: "I think it's just super; I want to get to the bottom of this, I want to get my life back." Having settled this, the OT eagerly turns to detailed advice on activity regulation, which Trond quickly supplements with suggestions of his own, interspersed with worries about the malpractice. The OT continuously tries to get him to focus on his resources and positive experiences that he must try to activate. The session ends in an atmosphere of emotional weariness. Trond appears exhausted from trying to explain himself again and again. However, he also tunes into, somewhat submissively, the offers he gets. Ultimately, he is on the verge of crying as he thanks the team for its assessment and help.

Trond's encounter with the team was dominated by distinct intensities in the clinical interaction. In the first part of the session, the possible constitution of a diagnosis was what mattered. The Canada criteria, especially activity reduction and advice on activity regulation, became the central discursive practice that helped create the diagnosis, enacted by the different human agents through the paradoxical affective atmosphere that dominated the session. The intensity of that atmosphere brought out different viewpoints, responses, and resonances, as well as shared perceptions of dealing with an overbearing male patient. Eventually, the activity reduction criterion was used to dismiss the CFS diagnosis together with cancer as an exclusion criterion even though there was initial disagreement on this. Overall, the notion of activity, both biomedical and colloquial, demarcated the boundaries of the ill body and the recovering and healthy body, emphasizing the agentic and active body as the endpoint of clinical concerns.

Hope, in this case, we suggest, is strongly evoked by Trond by making hope specific and determinate (Anderson 2006). At the same time as Trond hoped for medical support, solutions, and help, he repeatedly performed his "recovery potential", hoping for recognition through a persistent narrative of competence versus shortcomings. This, however, had a contradictory effect on the health professionals who focused on his high activity level rather than on his suffering. The health professionals transformed Trond's hopes by enacting a personhood that needed help, not by jointly enacting a diagnosis. This transformation was driven simultaneously by Trond's despair and hopes and the intensity in the room that depended on, and was changed by, the notion of activity as a biomedical criterion. As such, the diagnostic process drew on gendered, intersubjective, and affective attunements as much as on specific clinical affordances.

## Concluding discussion

We have invited the reader into the affective attunements and atmospheres of clinical encounters, making a point of attending to affects, including hope, fear, passion, and despair, which move forward and drive the setting of diagnosis and care—a setting that is always in the making. In our analysis, intensities, affective attunements, and atmospheres determined the course of the consultations and played a decisive role in enacting the relational encounters and negotiating mutual roles and practices. We thus may say that affect was the "felt reality of a relation" (Massumi 2002: 16), embodying diagnostic work (Goodwin 2010).

Some scholars, inspired by post-humanist approaches, have proposed to shift analytical attention to relationality as the core unit of analysis (e.g. Barad 2003; Kazimierczak 2018; May 2007). Attending to relationality goes beyond attending to dyadic interaction. Rather, it calls attention to relations that are ontologically prior to an interaction between self-contained selves and opens up for experience in the making (Manning 2013). Relationality accounts for the mutuality and immediacy of different agents, inter-relational dynamics, and resonances of which affect is central, affect being essentially relational. Adding to an analysis of affect such as we have proposed here, we follow Kazimierzcak who suggests that we need to understand "how different agents come to be articulated, enacted and materialized in relations and practices, which make these distributions and configurations possible" (Kazimierczak 2017: 9). Inspired by this, we see a link between the concept of "relationality" with its emphasis on situational immediacy and affect which is present in the diagnostic processes presented.

Investigating how relationality and affect may drive and generate diagnostic procedures seems inherent to analyzing the contingency of clinical encounters. For Anna, hope and fear remained open to what might come and they worked as modalities which moved the health professionals into empathetic resonances. Accordingly, the professionals attuned their clinical decisions to Anna's gendered performance of hope, strength, and competence as a caring mother (Young 2005), while simultaneously drawing on their professional ethos and passion to support her. The emergent hopeful atmosphere was shared, hope being a form of affect, and moved the diagnostic decision.

Trond also expressed hope, together with a sense of despair. However, Trond projected hope into potentialities and possibilities by attempting to present a narrative of competencies, his "recovery potential", to comply with what he thought was expected from him; however, his apparent well-run life made it difficult for the health professionals to attune to him. In this way, we might say that Trond himself transformed his hopefulness: Through being excessively eager to perform competence he appeared to seek to reconcile different forms of masculinity in health (Courtenay 2000; Nissen 2017). In Trond's case, the intensity of hope and despair is overwhelming and calls on the professionals first to negotiate their shared position and then to contain Trond. The diagnostic process entails Trond's affectivity, together with enacting specific agency, masculinities, and personhood as much as the health professionals' enactment of care and professional ethos in their diagnostic endeavor. Yet, no clear and definitive diagnosis was enacted.

According to Brown and Tucker (2010: 3202), there is "a material arrangement of relations between bodies that allows for certain potentials to act." In the cases above, the CFS diagnosis was a potential diagnosis from the outset, with its potentiality governed by the affectivity generated by moments, movements, and interaction-in-the-making of the clinical encounters, the relations between the professionals (i.e. three women professionals) as well as the hierarchical relations between their professions. The diagnostic outcome is partly determined and accomplished through affect, but it is the process of constituting bodies and affecting bodies, including affecting gendered bodies, that counts and shapes the diagnostic assessment, moving bodies from "here" to "elsewhere." But bodies do not move on their own. Potentiality in the case of CFS draws on guidelines, the morality of self-management, and the politics of healthy activity which requires patients "to do something." The dynamics of power are immanent in affectivity and help us to understand how bodies and subjectivities are being affected and by what. However, potentiality is ambiguous and always open-ended; it must be studied both locally and socially. Looking for its outcome requires sensitivity to what moves in ordinary worlds as well as attention to discourses (Wetherell 2012). Our analysis focused on how tensions, intensities, bodies, and sensations made parties participate, act, react, and move in a clinical setting. Attending methodologically to affective attunement and atmospheres to dissolve the dyadic clinical encounter foregrounds that, just as a CFS diagnosis is contested among patients and health professionals outside the clinic, it is also fluid and worked on in a clinic environment through and in response to the affectivities at play (Tessier 2018). Affectivity clarifies that being "under diagnosis" (Martin 2007) and working out a diagnosis or treatment advice is an arrangement of affect, policies and practices, relations, and participation in these relations, rather than merely a discursive and linguistic performance.

## References


Adams, Vincanne, Michelle Murphy, and Adele E. Clarke. 2009. Anticipation: Technoscience, Life, Affect, Temporality. Subjectivity 28(1): 246–265.

Addison, Courtney. 2013. Chronic Fatigue Syndrome/Myalgic Encephalopathy: A Knowledge-based Approach to an Indeterminate Illness. M.A. thesis. University of Auckland, Auckland, New Zealand.

Ahmed, Sara. 2004. The Cultural Politics of Emotion. Edinburgh: Edinburgh University Press.

Anderson, Ben. 2006. Becoming and Being Hopeful: Towards a Theory of Affect. Environment and Planning D: Society and Space 24(5): 733–752.

Anderson, Ben. 2009. Affective Atmospheres. Emotion, Space and Society 2: 77–81.

Barad, Karen. 2003. Posthumanist Performativity: Toward an Understanding of How Matter Comes to Matter. Signs: Journal of Women in Culture and Society 28 (3): 801–831.

Brown, Steven D., and Ian Tucker. 2010. Eff the Ineffable: Affect, Somatic Management, and Mental Health Service Users. *In* The Affect Theory Reader. Melissa Gregg and Gregory J. Seigworth, eds. Pp. 229–250. Durham and London: Duke University Press.

Büscher, Monika, Dawn Goodwin, and Jessica Mesman, eds. 2010. Ethnographies of Diagnostic Work. Dimensions of Transformative Practice. New York: Palgrave Macmillan.

Carruthers, Bruce M., Anil K. Jain, Kenny L. De Meirleir, Daniel L. Peterson, Nancy G. Klimas et al. 2003. Myalgic Encephalomyelitis/Chronic Fatigue Syndrome. Journal of Chronic Fatigue Syndrome 11(1): 7–115.

Chew-Graham, Carolyn, Christopher Dowrick, Alison Wearden, Victoria Richardson, and Sarah Peters. 2010. Making the Diagnosis of Chronic Fatigue Syndrome/Myalgic Encephalitis in Primary Care: A Qualitative Study. BMC Family Practice 11(1): 16.

Clarke, Juanne N., and Susan James. 2003. The Radicalized Self: The Impact on the Self of the Contested Nature of the Diagnosis of Chronic Fatigue Syndrome. Social Science and Medicine 57(8): 1387–1395.

Collu, Samuele. 2019. Refracting Affects: Affect, Psychotherapy, and Spirit Dis-Possession. Culture, Medicine, and Psychiatry 43(2): 290–314.

Courtenay, Will H. 2000. Constructions of Masculinity and Their Influence on Men's Well-Being: A Theory of Gender and Health. Social Science and Medicine 50(10): 1385–1401.

Gardner, John, Kevin Dew, Maria Stubbe, Tony Dowell, and Lindsay Macdonald
2011 Patchwork Diagnoses: The Production of Coherence, Uncertainty, and Manageable Bodies. Social Science and Medicine 73(6): 843–850.

Gardner, John and Clare Williams. 2015. Corporal Diagnostic Work and Diagnostic Spaces: Clinicians' Use of Space and Bodies During Diagnosis. Sociology of Health and Illness 37(5): 765–781.

Geertz, Clifford. 1993. Religion as a Cultural System. *In* The Interpretation of Cultures. Pp. 87–125, Fontana Press.

Goodwin, Dawn. 2010. Sensing the Way: Embodied Dimensions of Diagnostic Work. *In* Ethnographies of Diagnostic Work: Dimensions of Transformative Practice. Monika Büscher, Dawn Goodwin, and Jessica Mesman, eds. Pp. 73–92. London and New York: Palgrave Macmillan.

Hadolt, Bernhard. 2018. A Desire for Knowing: Ontological Uncertainty, Diagnostic Evidence and Generative Affectivity in Pre-symptomatic Genetic Counselling. *In* Diagnostic Fluidity: Working with Uncertainty and Mutability. Nina Nissen and Mette Bech Risør, eds. Pp. 129–147. Tarragona: Publicacions URV.

Hastrup, Kirsten. 2013. Scales of Attention in Fieldwork: Global Connections and Local Concerns in the Arctic. Ethnography 14(2): 145–164.

Hay, M. Cameron. 2010. Suffering in a Productive World: Chronic Illness, Visibility, and the Space Beyond Agency. American Ethnologist 37(2): 259–274.

Helsedirektoratet. 2015. Nasjonal veileder. Pasienter med CFS/ME: Utredning, diagnostikk, behandling, rehabilitering, pleie og omsorg. Oslo: Helsedirektoratet

Hydén, Lars-Christer, and Lisbeth Sachs. 1998. Suffering, Hope and Diagnosis: On the Negotiation of Chronic Fatigue Syndrome. Health 2(2): 175–193.

Kazimierczak, Karolina A. 2018. Clinical Encounter and the Logic of Relationality: Reconfiguring Bodies and Subjectivities in Clinical Relations. Health 22(2): 185–201.

Knudsen, Britta Timm, and Carsten Stage. 2015. Introduction: Affective Methodologies. *In* Affective Methodologies: Developing Cultural Research Strategies for the Study of Affect. Britta Timm Knudsen and Carsten Stage, eds. Pp. 1–22. London: Palgrave Macmillan.

Knudsen, Britta Timm, and Carsten Stage. 2016. Affektteori. *In* Kulturteori og Kultursociologi. Bjørn Schiermer, ed. Pp. 53–75. København: Hans Reitzels Forlag.

Laidlaw, John. 2010. Agency and Responsibility: Perhaps You Can Have Too Much of a Good Thing. *In* Ordinary Ethics: Anthropology, Language, and Action. Michael Lambek, ed. Pp. 143–164. New York: Fordham University Press.

Manning, Erin. 2013. Always More Than One: Individuation's Dance. Kindle Edition: Duke University Press.

Martin, Emily. 2007. Bipolar Expeditions: Mania and Depression in American Culture. Princeton and Oxford: Princeton University Press.

Massumi, Brian. 2002. Parables for the Virtual: Movement, Affect, Sensation. Durham, NC: Duke University Press.

Mattingly, Cheryl. 2010. The Paradox of Hope: Journeys through a Clinical Borderland. Berkeley: University of California Press.

May, Carl. 2007. The Clinical Encounter and the Problem of Context. Sociology 41(1): 29–45.

Mol, Annemarie. 2002. The Body Multiple: Ontology in Medical Practice. Durham and London: Duke University Press.

Moser, Ingunn. 2010. Diagnosing and Acting Upon Dementia: Marte Meo. *In* Ethnographies of Diagnostic Work: Dimensions of Transformative Practice. Monika Büscher, Dawn Goodwin, and Jessica Mesman, eds. Pp. 193–209. London and New York: Palgrave Macmillan.

Nissen, Nina. 2017. Men's Everyday Health Care: Practices, Tensions and Paradoxes, and Masculinities in Denmark. Medical Anthropology 36(6): 551–65.

Rasmussen, Erik B. 2017. Balancing Medical Accuracy and Diagnostic Consequences: Diagnosing Medically Unexplained Symptoms in Primary Care. Sociology of Health and Illness 39: 1227.1241.

Risør, Mette Bech, and Kjersti Lillevoll. 2021. Caught Up in Care: Crafting Moral Subjects of Chronic Fatigue. Medical Anthropology 40(5): 432–445.

Risør, Mette Bech, and Nina Nissen. 2018. Configurations of Diagnostic Processes and Practices: An Introduction. *In* Diagnostic Fluidity: Working with Uncertainty and Mutability. Nina Nissen and Mette Bech Risør, eds. Pp. 11–32. Tarragona: Publicacions URV.

Rosenberg, Charles E. 2006. Contested Boundaries: Psychiatry, Disease, and Diagnosis. Perspectives in Biology and Medicine 49(3), 407–424.

Sachs, Lisbeth. 2001. From a Lived Body to a Medicalized Body: Diagnostic Transformation and Chronic Fatigue Syndrome. Medical Anthropology 19(4): 299–317.

Sachs, Lisbeth. 2016. Making Sense of Unmeasurable Suffering: The Recontextualization of Debut Stories to a Diagnosis of Chronic Fatigue Syndrome. *In* Diagnostic Controversy: Cultural Perspectives on Competing Knowledge in Healthcare. Carolyn Smith-Morris, ed. Pp.107–126. New York and London: Routledge.

Seppola-Edvardsen, Tone, and Mette Bech Risør. 2017. Ignoring Symptoms: The Process of Normalising Sensory Experiences after Cancer. Anthropology in Action 24(1): 34–40.

Smith-Morris, Carolyn, ed. 2015. Diagnostic Controversy: Advancing and Competing Knowledge and Medical Inquiry. New York: Routledge Publishing.

Staiano-Ross, Kathryn. 2012. The Symptom. Biosemiotics 5(1): 33–45.

Staunæs, Dorthe, and Justine G. Pors. 2021. Strejfet af en tåre – at læse affekt gennem friktionelle begreber. *In* Eklektiske analysestrategier. Emil Husted and Justine G. Pors, eds. Pp. 39–62. Nyt fra Samfundsvidenskaberne.

Stewart, Kathleen. 2007. Ordinary Affects. Durham and London: Duke University Press.

Stewart, Kathleen. 2017. In the World that Affect Proposed. Cultural Anthropology 32(2): 192–198.

Swallow, Julia and Alexandra Hillman. 2019. Fear and Anxiety: Affects, Emotions and Care Practices in the Memory Clinic. Social Studies of Science 49(2): 227–244.

Taussig, Karen-Sue, Klaus Hoeyer, and Stefan Helmreich. 2013. The Anthropology of Potentiality in Biomedicine: An Introduction to Supplement 7. Current Anthropology 54(S7): 3–14.

Tessier, Laurence. 2018. From Evidence to Experience: The Diagnosis of Dementia in a US Clinic. *In* Diagnostic Fluidity. Working with Uncertainty and Mutability. Nina Nissen and Mette Bech Risør, eds. Pp. 105–129. Tarragona: Publicacions URV.

Thrift, Nigel. 2008. Non-representational Theory: Space, Politics, Affect. London and New York: Routledge.

Ware, Norma C. 1992. Suffering and the Social Construction of Illness: The Delegitimation of Illness Experience in Chronic Fatigue Syndrome. Medical Anthropology Quarterly 6(4): 347–361.

Ware, Norma C. 1999. Toward A Model of Social Course in Chronic Illness: The Example of Chronic Fatigue Syndrome. Culture, Medicine and Psychiatry 23(3): 303–331.

Wetherell, Margaret. 2012. Affect and Emotion: A New Social Science Understanding. London: SAGE.

White, Daniel. 2017. AFFECT: An Introduction. Cultural Anthropology 32(2): 175–180.

Young, Iris Marion. 2005. On Female Body Experience. Oxford: Oxford University Press.

# 12 Fighting for Recovery

## The Certain Uncertainty of Living with Locked-in Syndrome

*Lina Masana*

### Introduction

When I first began to familiarize myself with the phenomenon of locked-in syndrome (LIS), through written and audiovisual materials about people's experiences with the condition, I was surprised to learn that very few completely recovered their previous healthy functioning, and others never recovered at all. In between are different degrees of recovery, varying greatly from case to case. I wondered why this was, what sort of "luck" it is that makes it happen one way or another. The answer to this question falls primarily into the medical domain, as I will explain below. However, from an anthropological perspective, I wondered how people with LIS perceive the fact that some recover completely and others not at all. Are they (made) aware of it? How much information do they have about recovery? What do health professionals tell them? What are their thoughts, expectations, wishes, hopes, or fears regarding recovery?

In this chapter, I will elaborate some provisional answers to those questions with the aim of shedding light on the paradox of what I call the *certain uncertainty* of living with LIS. First, I will explain the particularities of the syndrome from a medical point of view, what types of LIS exist, and the clinical classification of degrees of recovery. Then I will describe the illness trajectory for people with LIS and their perceptions and experiences regarding recovery. Finally, in this chapter I intend to show how "fighting" for recovery is a controversial notion for cases of LIS, because it starts from a medically created certainty grounded on uncertainty: scarce and random possibilities, misinformation or lack of information, and, sometimes, misleading or unrealistic expectations.

## Locked-in syndrome

Locked-in syndrome (a term coined by Plum and Posner 1966) is a rare condition usually resulting from a stroke in the brainstem (53 percent of cases are of vascular origin; this is predominantly the kind I will analyse in this chapter) or appearing in the advanced stage of a neurodegenerative disease such as amyotrophic lateral sclerosis. A few cases have been reported due to trauma (e.g., accident or concussion) or infection (e.g., listeria or meningitis). People with LIS cannot move (quadriplegia) or speak (anarthria), but they are conscious and cognitively able, can see and hear, and retain bodily sensation (e.g., touch, temperature, pain, pleasure). Interpersonal communication is laborious. Persons with LIS communicate by multimodal means: through vertical eye movements or blinking or spelling using an alphabet board or technological system (a tablet or computer). Some can only communicate through an interpreter (family member or professional), others manage to do it also autonomously (see the issue of communication for persons with LIS in Masana and Vidal in press; n.d.).

There are three forms of LIS according to the medical classification (Bauer, Gerstenbrand and Rumpl 1979): in *classic LIS* vertical eye movement or blinking is preserved; in *incomplete LIS*, aside from eye and eyelid movement, the individual can voluntarily move a part of their body (e.g., finger, neck, head, mouth) enabling them, for example, to manoeuvre an electric wheelchair or communicate autonomously using technological devices (tablet, computer), e.g., by using a joystick or an adapted gadget. *Complete or total LIS* entails full immobility (including eye mobility). In all cases, "the course and prognosis vary widely, even among patients with pontine [brainstem] stroke" (Bernat 2020: 231).

Five stages of motor or functional recovery have been clinically described in patients with LIS (Patterson and Grabois 1986: 761), based on the absence or presence of motor return and degree of dependence on caregiving for daily living. *No recovery* refers to patients with no motor return and total dependence on care; *minimum recovery* refers to those with minimal voluntary motor return (e.g., finger, mouth, neck) but still complete dependence on care; *moderate recovery* entails significant motor return which allow patients independence in some but not all their daily activities; *full recovery* refers to patients who gain independence in all daily activities but still have some minimal neurological deficit; and *no neurological deficit* refers to patients who recover completely, without residual neurological deficit.

The few existing longitudinal medical studies of the evolution of motor recovery for patients with LIS show significantly varying rates. For instance, a study by Patterson and Grabois (1986) finds full recovery rates of 7 percent while Casanova et al. (2023) find 34 percent. These data cannot be explained: not why, how, or to what extent some recover moderately or fully, and others minimally or not at all. What these studies agree on is the importance of intensive early rehabilitation (from one month after the stroke) as this, it is believed, reduces mortality and increases the chance of recovery. This is now the protocol in most hospitals and rehabilitation centres for persons with severe disabilities after stroke.

It is worth mentioning that LIS is not a disease but a severe disabling condition, a physical state that entails physical and functional disability, but not sensory, cognitive, or intellectual disability. People with LIS do not die from the condition itself, but usually from respiratory complications (35 percent of deaths according to Patterson and Grabois 1986). They have long life expectancy: studies find that 83 percent live ten years and 40 percent live 20 years, and others live for decades (Bruno et al. 2008; Doble et al. 2003; Halan et al. 2021; Hocker and Wijdicks 2015; Rousseau et al. 2015; Smith and Delargy 2005). Living with LIS, therefore, can be a lengthy journey, as is recovery.

## The illness trajectory of LIS

The illness trajectory for people with LIS of vascular origin in Spain or France (the settings of our research) usually follows a pattern. After the stroke, they spend one or two months in an induced coma in an intensive care unit (ICU). This is a crucial period in which death may occur: 87 percent of deaths occur within the first four months after the stroke (Casanova et al. 2003; Patterson and Grabois 1986; Rousseau et al. 2015). After coming out of the coma, they are sent to a neurology unit at the hospital where an initial assessment is carried out to discern whether they have LIS or are in a vegetative state. From then on, a physiotherapist comes daily to carry out basic respiratory physiotherapy (most have a tracheostomy) and to move the individual with LIS to avoid pressure sores and limb deformities, and to ensure that the joints do not stiffen. In certain hospitals a post-intensive-care rehabilitation team will take over to provide early rehabilitation care for patients suffering from serious neurological conditions. This is a bridge between intensive care and the rehabilitation centre.

After patients have spent about six months (on average) in the neurology unit, they are transferred to a rehabilitation centre or a long-term hospital with a specific rehabilitation unit. This period is crucial for people with LIS, and usually involves a stay of 6–9 months. Afterwards, some return to live at home with their families. For this, it is necessary to first adapt the home to their new needs, and to have family or professional caregivers who can provide 24/7 assistance. The services of other professionals, such as physiotherapists and speech therapists, are also required to continue the rehabilitation process. Other people with LIS instead go to live at a care home for persons with disabilities and receive daily motor and functional rehabilitation services and other treatment (speech therapy, psychology, etc.). In some cases, patients also have to pay for external professional services.

Both France and Spain have several specialized care homes for persons with disabilities. Additionally, since 2016, there is a specialized centre for persons with LIS in France. There is no such centre in Spain. France also has a well-established association for people with LIS and their families (Association du Locked In Syndrome, ALIS),[1] with about two hundred members. The association provides valuable information about resources, professionals, and facilities, and engages members in activities. There is no such association in Spain.

Both the Spanish and French health-care systems are tax-based and cover care services for dependent persons with severe disabilities, but do not cover everything. Whether living at home or in a care home, affected individuals or their families have to bear certain expenses. This can be a significant economic burden. While I will not deal with the economic problematic in this chapter, it is worth noting, as people with LIS and their families are told that recovery (if possible at all) can only be achieved with intensive early rehabilitation followed by continued rehabilitation over time. While the former is available in both the Spanish and the French health-care systems, neither fully covers the latter over the years. Therefore, there is an economic inequality regarding access to services and resources for people with LIS.

Fighting for an uncertain recovery, therefore, has financial, emotional, and moral costs. It implies having technical resources (aids) and continued and specialized professional care for years, as well as perseverance and personal dedication on the part of the affected person—all this without certainty of what the result of so much investment will be.

## Methods

This chapter's contribution comes from postdoctoral research (2019–2023) conducted as part of a larger project entitled *Anthropology and Phenomenology of the Locked-in Syndrome*, at the Medical Anthropology Research Centre (MARC) of the University Rovira i Virgili (Tarragona, Spain).[2,3] The overall purpose of the study was to learn about the lived experience of LIS from those suffering from it, and its impact and implications for their close relatives and professional caregivers

1 https://alis-asso.fr

2 This work was supported by the Spanish Ministry of Science and Innovation under Grant PID2019-106723GB-I00, granted to the principal investigator, Fernando Vidal.

3 This research has been performed in accordance with the principles stated in the Declaration of Helsinki and obtained the ethical approval of the Ethics Committee of the Department of Anthropology, Philosophy and Social Work (DAFiTS), of the University of Tarragona (URV), Spain, where this research was conducted.

(Masana and Vidal 2020; Vidal 2020). I was responsible for the ethnographic research—qualitative methods, fieldwork, data collection and analysis—among other tasks. The data presented here were analysed solely by me.

The data were drawn from written narratives gathered through a qualitative questionnaire specifically designed for the above-mentioned research, together with oral interviews with two participants with LIS who regained speech. These primary data are complemented with the publicly available autobiographical accounts of persons experiencing LIS, such as published books or audiovisual materials on the internet. The names of research participants are pseudonyms to preserve their anonymity, except where I rely on public accounts.

The research participants are persons with LIS from Spain (n=5) and France (n=11). In most cases (14 out of 16) their LIS has a vascular origin. All participants have incomplete LIS, except two with classic LIS. Those with incomplete LIS have regained mobility and speech to different extents. They constitute a heterogeneous group of individuals differing in several factors, such as age, sex, gender, type of LIS, time with LIS, degree of disability, family situation, place and type of residence, and cultural and socioeconomic background. Despite this heterogeneous and non-representative sample, I encountered several commonalities in their narratives regarding the lived experience of LIS in general, and with regards to the certain uncertainty of the prognosis for recovery.

Fieldwork was conducted online—by e-mail or videoconference—between September 2019 and July 2021. Spanish participants were recruited using snowball sampling from a first key participant who had published a memoir about living with LIS. French participants were recruited through ALIS which issued a call to its members, providing information about our research project and its contact details. People willing to participate contacted the project directly by e-mail. All participants in Spain and France received and answered autonomously the same qualitative questionnaire (in Spanish or French). This consisted of 34 open-ended questions about the personal experience of living with LIS and its impact on their life. The participants sent their responses back by e-mail. I followed up on certain responses that needed clarification or asked for further details. I have discussed elsewhere the methodological challenges encountered when designing and conducting ethnographic research with people with LIS (Masana in press; n.d.).

For various methodological reasons, a specific question about the participants' certainty or uncertainty about their prognosis for recovery was not included in the qualitative questionnaire. However, the questionnaire did ask about issues that indirectly refer to the topic, such as the most important things in their lives, their expectations for the future, their experience of immobility, the evolution of their mobility over time, and their quality of life.

It is worth mentioning that regaining speech is key for persons suffering from LIS. It entails lengthy and intensive speech therapy to be able to talk (if possible at all), but also to recover other related functions, such as swallowing and chewing. In this chapter, I focus only on motor recovery, as I have dealt elsewhere with regaining speech and communication in LIS (Masana and Vidal in press; n.d.).

## Findings

The findings point to four situations regarding recovery from the point of view of those affected with LIS: *fatal prognosis, no recovery, partial recovery*, and *full recovery*. These are distinct from, though overlapping with, the medical stages of functional recovery described earlier in this chapter. In each situation, I encountered common narratives that were expressed similarly by different participants.

### Fatal prognosis: "They gave me two months to live"

After a stroke in the brainstem, our research participants spend between one and four months in a coma in an ICU. Once they "wake up" or "come out" of the coma (as they say in Spanish and French), and are diagnosed with LIS, the situation is critical from a medical point of view. As mentioned earlier, mortality is high in those early stages. Because of this, the initial prognosis is fatal, and clinicians tell relatives of persons with LIS: "be prepared for death, they could die at any moment". This is a preventive communication strategy used by clinicians to prepare families for a fatal outcome. Another version reported is "they would be better off dead" when doctors realize the extent of brain damage and that the patient will be locked in "forever". This phrasing illustrates the notion of the *disability paradox* (Albrecht and Devlieger 1999), where health professionals, relatives, and other external observers believe that a life with LIS is not worth living: there is no quality of life. In our research, those messages were only given to family and relatives, not to patients themselves who were just awakening after being away for several weeks or months. This is what happened to George.

George is a married man aged 58 years who lives with his wife and two children (now aged 22 and 20 years) in a residential neighbourhood of a small city in the north of Spain. He had a stroke in 2004 when he was 39 years old. At that time, the children were three years and nine months old respectively. George followed the usual illness trajectory for a person with LIS: a month and a half in the ICU, four in the neurology unit of the hospital, and six at a rehabilitation centre, and then back home. Today, he loves music and goes to the gym every day, he says, "to maintain all the achievements I have accomplished".

After the stroke, however, when George awoke from the coma and was diagnosed with LIS, his wife was given the initial fatal prognosis that he might only live two months. Today, 19 years later, he is alive, and his recovery is significant: he has experienced almost full recovery. George himself did not know about the two-month prognosis doctors gave initially. Now he knows, and uses the same narrative which he reconstructed afterwards: "They gave me two months to live, and look at me!" Indeed, patients are usually not made aware of the initial fatal prognosis until much later, when relatives reveal to them what they were told. This means that such persons with LIS could not knowingly, consciously, or voluntarily, do anything to improve their health condition and beat those fatal odds. And yet, George, and others like him, repeat their doctors' fatal prognosis with a sense of having fought it and of achieving victory over their own death.

Coincidentally, George lives in the same neighbourhood as one of the doctors who cared for him in the ICU, in fact the same one who gave his wife that terrible prognosis. George says that, one day, he and the ICU doctor met at the neighbourhood supermarket and recognized each other. George approached the doctor and asked: "Why...?". George explains that the doctor apologized and said he was terribly sorry, and acknowledged that "we did not know, we could not know". Thus, there is also clinical uncertainty around LIS: professionals know that they do not know certain things (e.g., the prognosis), but it may be difficult for some to acknowledge this as it challenges their professional knowledge and status. This is why most choose the preventive communication strategy of "no hope" to prepare relatives for a short life expectancy and their relative's death.

On another occasion, the same ICU doctor met George's wife at the supermarket, and said "Oh dear me, the things we told you!" She explained to him how autonomous George is nowadays, all the things he can do by himself. The doctor responded: "I cannot believe it, how lucky you have been!" I opened this chapter by wondering what sort of "luck" makes recovery happen one way or another, and here it is luck to which the doctor turned to explain or justify (to himself or to George's wife) George's incredible recovery, which he had believed, or said he believed to be impossible. In this case, the use of the expression "being lucky" is founded on a comparison with other persons with LIS who could not recover, and contrasts with the poor clinical prognosis for recovery. The notion of luck is recurrent in the experience of illness and in the medical narrative. Luck with the health professionals who care for you or with the patient you had; luck with the treatment efficacy; luck with the condition itself and its evolution; luck with relatives and friends' responses to illness, disability, or dependency; luck with recovery. Talking about good or bad luck is a culturally and medically framed discourse used by both doctors and patients to avoid talking about disagreements and disappointments, especially in the face of a poor prognosis and uncertainty.

As already noted above, people with LIS with vascular origin who beat the two-month prognosis have a long life expectancy. At the time of writing (2023), the Spanish participants had lived with LIS for between 12 and 37 years, and the French participants for between 4 and 32 years. Living two, three, or almost four decades in classic or incomplete LIS is an achievement in terms of survival, but not in terms of recovery. Life expectancy is a medical measure that is relevant when dealing with a life-and-death situation. Once survival is certain, what matters to people with LIS is the extent to which they can recover their bodily functions and lead an autonomous life. We asked our participants about the evolution of their condition over the years and decades.

## No recovery: "No future"?

Only two of all the participants—Phoenix and Calvin—have had classic LIS for extended periods (38 and 11 years respectively) and have not experienced any motor recovery. They only move their eyes and eyelids to communicate, are fed by gastric tube, and breathe via tracheostomy. Their answers to the qualitative questionnaire are brief and do not tell us much about uncertainty, although they do tell us about the absence of expectations for the future and for recovery.

Phoenix is a 66-year-old man who has been married for 40 years. He has two children (now aged 38 and 32 years) and two grandchildren (twins, almost three years old). He lives at home with his wife in a house in a small village in east France, in a quiet area surrounded by nature: "well-flowered and woody", he says. One of his sons, the father of the grandchildren, lives a kilometre away, while the other lives far away (950 kilometres). In 1986, when Phoenix was 28 years old, he was in a car accident which caused brainstem trauma. At that time, one of his sons was one year old. The second was born five years after the accident, when he already had LIS. Phoenix has been in classic LIS for almost 38 years since the accident, with no improvement or motor recovery at all. He can only move his eyelids and eyes to communicate by blinking and using an alphabet board. He uses assisted communication technology (eye-controlled human-computer interface) with a special tablet and computer, and used it to answer the questionnaire autonomously. His answers are very brief, partly because, as he explains, he had a heart attack six years ago and, since then he feels very tired and has difficulty expressing his thoughts. Besides, he says, communicating through the computer interface is tiring for him.

Phoenix had a different illness trajectory than the usual pattern described above, probably because he had a car accident and not a stroke. He spent less than a week under sedation in the ICU, and two years and nine months hospitalized before he could return to home, where he has lived ever since. He describes being in LIS as a "very heavy handicap...". In several of his responses he emphasizes the issue of dependency, and that "being dependent for everything brings no quality of life". In fact, he reports being in complete LIS (instead of classic LIS), which is not the case according to the medical definition, but from his bodily perception. Although he acknowledges receiving very good care from professionals, he does not see room for improving his quality of life "I'm getting older and don't want much anymore." He does not talk of, nor consider, recovery: not for him nor anyone else (family or professionals). He enjoys his family life; spending time with her wife, children, and grandchildren: the most important things in his life. He says that what helped him most for living with LIS is: "my faith in God, the support of my religious community, my family". He attends religious services online or by phone and receives visits from his community at home. His narrative combines what we could call peaceful acceptance with bitter resignation to his condition, with no expectations or projects for the future, but seemingly content with the present. When asked about the future he responds "???", followed by "I don't know, I am a little fed up...".

Calvin is a 59-year-old married man who suffered a stroke when he was 38 years old. He lives in a specialized care centre for people with LIS in France, together with 22 other residents. His wife visits him weekly. Since the stroke 11 years ago, Calvin has had classic LIS. Like Phoenix, Calvin uses assisted communication technology and answered the questionnaire autonomously. His answers are also brief. In the years since his stroke, he has not had any improvement or motor recovery, despite receiving daily physiotherapy. Like Phoenix, recovery is not even considered, yet Phoenix has had LIS for 38 years and Calvin for 11. However, unlike Calvin, other participants with LIS have continued to fight and hold out hope for recovery through similarly long durations (as we will see in the next section). Calvin loves listening to music, watching police serials, receiving visitors, and having conversations with people. His narrative, though, seems bitter and dark. He describes being in LIS as "I have the feeling of being good for nothing", a sense of uselessness and powerlessness which Frank (1995) already described in *chaos narrative*. In his questionnaire responses, Calvin also explicitly writes that LIS is "extremely difficult to live with, why did they save me?", suggesting that letting him die would have been better. This points to the deep suffering experienced by some people with LIS and is consistent with the notion of *disability paradox* as presented by Albrecht and Devlieger (1999). Regarding mobility, he explains he cannot move anything (apart from his eyelids), that he cannot do anything, and that he feels "degraded". "I no longer consider myself a man," he says. As for his expectations for the future, Calvin is explicit and concise: "no future", "no expectations". He wishes only that he could travel to Marseille to see his father.

When analysing the data, another participant, Francis, also seemed to have classic LIS (i.e., no recovery) like Phoenix and Calvin, and explicitly answered the question about the evolution of his mobility and motor recovery as "no evolution". However, I found an online publication—the annual newsletter of ALIS (2017)—and realized that he could move his head, neck, and mouth, and that he has regained the ability to speak. Under the medical definition, therefore, he does not have classic LIS but incomplete LIS, and has experienced minimum recovery. As with Phoenix, Francis' story appears a mismatch between the medical classification of the degree of motor recovery and his personal bodily experience. Francis can move his head, neck, and mouth, and with a special joystick, to manoeuvre his wheelchair and use the computer and home automation devices autonomously. In the ALIS newsletter he says:

> When my daily care [washing, dressing] is finished [by caregivers] and I am put in the chair, I am totally independent! [...] I can do everything with my computer, and more importantly, I am free. (Francis, 21 years with incomplete LIS)

Here, Francis is talking about being free, a significant term that could be understood as the highest level of control regained over his life given his severe disability. Yet, in the questionnaire, he states there has been "no evolution". A possible explanation for this underreporting of his functional abilities is that he expected to improve and regain more mobility and, therefore, considers his present state of minimum recovery to be equivalent to "no evolution". But there could be other explanations, such as the moment—the mood, time, day, or circumstances—in which he responded to the questionnaire, or the image of himself he wanted to present, whether in the questionnaire or in the association newsletter, which were aimed at different readers. In other words, the perceived difference between the reality of illness, in this case of disability, by health professionals or by patients, highlights how their explanatory models differ (Kleinman 1988), as well as their expectations of recovery.

## Partial recovery: "You have to work hard if you want to recover"

Only some individuals with LIS will, over time, regain partial motor recovery, though nobody knows beforehand the extent to which they will recover, if at all, and which part of the body might recover. Partial recovery is the lay, emic term covering the medical classifications described earlier, of minimum and moderate recovery. Most of our research participants have experienced minimum recovery (minimal voluntary motor return e.g., finger, mouth, head, or neck, but still complete dependence on care).

What is certain in LIS is that recovery requires an enormous investment in rehabilitation (physiotherapy, respiratory, swallowing, and speech therapy). While, nowadays, most hospitals and rehabilitation centres initiate early intensive rehabilitation, this was not always the case. Some health professionals failed to do so, because they did not believe in their patient's chances of recovery, or simply did not know it was needed. As one participant writes in his memoir:

> It is not that I resent him [doctor] for not having been able to recover some more movement (which I am convinced would have been possible), but I will never be able to forget that, in depriving me of that care [early rehabilitation], what he really did is to abandon us, my family and me, to the deepest ignorance [that he

> might be able to recover to some extent] (Carballo 2005: 34; 24 years in incomplete LIS).

The onset of LIS in some of our participants (as in the example quoted above), and in some of the memoirs, dates back to the late 1990s and early 2000s, when little was known about the condition, and health professionals did not know of, or trust, the possibility of recovery, due to its initial severity (quadriplegia and anarthria). I was interested in knowing how much information people with LIS have about recovery, and what professionals tell them about it. Analysing the data, and as the example above shows, little or no information was available at that time. Clinical uncertainty and lack of belief in the possibility of recovery had severe consequences for patients with LIS, both on a motor and moral level. On the one hand, they did not receive the care that would give them a chance to recover; on the other hand, they experienced feelings of abandonment and betrayal by medical professionals who gave up on them in the face of the severity of the condition.

And yet, the uncertainty of recovery is not just a matter of investment in rehabilitation and personal effort, although it is usually presented as such. A common narrative we heard from participants is: "you have to work hard if you want to recover". This came from participants who have regained mobility and speech to some extent (however limited), not from those who are still trying (or not) and have not experienced any motor or functional recovery. The narrative is not free from judgement, since it puts the blame on those who have not made it (yet?), as if they have not worked hard enough. Failure to recover is interpreted as a moral failure. It can also be a source of frustration, despair, and hopelessness (like in Frank's *chaos narrative*, 1995). In the cultural discourse, the popular notion of the "culture of effort" values a "fighting attitude". This was shared by Spanish and French participants and is found in the memoirs of people with LIS from other countries. It involves fighting for your goals actively, daily, with perseverance and discipline.

With LIS, physical and functional changes happen very slowly, if at all. Persons with LIS explain that is a very long and slow process:

> Through a tremendous amount of hard work and perseverance I have gained ever so slowly since my accident and still continue to make gains now (they seem huge gains to others, but they seem far too slow for me—I've got to live through it all), with the much-appreciated help and support of others and a copious amount of extremely hard work and sometimes pain. (Chisholm and Gillet 2005: 94; 23 years with incomplete LIS)

Some persons with LIS can live 10 or more years with no physical improvement at all but, continue investing time, energy, and resources fighting for an uncertain recovery. Others, like Calvin, may not. What drives the former to fight for recovery is puzzling, since we learn from their narratives that they are not very aware, nor informed, about the level of recovery they can achieve. As Conrad explains:

> My relatives, I think rightly, at that time they did not tell me the truth, that I was going to be like this [locked-in, immobile] forever; then I think I would have given it up too soon. For example, the communication programme I'm writing with requires a click, and they told me that if I wanted to use this programme, I had to move a finger, and from then on, with a lot of willpower, I began to constantly try to move my finger until I finally managed to move my finger. (Conrad, 24 years with incomplete LIS)

Knowing the tremendous effort that recovering entails, it is common for every improvement to be valued and to give hope for further recovery: "the moment I started to move my toes (minimally) I already felt that everything was going to change", says George (19 years with incomplete LIS). For some participants, no matter how minimal or partial their recovery is, it is perceived as a victory over the body's limitations and a reward for personal effort, investment, time, perseverance, and discipline, led by the sense of "I can" or at least "I am trying". As Patricia says: "I am very proud of myself, of what I have achieved".

Patricia is a 54-year-old woman, who has been married since 2020 to her long-term partner. She lives in a care home for persons with severe disabilities in a quiet village in the south of Spain. Her spouse visits her once a month and they go out for the weekend to the family house or to the beach, which are about 200 kilometres away. In 2008, when she was 28 years old, she had a stroke. She spent 10 years with classic LIS (no recovery) and only started experiencing motor improvements during the last five years. She can move her head, mouth, fingers, hands, arms, legs (she can walk few steps), and has recovered speech (and is still working on it). Patricia drives her wheelchair autonomously and loves to go into town to shop, visit the hairdresser, go to the movies, and do other activities, alone or with someone. She can autonomously write with a special tablet and computer. She answered the questionnaire by herself and is a profuse writer: aside from the questionnaire, she sent us additional writings about her lived experience with the condition. She started working on her recovery soon after the diagnose of LIS:

> The doctors told my family that I suffered from a rare disease called Locked-in Syndrome, that I was going to be bedridden for life, and they advised them that they could now go find me a care home to put me in. [...] And by trying very hard, based on hard work that I imposed on myself, and thanks to the great support of my partner and help, I have managed to become INDEPENDENT (something unthinkable for me!) and thanks to my perseverance, encouragement, and desire to live, I'm still moving very very slowly, but I'm going against all odds! (Patricia, 10 years with classic LIS and five with incomplete LIS; capitalization in the original).

Again, we find a mismatch between individual body perception (disability reality) as functional and independent—she emphasizes this in capital letters—and the medical reality that she still needs continued care for the basic activities of daily living. Aside from the mismatch in explanatory models (Kleinman 1988), we must consider the lens through which we assess disability and recovery. If we only take a functional view and define recovery in terms of the activities persons with LIS can perform or if, through a social lens, we consider the conditions in the social environment that prevent or enable participation in society for persons with LIS. The sense of independence and autonomy, therefore, varies depending on who is assessing it. And yet, Patricia, like others, recounts her achievements with a sense of victory and having fought the odds, that is, against the certain and uncertain poor prognosis of LIS.

Another excerpt illustrates the kind of "hard work" Patricia refers to. She walks us through her daily life in the care home:

> They wake me up every day at 7 a.m. in the morning, I go to the patio for silence and meditation [...]. Then I have breakfast and at 10 a.m. the workshops begin, we do read and writing, mental calculation, cognitive stimulation, sports training, manipulative therapy, musicotherapy, recreational activities, computers, and outings. All this is spread throughout the week in the morning and afternoon. In between I stand up for an hour each day on my standing frame, plus one hour of physio and one hour of speech therapy every day. At 1:30 p.m. I stop to eat and then I go out to the patio to lie down in my chair and to stretch my legs (I have my chair adapted with those functions). At 3 p.m. I continue with the workshops until 5 p.m. I get on an adapted automatic bike, and it moves my legs and arms, I do 20 to 25 kilometres a day and I It feels great, especially on my legs. I'm pedalling until dinner (7:30 p.m.). I take advantage of the mirror in the living room and do the speech therapy exercises, gesticulate, and vocalize, all every day. So, when I fall into bed (I fall dead) I only turn on the TV to watch the news, and that hour of TV, I use it to do breathing exercises with a respirator to strengthen my lungs. At 11 p.m. they put splints on my hands and feet, so they don't become deformed (I look like a robot) and it's uncomfortable. As you can see, I lead a very busy life, and I dedicate the weekends to myself, on Saturdays I go to a private physio for two hours to get massages on my back, lumbar, neck, etc. and the shopping, going to the bar, etc. (Patricia, 10 years with classic LIS and five with incomplete LIS).

As Kleinman (2006: 6) points out: "We employ a variety of strategies to deal with the profound sense of inadequacy and existential fear bred by the limits of our control". In LIS, people lose complete control over their bodies, which results in loss of control over their lives. Staying active and busy working for recovery, as Patricia does, is an attempt to regain some control over her live and fate in a pragmatic way when facing misfortune and uncertainty. It is also a way to show value, power, personhood, and social identity (Whyte 1997). Indeed, her daily hard work is perceived as such, daily work like ordinary people, leading also "a very busy life". Proof of that is when she says: "and I dedicate the weekends to myself". Paradoxically, the constant work she does from Monday to Friday for her recovery is not conceptualized as dedicated to herself, that is, she clearly differentiates between work (working toward recovery) and free time for herself (for leisure activities).

## Full recovery: "The power of the will"

There was no case of full recovery among our participants, although George, whom we met earlier, comes the closest: he was given two months to live and, against all odds, improved significantly over the years. He explains that he started by moving his toe several months after the stroke and now, 19 years later, leads an autonomous life, saying: "I lead a more or less 'normal' life". He can walk and talk, take care of himself and perform basic daily activities such as washing, dressing, cooking, eating, etc. He goes out and about by himself, shopping, going to the gym daily, meeting friends, etc. He uses a wheelchair and crutches when needed, since he still has balance problems, and complains that he does not "speak well" yet, and that some people have problems understanding him or refuse to talk to him.

As already mentioned, full recovery from LIS is very rare (Bernat 2020; McCusker et al. 1982; Hocker and Wijdicks 2015). A case that caught my attention, and perhaps triggered this chapter, is that of a British woman called Kate Allatt who recovered completely from LIS of vascular origin, and wrote an autobiography entitled *Running Free: Breaking Out from Locked-In Syndrome* (Allatt and Stokes 2011). In 2017, Kate was interviewed on a morning television show (*Good Morning Britain*)[4] and talked about "her incredibly recovery" (as it was presented on the show). When the journalist asked: "How do you physically manage to go from that state to actually being able to walk out of the hospital?", she responded:

> You know, I'm really glad you asked me that because I didn't know about neuroplasticity [...] I just knew I had the will to be home with my kids. (Kate Allatt, BBC *Good Morning Britain*, 08/02/2017)

Kate's spontaneous response is striking and informative. Her will to be home with her kids, though not a guarantee of recovery, is what motivated or helped her to work toward recovery. When losing total control over their bodies and lives, people with LIS point to the most important things in their lives. In her book, Kate also lists other

4 BBC, *Good Morning Britain*, 08/02/2017, Woman With Locked-in Syndrome Talks About Her Incredible Recovery: https://www.youtube.com/watch?v=F8pNAbmwIfA

factors she believes contributed to beating LIS: her fitness, support from her family and friends, her will, disciplined therapy, setting goals, among others (Allatt and Stokes 2011: 209). On the TV show, as Kate described her will to be home with her children, her doctor (who was also on the show), interrupted her to say that full recovery is extremely rare in cases of LIS, and that the medical profession is learning a lot from Kate's case. He reinforced the *power of the will* message by saying:

> We are learning that, we are talking about neuroplasticity here, the ability of the will to relentlessly pursue getting the voluntary movements back is often down to the patient, and you [looking at the patient] would determine to recover. (Kate Allatt's neurologist, BBC *Good Morning Britain*, 08/02/2017)

Can willpower beat clinical uncertainty and a poor prognosis? It is risky and dangerous to correlate such things, not only because it might not be true or feasible, but because it puts blame on those who cannot make it, as if their will is weaker. Although the doctor repeated several times that recovery is extremely rare, the message of the power of the will was served and reinforced. Nor is this exclusive to Kate's case. Patricia also speaks of the power of the mind for healing.

Such stories are usually presented in the media, either on official channels and programmes or through personal social media, as inspirational: "If she could, others can", or "If I could, you can". In the case of Kate Allatt, the BBC programme presents her as an extraordinary woman with an extraordinary recovery, who beat LIS and its poor prognosis by the power of will. In the case of Patricia, through her Facebook account, she portrays her perseverance, hard work, and power of the mind, and is admired by her followers: "Those who know me say I am an example to follow", she says.

In the social presentation of persons with disabilities in the media (TV, press, magazines, blogs, etc.) it is common to find extraordinary examples of persons who are presented as heroes that beat, endure, and cope with physical constraints and functional disabilities, following the *supercrip* model or stereotype of disability. Those extraordinary examples might be inspirational for some, but may also be a source of frustration and feelings of failure for others who, despite their own will and hard work, could not recover. As with many other chronic conditions, and the paradigmatic example of cancer, the cultural discourse values a fighting attitude, maintaining the hope and positivity associated with getting better (Good et al. 1990; Lupton 1994; Saillant 1990). This notion of willpower or mind power for healing is a social and cultural discourse embedded in a neoliberal context, in which sick persons must do their best to recover and become productive again (Hay 2010; Masana 2011; Parsons 1991). In both the medical and the social spheres, the *restitution narrative* (Frank 1995) is promoted as the preferred cultural option. However, people with LIS might have no option to recover, whether partially or completely. Frank has previously noted that the restitution narrative no longer works for certain chronic illnesses (Frank 1995). And, I add, it is much less applicable for severe disabilities with an uncertain prognosis like LIS. Precisely for this reason, the culturally, socially, and medically promoted discourses of hard work and willpower to recover from LIS are nothing more than a fallacy that adds moral suffering to people with LIS.

## Final considerations

As we have seen, the *certain uncertainty* of LIS recovery works as follows: even without proper knowledge and a guarantee of recovery, some individuals choose to work hard and tirelessly to recover (without knowing to what extent), while others do not. The reasons are varied: their personal and health situation, professional help, resources, family support, living circumstances, financial situation, etc. Therefore, each case must be analysed individually; there is no common rule, despite a dominant cultural and medical discourse that promotes fighting to recover, or at least to improve the health condition. Fighting for recovery is, in a way, fighting uncertainty, fighting the odds, fighting doctors' knowledge: "Sometimes I felt like my recovery was one continual fight: me against the medical profession", Kate writes in her memoir (Allatt and Stokes 2011: 150). It is an attempt to prove to oneself or to others that one was right and others were wrong: "I want to prove wrong the persons who have written me off!" (Allatt and Stokes 2011: 108). In other words, it is to regain some control over their bodies and lives that have been, altered, shattered, disrupted by LIS. However, those victory narratives can be and are only written afterwards if recovery was successful.

Seeing the lack, or misleading nature, of information on recovery that patients and families receive, recommendations for good professional practice could include advising health professionals to carefully consider what information they share with their patients about the possibility of recovery: sustaining hope for recovery, not giving too much hope, or none at all. They should also be extremely careful when disclosing, or not, other patients' partial or full recovery. To my knowledge, and according to the data, most patients and families are not aware that full recovery is an option. In fact, what people with LIS (and their relatives) are told about recovery is crucial and has to do with ethical medical practice (caring for and sharing information with patients) and with the issue of decision-making for both professionals and patients (Bernat 2020). How can patients and their families take decisions concerning their care and future lives if they are not aware of their possibilities or probabilities of recovery?

As with many chronic conditions, LIS cannot be cured, and most persons will not recover. In pursuing recovery, we could say that some do not abandon hope: hope to gain access to the *kingdom of the well* (Sontag 1977), hope toward restoring their life before the illness (Frank 1995). Curiously, their narratives are centred on recovery and not on the notion of hope, as I had initially thought. This does not mean that they are hopeless. On the contrary, they keep hoping, but do not express it in a direct way. Paradoxically, this desire or expectation to recover, that would fit the restitution narrative model, does not always work, as it does with many chronic conditions, "because it sets up expectations that are unlikely to be met" (Garret 2001: 100): the restitution narrative is for acute conditions, not for chronic ones. Therefore, with chronic LIS, as with other chronic conditions, hope for recovery could be considered a "false hope" (Garret 2001) and it resembles what Mattingly finds:

> [...] cultivating a hopeful stance is paradoxical; it involves an ongoing conversation with embittered despair. To hope is to be reminded of what is not and what might never be. (Mattingly 2010: 3)

For people with LIS, if *certain uncertainty* is sustained, hope for recovery remains a possibility, however faint. Indeed, certainty would crash hope and all possibility.

## Acknowledgements

I am very grateful to the research participants for their valuable contributions. I am also grateful to the colleagues at the *MAAH XI conference* (2021) for their comments to a previous shorter draft of this manuscript, and to the editors of this volume, Bernhard Hadolt and Andrea Stöckl, for their support and insights into the final manuscript. My gratitude to Fatima Raja for her dedicated proofreading of this chapter.

## References

Albrecht, Gary L., and Patrick J. Devlieger. 1999. The Disability Paradox: High Quality of Life Against All Odds. Social Science & Medicine 48: 977–988.

ALIS (Association du Locked-in Syndrome). 2017. Les 20 ans d'ALIS. La lettre n° 29 d'ALIS (November). Available at: https://alis-asso.fr/wp-content/uploads/2019/03/Lettre_d_alis_29.pdf

Allatt, Kate, and Alison Stokes. 2011. Running Free: Breaking Out from Locked-In Syndrome. Bedlinog: Accent Press Ltd.

Bauer, Gerrit, Franz Gerstenbrand, and Erik Rumpl. 1979. Variables of the Locked-in Syndrome. Journal of Neurology 221: 77–91.

Bernat, James L. 2020. Medical Decision Making by Patients in the Locked-in Syndrome. Neuroethics 13: 229–238.

Bruno, Marie-Aurélie, Frédéric Pellas, Caroline Schnakers, Philippe Van Eeckhout, Jan Bernheim, Karl-Heinz, François Damas, Marie-Elisabeth Faymonville, Gustave Moonen, Serge Goldman, and Steven Laureys. 2008. Le Locked-In Syndrome: La Conscience Emmurée. [Blink and You Live: The Locked-in Syndrome]. Revue Neurologique 164(4): 322–335.

Carballo, Jose Carlos. 2005. El síndrome de cautiverio en zapatillas [The Locked-In Syndrome in Slippers]. Burgos: Rico Adrados SL.

Casanova, Emanuela, Rosa E. Lazzari, Sergio Lotta, and Anna Mazzucchi. 2003. Locked-in Syndrome: Improvement in the Prognosis After an Early Intensive Multidisciplinary Rehabilitation. Archives of Physical Medicine and Rehabilitation 84(6): 862–867.

Chisholm, Nick, and Grant Gillet. 2005. The Patient's Journey: Living with Locked-in Syndrome. *BMJ* 331: 94–97.

Doble, Jennifer E., Andrew J. Haig, Christopher Anderson, and Richard Katz. 2003. Impairment, Activity, Participation, Life Satisfaction, and Survival in Persons with Locked-in Syndrome for Over a Decade: Follow-up on a Previously Reported Cohort. The Journal of Head Trauma Rehabilitation 18(5): 435–444.

Frank, Arthur W. 1995. The Wounded Storyteller: Body, Illness and Ethics. Chicago: The University of Chicago Press.

Garret, Catherine. 2001. Sources of Hope in Chronic Illness. Health Sociology Review 10(2): 99–107.

Good, Mary-Jo Del Vecchio, Byron Good, Cynthia Schaffer, and Stuart E. Lind. 1990. American Oncology and the Discourse on Hope. Culture, Medicine and Psychiatry 14: 59–79.

Halan, Taras, Juan Fernando Ortiz, Dinesh Ready, Abbas Altamimi, Abimbola O. Ajibowo, and Stephanie P. Fabara. 2021. Locked-In Syndrome: A Systematic Review of Long-Term Management and Prognosis. Cureus 13(7): e16727. https://doi.org/10.7759/cureus.16727

Hay, M. Cameron. 2010. Suffering in a Productive World: Chronic Illness, Visibility, and the Space beyond Agency. American Ethnologist 37(2): 259–274.

Hocker, Sarah, and Eelco F.M. Wijdicks. 2015. Recovery from Locked-n Syndrome. JAMA Neurology 72: 832–833.

Kleinman, Arthur. 1988. The Illness Narratives: Suffering, Healing, and the Human Condition. New York: Basic Books.

Kleinman, Arthur. 2006. What Really Matters: Living a Moral Life amidst Uncertainty and Danger. New York: Oxford University Press.

Lupton, Deborah. 1994. Medicine as Culture: Illness, Disease and the Body in Western Societies. London: Sage.

Masana, Lina. In press; N.d. Methodological Challenges When Conducting Ethnographic Research with Persons that Cannot Talk or Move (provisional title).

Masana, Lina. 2011. Invisible Chronic Illnesses Inside Apparently Healthy Bodies. *In* Of Bodies and Symptoms: Anthropological Perspectives on their Social and Medical Treatment. Sylvie Fainzang and Claudie Haxaire, eds. Pp. 127–149. Tarragona: Publicacions URV- Col·lecció Antropologia Mèdica.

Masana, Lina, and Fernando Vidal. 2020. Antropologia i fenomenologia de la síndrome de captiveri [Anthropology and Phenomenology of the Locked-in Syndrome]. Arxiu d'Etnografia de Catalunya, Notes de Recerca 21: 224–230.

Masana, Lina, and Fernando Vidal. 2023. The Lockdown of the Locked-in: Experiences of Persons with Locked-in Syndrome during COVID-19 Pandemic. Disability & Society. https://doi.org/10.1080/09687599.2023.2279484

Masana, Lina, and Fernando Vidal. In press; N.d. Communicating Through Persons and Devices in the Locked-In Syndrome.

McCusker, Elizabeth A., Richard A. Rudick, Gerald W. Honch, and Robert C. Griggs. 1982. Recovery from the 'locked-in' syndrome. Archives of Neurology 39: 145–147.

Mattingly, Cheryl. 2010. The Paradox of Hope: Journeys through a Clinical Borderland. Berkeley: University California Press.

Parsons, Talcott. 1991 [1951]. The Social System. London: Routledge.

Patterson, James R., and Martin Grabois. 1986. Locked-in Syndrome: A Review of 139 Cases. Stroke 17: 758–764.

Plum, Fred, and Jerome B. Posner. 1966. The Diagnosis of Stupor and Coma. Philadelphia: FA Davis.

Rousseau, Marie-Christine, Karine Baumstarck, Marine Alessandrini, Véronique Blandin, Thierry Billette de Villemeur, and Pascal Auquier. 2015. Quality of Life in Patients with Locked-in Syndrome: Evolution over a 6-Year Period. Orphanet Journal of Rare Diseases 10: 88. https://doi.org/10.1186/s13023-015-0304-z

Saillant, Francine. 1990. Discourse, Knowledge and Experience of Cancer: A Life Story. Culture, Medicine and Psychiatry 14(1): 81–104.

Sontag, Susan. 1977. Illness as Metaphor. New York: Farrar, Straus and Giroux.

Vidal, Fernando. 2020. Phenomenology of the Locked-in Syndrome: An Overview and Some Suggestions. Neuroethics 13: 119–143.

# 13 Figurations of Feasting on Fermented Food in Four Remote Regions of Switzerland

## With Hope, for Health, at Home

*Elisabeth Hsu*

## Preamble

In the opening scene to his monograph *The Pasteurization of France*, Bruno Latour (1988) presents us with the military "genius" of the Russian general Kutuzov who won the battle in Tarutino over the *Grande Armée* led by Napoleon in 1812 (ibid.: 3). In other words, a military metaphor underlay medical success in the 19th century, and the military target of combating microbes quickly became the predominant metaphor for the biomedical control of acute infectious disease. The 21st century, by contrast, is riddled by chronic conditions (Manderson and Smith-Morris 2010; Fainzang and Haxaire 2011; Nissen and Risør 2018), to the effect that differentiating between infectious and non-infectious disease has become obsolete, both in the northern and southern hemisphere (Whyte 2012; 2014). Chronic conditions require care (Mol 2008), not necessarily self-medication (Fainzang 2017), but social care, which paradoxically is delivered increasingly through technological devices (Pols 2014).

So, germ theory advocated the combat of microbes in order to unspecifically prevent and specifically treat acute infections. Yet current health care is encumbered by chronic conditions. This requires a rethinking of medical principles. As research on the microbiome has shown (e.g. Hendy et al. 2021), fermented food has long been recognised as tasty and nutritious (due to a co-evolution of the human gut and specific microbes in its host's habitat). Furthermore, as will be argued here, fermented food is often psychotropic and modulates affect as well as atmosphere. This means it can be affectively uplifting, making people "feel lighter" (Hsu 2012), which is a "somatic mode of attention" (Csordas 1993) that can result in dispositions experienced as health-enhancing. To be sure, no claim is made here that feasting on fermented food is the one and only universal formula for treating and preventing 21st century chronic conditions. Rather, we merely can hope to preliminarily explore which features of the sociality that feasting on fermented food generates are experienced as health-enhancing by the people who do so.

In Hendy et al. (2021), some authors foreground the interlocking of temporalities as essential to fermentation, others point out the multiple materialities that need to be mutually attuned to effect place making. In both cases microbial cultivation is known to be fraught with uncertainties as is any artistic co-creation. Uncertainty is in the case of fermentation generally experienced less as a threat than as a challenge that invites "trying out", playfulness and gentle probing. After some general reflections, we shall focus on those "figurations of fermentation" that can provide care for chronic conditions as an "art of the hearth".

## Government-instigated health promotion: Initial reflections

In January 2013 I was struck to see in one of Lucerne 's public busses, a governmental health promotion that advocated socialising as preventive health measure, advertising weekly singing in choirs and dancing classes, all for free. The advert was issued by the Swiss Ministry of Health (BAG) which is staffed mostly by medical professionals. I was intrigued to see that they promoted socialising as preventive medicine—not just any odd socialising but a socialising through rhythms of movement and music. What a sensible health measure against conditions like chronic back pain, I thought, as they are known to be aggravated through isolation and loneliness (e.g. Honkasalo 2001).

A comparable concern, specifically targeting rural communities, was at the time aimed at preventing social fragmentation. It was launched not by the Ministry of Health but by the Bureau of Tourism. Among the communal activities it encouraged were events of socialising during the four weeks before Christmas in the *Adventszeit.* It was those convivial events that were marked by a particular sociality which was brought about, not least by feasting on fermented food. To be sure, feasting on fermented food was not advertised by the BAG as healthful. On the contrary, excessively snacking and drinking beer, wine and liquors is known to cause health problems such as overweight. And yet, there are aspects of cultivating and consuming microbes central to what we shall call "figurations of fermentation" which have a health-potential for everyone involved, also those suffering from chronic conditions. Before examining this claim with circumspection, the term "figuration" needs to be explained.

## Figurations of fermentation: Some theory

Why speak of "figurations" rather than of "social structures"? The latter describe a synchronous socio-political order, while Norbert Elias's (1937) notion of figuration aims to foreground people's affective engagement, as instigated through specific bodily routines. Elias was trail blazing in this regard, being interested in how individual bodily urges like eating, sleeping, and defecating, and the strong affective drives that accompany them, became socialised. The notion of "figuration" which he coined would account for trends in historical developments of how people's "psychic household" changed over several hundred years. While his work has recently been taken up by medical anthropologists who speak of "transfigurations" (e.g. Mattes et al. 2020), "fermentation" has not been discussed as an aspect of his figurational sociology. In fact, it has barely been discussed in medical anthropology (one notable exception is Devish 1993), apart from science studies on the microbiome (e.g. Paxson 2013). In contrast to the notion of culture, speaking of "figurations of fermentation" foregrounds affective processes and the atmospheric, and in so far they also pertain to changes in the "body ecologic" (Hsu 1999: 78; 2002). [1] Fermentation is then a mode of interconnecting with the locality and its specific materialities (inclusive of microbes), and towards the making of place that can generate feelings of belonging (Feld and Basso 1996). However, given the many uncertainties inherent to any process of fermentation, their outcome is also uncertain. Figurations of fermentation have thus affinity with "ritual terroirs" (Chau 2021), which are not unchanging, but always already in the course of being transformed precisely through the ritual practices that connect them to the locality. In the *Adventszeit* social relations would be expected to be experienced, in figurations brought about by feasting on fermented foods, through a celebration of locality in a jolly and joyful manner.

Medical anthropology has furthermore been affected by the ontological turn (Henare et al. 2007; Holbraad and Pedersen 2017: 1–29). When investigating "figurations of fermentation", we shall therefore be particularly attentive to specific materialities of the locality. In general, feasting on fermented food involves body techniques and social practices arising from a long-term hands-on engagement with the locality one inhabits, and hence is bound to reinforce one's "emplacement" (Howes 2005) or "empotment" into it (Hsu 2022: chapter 3). Yet, the very processes that enable emplacement and empotment have also the potential, as Chau (2021) shows vis-a-vis "ritual terroir", to completely transform the locality. Relevant for us here is merely that some of these "doings" ultimately can be health-affirming.

1 The body ecologic, like the body politic, does not have the clearly drawn out boundaries of the representative classical Greek body (Hsu 1999: 83), but comprehends social practice in terms of a body moving through space, enskilling into and becoming entangled with an ecology that it both shapes and is shaped by (see also Laplante 2016).

Yet the growth and cultivation of microbes that enable fermentation, which is a regulated process, is always accompanied by a tickle of uncertainty.

## The argument: From the militant combat of microbes ...

When thinking today about microbes, Bruno Latour's (1988) first monograph comes to mind. It was based on his doctoral thesis. His method was traditional: it was concerned with semiotics. Yet the results of Latour's study were revolutionary: "... [S]ociologists of science think they are very clever because they have explained hygiene [i.e. the social movement of the hygienists] in terms of class struggle, the infrastructure and power ...", Latour said, while pointing out that, "the exact sciences elude social analysis not because they are distant or separated from them, but because they revolutionize the very conception of society and of what it comprises" (ibid.: 38).

"We cannot form society with the social alone. We have to add the action of the microbes," Latour continued, "... millions of omnipresent, terribly effective, often dangerous, and quite invisible microbes" (ibid.: 35 and 38). He reinforced this by saying: "Society can exist, live, and survive only thanks to the constant intervention of microbes ..." (ibid.: 37). In a medical encounter there is not merely patient and practitioner, there is also a *tertium quid* participating in this social event. This *tertium quid* is the microbe.

Pasteur's contribution was a fulcrum: He made the enemy visible (ibid.: 34): It was the microbe. As Latour (1988: 43, 47, 48) puts it: "The hygienists had been at war and were fighting on all fronts, ... They were everywhere, but were everywhere weak ... The hygiene that took over the doctrine of microbes became stronger and simpler, more structured."

Bruno Latour famously claims how in the 19th century Pasteur's focus on the microbe not merely led to the preventive medical practice of the pasteurisation of milk, but also to the 'pasteurisation of France' in so far as the study of microbes was not only to become central to the natural sciences, but actually transformed the understanding in the social sciences of what society was. Accounting for the microbe as a *tertium quid* gave rise to an understanding of society as an association. Sociology should be "not the science of the social, but of associations" (Latour 1988: 40).

## ... to figurations of fermentation

> Biologically, fermentation is ... defined as a process of anaerobic digestion and decay. It differs from combustion in that it involves micro-organisms [e.g. yeast] whose metabolism does not require oxygen to break down large organic

> molecules into smaller ones [e.g. sugar is metabolized into alcohols and carbon-dioxide] (Latour 1988: 40; information in square brackets added by author).

However, to understand the role of fermented foods when feasting—with hope, for health, at home—, Emile Durkheim's understanding of fermentation may be more relevant, and his understanding of the "collective effervescence" that feasting on fermented food and drink causes. Fermentation is here associated with a bubbling sense of life and effervescence (Durkheim 2015; Hsu 2019).

Like all organic matter that rots, fermented foodstuffs have strong odours and a distinctive taste that people either like or dislike. The predilection for specific fermented food stuffs is an acquired taste (Bourdieu 1984). Yet, rather than suggesting that the strengthening of national identity and nationalistic sentiment were health-enhancing, Ingold's (2000: 349–61, chapter 19) concept of skills and enskilment foregrounds the hands-on and technical facilitation of fermentation. This frames fermentation as a practice of enskilling oneself into the environment. As Ingold (2000: 197) puts it, agency is found in "rhythm" or in "the successive building up and resolution of tension" (Langer 1953: 126, quoted in Ingold ibid.), "a complex interweaving of very many concurrent cycles" (ibid.). In summary, rhythm interlaces a network of interdependent tasks, each with its specific resonances, that are embodied, and part of a generative field (ibid.: 200). It is not a matter of one adapting to another, say, people adapting to place. Rather, agency resides in an interdependent rhythmic entanglement.

By framing fermentation as a culinary art that prepares local food eaten by locals, people are seen to be enskilling themselves into their "body ecologic" and becoming part of its materialities, its taskscapes, its locality-specific spatial rhythms and resonances. The water quality matters, the inorganic mineral composition of the soil, the plant and animal species that this locality accordingly attracts, the microbes and microclimates they produce, the temperatures, the smells and tastes all matter. Culinary techniques for preparing fermented food differ accordingly in different places, and resist standardisation. To be sure, this attentiveness to locality-specific natural and ritual terroir applies also to the body politic of locally-produced fermented foods, which in the past was not merely locality-fixated. Rather, precisely due to their local specificities the locality became enmeshed with trade connecting into the wider world.

So, the genius of the [male] military strategist at the apex of a hierarchical body politic is no longer in the limelight. Rather, interdependent rhythms and resonances, finely interlaced, secure well-being. Chronic conditions become manageable, less through boundary control and the will to exterminate all microbes but more through the recognition that long-term care for the other, involves an intercorporeal sharing, which in the case of fermentation would be in accord with an artful regulation of the proliferation of some local microbial populations.

## Figurations of fermentation

In what follows, four vignettes are presented that relate the lived experience of how people participated in different processes of producing and consuming fermented foods in remote parts of Switzerland. As argued here, they thereby "empotted" themselves into a locality in ways that are conducive to health. The notion of *empotment* (Hsu 2022: chapter 3) elaborates on that of *emplotment* (Mattingly 1998; 2010) in so far as both put single measures of treatment in wider perspective, through narration and/or negotiations over the texturing of the surrounding spaces: empotment highlights person-to-place interdependency. The focus is on "cultivation", both self-cultivation and the cultivation of the bacteria enabling fermentation processes.

The following ethnographic vignettes reflect on my visits of my *Aussteiger* (non-careerist) friends who settled in different language-speaking communities in rural, if not remote parts of Switzerland (remote in so far as they were outside the reach of the national railway, the *Schweizerische Bundesbahn*, SBB, but they could be accessed by the *Postauto* or local trains, and, of course, the private car). These vignettes report on chance encounters, and they should not be read as resulting from a carefully designed research project. Hence, they will not be subject to a strict comparativist analysis. The question we examine is what is specific about the diverse ways in which culinary techniques that facilitate fermentation create socialities that have salubrious potential.

Admittedly, the methods underlying this research are unusual, but they are in keeping with other anthropological fieldwork. In their introduction to *Search after method*, Laplante, Gandsman and Scobie (2020) call into question the usefulness of "method" for anthropological fieldwork and, instead, advocate "ways of doing anthropology as an improvisatory joining in with normative processes" (ibid.: 4).

So, the four vignettes are based on findings derived from a professionally learned attitude of being ethical and reflective as anthropologist, and they are also methodological insofar as these encounters have been submitted to criteria of ethnographic rigour. They are personal reflections on the question of what makes some of the figurations of fermentation so distinctive. What kinds of health-enhancing potential is contained in these recently revived, yet partially age-old practices? If they do celebrate the local body ecologic and, as we will see below, an egalitarian body politic, are they more of a problem than a welcome addition to the hierarchically structured health regimes of modern nation states?

The first vignette is from the Italian-speaking canton Ticino in southern Switzerland. It requires the reader to infer from the photos of material culture the forms of social relatedness that shaped the production and consumption of fermented foods. The two following vignettes are about an initiative launched by a semi-governmental agency to revitalise the rural parts of French- and Romansch-speaking Switzerland by [re-]introducing *Adventssingen*. Finally, the fourth vignette from the German-speaking canton of Appenzell presents an encounter where no fermented foods were eaten.

## 1. Wine and cheese from cool caves in the Ticino

My attention was for the first time drawn to fermentation as a process that straddles the interface of "nature and culture," while looking at the black and white photographs selected for publication on "peasant art and architecture" in *Grotti, Splüi, Cantine* by Ralph Hut and Thomas Burla (1995). This publication was made possible only after the authors roamed for many years the steep mountain slopes that were covered by chestnut forests and interspersed with small meadows, some terraced, testifying to intense agricultural activity in the past. The photographers spent hours, if not occasionally an entire day, together or on their own, in front of an object, just to get the "right light".

Looking with one of the authors at these photos of now deserted cellars and caves triggered conversation about how, in the 19th century, wine and cheese would be enjoyed on Sunday after mass when villagers would migrate from the church to the outskirts of the village and congregate by the *grotto*. If a party became particularly jolly, they would start dancing. The granite dance platforms, stone benches and tables were providing a sadly silent testimony of this today. These festival platforms occupied, at the margins of often completely deserted villages now, a liminal space between the village and the forest. Their architectural structures reinforced this sense of liminality by artfully complementing the natural rock formation with stone masonry. This secured the "culturally"-monitored "natural" conditions for the fermentation process. In these cool, dark, and hidden spaces of the *grotto* constancy was cultivated, a constancy of a certain humidity and temperature that fosters life, namely, the many generations of bacterial lives that must be maintained throughout many years to mature both cheese and wine. These processes were monitored in subtle ways. They involved, in particular, body techniques effecting ultimately Ticino farmers' enskilment into their environment. For measuring the right temperature and humidity, for instance, no thermometer and no hydrograph was necessary. Observation of qualitative indicators sufficed—a certain spider species for instance, or rather, its traces, the much-welcomed spider webs at the entrance of a grotto—as an old man had revealed in a conversation with one of the photographers in broken Italian. Given their psychotropic and nurturing effects, these carefully monitored slowly fermenting products from the cool spaces of the *grotto* no doubt generated social heat in affectively intense transitional moments on the village's periphery.

This village-wide sociality of feasting on fermented foods when celebrating liminality, has now been discontinued. Yet the architectural remains testify to a figuration of fermentation of a once densely populated valley that thrived on people cultivating bacteria in the dark, yet due to decay, fecund spaces between granite rock and artful masonry.

## 2. "La goutte" dans le Petit-Val: The dew-drop that effects social heat

More than fifteen years later, in 2010, I was to experience such village-wide social heat that fermented food can generate. On the French-speaking borders in the region of the Jura, Paul, who after graduation in biology became a non-careerist, fetched me at the federal train station a fifteen-minute car drive away from the remote village in which he had built up an ecological mushroom farm but that, a decade later, he decided to sell for the sake of pursuing his interest in biology which led to a career, after all, in Basel's *Life Science* industrial complex. As he parked the car in front of his neighbour's house, he said: "Today, we are not cooking, you'll have to feed yourself on snacks". Little did I know that the "snacking" would consist of a feasting on fermented foods. We entered a large, old, stone built Jurassian farm house through a dark, narrow corridor that led us past the front room, i.e., the old living room, and the kitchen, and that opened into a large new dining room. About twenty people—men, women, adolescents, and few children—were busily chatting and laughing, drinking, and eating. The hostess had baked fresh white breads, one sweet, the other salty. This fermented staple was offered together with cured meats: this year's juicy *jambon*, two different kinds of lard, and then the fumigated *jambon* from a previous year, a true delicacy. Once the white breads were eaten, black bread was offered, and fresh fruits, then Christmas cookies. I had accepted a cup of hot and spicy tea, made of fermented leaf, from the hostess, but soon switched to the *Schnaps* that the host was offering, unaware that most guests had the courtesy to decline his servings; they left shortly before nine o'clock but, hours later, I found myself among a group of die-hards still sitting on the sofa.

One bottle after the other was brought out of the cellar. The host's father had been the only one in the village who had had a license to burn *Schnaps;* the villagers today all had to go to a distillery in a neighbouring village. We had started with *plumes*, then came the *poires*, the *apricots*, the *quinces*, the *pommes* and the *damassines*. These *gouttes* were *de vraie bio* (real organic-produce)—no one went through the trouble to spray the orchards with pesticides as they were considered "too unproductive".

Unlike fermented beers, these distilled drinks that were made of fermented produce from the orchard, had a high alcohol content, well of over 50 percent, as the old Jämy had once impressed on me (see photo in Brahier 1988: 45). Here in the Petit-Val, in which there was not even a church, villagers had their own ways of doing things, even if it went against "the laws made in Bern".

It must have been past mid-night when the host opened a particularly cherished bottle, and offered us a prohibited drink, a liquor made from the potato! As the potato was the main staple, its distillation had been prohibited by law at least since the two world wars, and the prohibition has not been lifted since. The host praised its refined taste: "It has a fineness that cannot be obtained from fruits".

While up to 1988 the municipality (then numbering 114 residents in total) was still predominantly inhabited by agriculturalists (15 houses out of 36 inhabited ones) and, generally speaking, milk production had steadily increased in the previous fifty years (Brahier 1988: 61), only two farmers were still in the village in 2010 (and six in the municipality as whole).[2] Switzerland has a policy of paying farmers at highly subsidised rates (a policy that would instantly stop with its becoming part of in the EU). Some consider this policy to reflect environmentalist considerations, and they support it, emphasizing the role of the 21st century farmer as "landscape gardener" (rather than as agricultural producer), others sigh about the conservatism of the Swiss farmer's union, interested only in getting ever more subsidies.

So, how exactly was the *goutte* made? Paul took me to the owner of a large old-style Jurassian farmhouse that one entered through a large hangar-like space. In this one space were shoe racks and pots of geraniums, bicycles, and skis, and a newly installed 5000 litre tank for storing hot water (from the solar panels on the roof). It was in this un-heated liminal zone between the freezing cold outside and the lived-in parts of the house that fermentation happened. We were shown several blue and grey plastic tons and half a dozen of very large balloon-shaped jars, and these fifty-litre bottles were filled with a transparent liquid.

Out of a one-hundred-litre blue plastic ton filled with damsons that were chopped up and stirred from time to time, to make sure the yeast was well distributed, people expected to distil 6–7 litres. It was local yeast that grew on the fruits, I learned later, no industrial yeast would be added. The fermentation of the damsons took perhaps six weeks at the relatively low temperatures of the Petit-Val. Then its container was closed to make the milieu in it completely anaerobic, before taking it to the distillery.

"Try some *gentiane!*" Our neighbour who had been showing us around his premises now uncorked one of the balloon-shaped bottles. *Gentianea lutea* is on the list of endangered species in Switzerland, but since it was a weed on the Jurassic

2 Most of the ca 90 villagers living in about 30 households were in employment in a nearby township, many had immigrated from other places, mostly from German-speaking cantons, but also from France (Bretagne), Germany, Turkey, Italy, and elsewhere. The foreign nationals constituted about one fifth of the current residents, not much different from the Swiss national average. One of the main employers of the commuters was the hospital in the nearby township.

meadows up there on the hill, he had obtained special permission from the municipality to dig them out. Three hundred-litre-tons could be filled by the washed and chopped root materials dug out in an afternoon; but each ton resulted in merely one litre of this most cherished liquor. *Gentiane* had a special taste, he said; it was very bitter, like a medicine. In fact, it was a medicine!, used both as a therapeutic and preventive home remedy.[3]

That evening, we went to a *fenêtre* (window) of a bungalow at the far end of the village. It was a newly invented tradition that each villager decorated a window of their house and light it for the first time on the day of hosting the villagers, and thereafter daily up to Christmas. It was a recent government initiative for revitalising remote areas. The window today showed a snowman amid nicely arranged pine twigs, and it showed the date, 6th December; the window on the following day showed a fairy-tale snow landscape made of fluffy cottons, through which cursed a small electric train; yet another one showed a sun set on a palm beach in the Indian ocean. Each window was different and distinctive.

Paul, his partner Regula and I were the first. The hosts were a recently remarried couple from German-speaking Switzerland; he had been a widower, she a divorcee. They hosted us in their garage; a dozen of white plastic chairs was arranged around a gas lamp and a plastic Christmas tree. "It cost only 15 francs in Aldi's" (ca 12 Euros), the hostess chided. Food was neatly arranged on a table, ranging from canapés and biscuits to nuts, mandarins and pralines, all from Aldi's, and a home-made cake. A large thermos flask provided hot tea, and since our hosts had heard about the jolly drinking party the night before, they soon started offering a newly bought bottle of *Kirsch* (cherry liquor) to those who took coffee. The guests were fewer in number this evening; some were familiar faces, others new. Gradually the garage filled with the chatter of conversation, allowing us an hour later to slip away unnoticed.

The following evening the house next door was host, it had snowed overnight, and temperatures had plummeted to minus fifteen degrees Celsius. Meanwhile, the feting house was brimming with vitality, hot and loud, with hordes of children and many new faces. Sweet hot punch was served, home-made bread and an oven-warm *quiche*. The complex flavours that the culinary art of fermentation produces were well on course of being side-lined by a predilection for sugar. Home-made Christmas cookies followed, and other sweets, after we had already left, as we stayed for a little less than an hour.

When Paul and I thereafter sat at the kitchen table of his house, I marvelled over the explosion of social heat in this village which otherwise looked rather quiet. We were nibbling on a dark bread and a hard cheese and shared a bottle of red wine. Evidently, these were fermented foods too, but ordinary ones of the everyday, rather than the high quality, freshly prepared fermented food offered when feasting. Red

3 Today, there is a shop in his house that sells precisely such liquors: https://gagygnole.ch/

wine and bread are also the meal of the sacred communion, I thought in this context; in this respect Christian faith accommodates to the modest means of the commoner. Until late that evening Paul and I talked about village life, inclusive of problems with neighbours and land disputes.

Nevertheless, when in the following year, as I visited Paul shortly after Christmas and inquired about the feting, he remarked that the atmosphere in the village had changed. Disputes over ridiculous issues had divided it. Only six families had made a *fenêtre* and hosted villagers in the period before Christmas. It was an invented tradition anyway, Paul added. 2010 had been the first year they ever practised it.

This vignette highlights that a psycho-tropically-enforced social heat is an important aspect of figurations of fermentation. Notably, the affective states of heightened gaiety often had a rebellious tinge, celebrating autonomy in a remote locality. The fermented food that was home-made was considered particularly tasty, and also healthy, while the human warmth and humorous banter around the hearth was both relaxing and uplifting.

## 3. Nus colliains (we hold together)—Engadin mobil

It was in the week before Christmas in 2011 that the long-awaited snow finally fell. Twenty centimetres of snow had fallen at night and another twenty throughout the day. Yet, rather than enveloping the village in silence, as new snow typically does, a frenzy of activity reverberated in it as the loud motors of Lazzarini trucks with frighteningly huge wheels, the height of an adult, pushed the snow around. "War on snow", I commented, as Miranda met me at the local train station of the RhB (Rhätische Bahn). Indeed, on that very day a woman had been killed by one such truck in the administrative centre of the region, she said as we were walking to her house at the upper end of the village.

Her three children were waiting for us in the hall of their three-storey high refurbished traditional stone house, ready to go to the *Adventssingen*. They knew me from the year before, and I invited myself for the day it happened this year. "It is an invented tradition," Miranda warned me on the phone. The woman in the village who had overseen tourism had initiated the *Adventssingen* some ten years ago. This woman had retired this year, and now the tourist bureau in the nearby township arranged these village events. So, rather than singing every evening in front of a different house that lit a "window", as the villagers did last year, only three gatherings had been scheduled for this year. The third one, which I attended, was coupled with the apparently first Christmas market the village ever held. This was a "German thing" I was told, overriding in an era of global commercialism the more traditional figurations of celebrating the *Adventszeit*.

When we reached the village square, it was snowing again. Enclosed by several-storey high, large traditional stone houses, the square looked rather picturesque, even if one could not see from there, as otherwise, the nearby alpine peaks. The "window" in front of which we gathered to sing was a rather plain front door. It was decorated with light bulbs shining through small colourful felt lamp shades. The hostess was embarrassed not to have gone into more trouble. On the outside of the door, along the window's bottom edge, she had fixed several bunches of red rowan berries. I noted this with delight. "They get eaten by crows", the hostess replied, and Miranda agreed. Then, a man chipped in saying it had been a heathen custom to make use of them; the church claimed they were poisonous, which they were not. Another villager spontaneously said the same on a later occasion. The mighty church was presented as the supra-regional institution that cheated the locals who however saw through her power game, and resisted her incursions, by continuing to practise their local custom. I noted here a comparable spirit of resistance to the one encountered in the Petit-Val.

In the meantime, a group of people had gathered in front of the inconspicuous house door, whom the hostess each gave a song booklet. We were about fifteen women, some toddlers, a very quiet couple that was not from the village (tourists perhaps?) and one middle aged man. Miranda's eleven-year-old daughter stood next to her but did not sing as she had a sore throat. The first song, no. 5, sounded a bit hesitant. We then sang no. 1, then nos. 10 and 11; they were all in Romansch. Then, suddenly, as the one man in the group was joined by another one, they initiated a song for which the booklet had only text. "Oh no", I heard Miranda saying, "there are no scores." No one cared. The two men then initiated the singing of another song for which the booklet had only text and no scores, and again, they were heartily joined by the others, who evidently knew it well. Life had come into the group! Yet in this moment the hostess decided to collect all booklets and within less than fifteen minutes the singing was over. I was a bit disappointed. Not only had we not sung every refrain of the songs, but the singers had also not been offered any fermented drinks, and the plastic cup of mulled wine on offer cost as much four Swiss francs.

There were now about fifty people on the square, and in the following hour it filled up even more. Some villagers had put some old furniture on sale, others had brought food, one made Belgian *gauffres* over a little camping gas fire, the other served barley soup out of the thermos flasc. "It is typical for this locality", Miranda said, "they do not buy food off each other but each family eats their own". The prices were forbidding, also for the foreigner. Village folklore was evidently on its way to being commercialised, and the ambiguous complexity in taste that fermented food and drink often has, was replaced with either sweet dishes or salty drinks, and vice-versa.

Ten years ago, Miranda explained, when the singing was first introduced, villagers had apparently not known how to handle it. They had outdone each other, and apparently, before long, too much of the cured meat and liquor had been consumed before Christmas. So, the municipality recommended that people only gather to sing in front of a "window", and no one was obliged to host the singers inside the house.

On my visit a year earlier, it was a delight to see that neighbours, i.e., the German-speaking *Zuzüger* (settlers) and the Romansch-speaking locals, were committed to singing together. They sung a variety of tunes out of the song booklet for some good twenty minutes, before gladly accepting the hot fruit tea Miranda had prepared, to which her husband added, for those who so desired, a drop of liquor. To be sure, it was not the best vintage out of the cellar, as I had been offered in the Petit-Val, but a rather bad brandy, as he told me later, a business gift he had received and could not otherwise get rid of. Since it was absolutely freezing cold, around minus twenty degrees Celsius, its warming qualities were very much valued and trumped over its awful taste. The entire event was over within the time of an hour. Teacups and song booklets were packed into the house and the children put to bed (or rather, in front of the TV, with their promise to go to bed an hour later), while the parents and myself jumped into their car to get to an experimental theatre musical—*Roti Roesli* (little red roses)—in the neighbouring village.

"The first time I came across this practice", Miranda explained, "was in Mexico. I used to stay in a convent, gathering strength—and restoring my health—before returning to the field. Throughout the month of December up to Christmas, the nuns sang every evening in front of a different door. It is a catholic tradition, really, but in the villages of the Unterengadin, except for Tarasp, which is already very Austrian and catholic, we are reformist". Miranda also pointed out that there had been a very old, presumably heathen tradition of singing on three evenings before New Year, rather than before Christmas, undertaken by adolescent girls and boys (Claglüna 2001: 44, "Sitten und Bräuche").

The village history also spoke of the villagers' spirit of resistance: "Wie sich die Ardezer Bauern 1918 einem sinnlosen Diktat aus Bern zur Wehr setzten" (ibid.: 29–34). Some courageous villagers had joined forces against the irrational imperatives from Bern (the federation's capital) and Chur (the canton's capital) to slaughter their cattle that had contracted foot and mouth disease. These village heroes deserve to be named, says the chronicler: "Claglüna, Fimian, Fratschül, Huder, Mengiardi, Marugg, Schucan and Vonzun", and gives their names in bold in the local history text, such that they spring to the eye of any casual reader.

In this context, Heiri Felix came to my mind, a now retired railway builder whom I had met the year before over several beers in one of the Engadiner cellars, as he too had resisted "those in Chur". He had refused to introduce audit culture into his group of workers. As supervisor of some twenty railway workers, he was expected to write a report on the performance of each of them, along a scale from one to six. When he gave them all the best possible mark, his superiors were puzzled and asked him to revise the report. "We are all equal when we work together", Heiri retorted. Only for himself he gave another mark, the lowest possible one. "Why?", his superiors queried. "Were they really no longer aware of the code of honour that was part of the culture among honourable men [in this place]?" Heiri retorted. The egalitarianism of fellowship engendered self-respect.

By singing together—in an egalitarian manner—in front of a window enjoying each other's company and making new acquaintances, the relations between the German and Romansch-speaking, *Zuzüger* and local inhabitants were strengthened. It was expected to facilitate the "empotting" of new and old villagers into their locality. However, in this village commercialised considerations reminiscent of a German *Weihnachtsmarkt* were on the verge of generating sociality primarily through the circulation of money in the public sphere. However folkloristic the Tourist Bureau's recent initiative may have been meant to be, it worked in this village towards a commercialisation of social relations, and a monetised form of relatedness, and discouraged the sociality of *Adventssingen*, which initially had involved the serving of the delicacies resulting from a fine-tuned cultivation of local microbes.

## 4. A baked cake in place of a braided white bread

It was in the morning of Swiss National Day (1st August) in 2012 that I arranged to meet Rebecca and her husband on my way to a family reunion in the canton of Appenzell. I had inherited some twenty-five years earlier from my grandmother a loom that her neighbours held in custody but given that they themselves had reached retirement age and had sold both the house and the land of their farm the year before, space had become scarce. Our conversation centred on a deeply felt attachment to the locality, but fermented food was not offered on this occasion.

I had arrived an hour earlier than expected due to fabulous connections of the local train that had helped transform a once remote place into a suburban area. As Rebecca opened the house door, a waft of a fresh bakery greeted me, which she offered together with an entirely unexpected wave of human warmth. I was sat with my hosts into the cosy *Stube* and made to enjoy the oven-fresh *Gleichschwer* (cake made of equally weighted ingredients), and the coffee, which came with a *gutsch Schnaps* (a drop of liquor). My hosts were ever so grateful to a close relative of mine who had helped them keep the meadow intact that lay in front of their house. The previous owner had sold that land to a land developer, a firm that was to transform the meadow into an apartment block for commuters.

"Can you imagine", said Rebecca, "we fought the village government for over a decade!" They had provided support to a neighbour who went from the municipal to the cantonal, and even to the national level of justice, when finally, their legal process was successful. Thanks to an easement that had been granted to the owner of this neighbour's land in the 17th century, they were finally heard at the national level of justice. However, throughout this time, Rebecca and her husband were outcasts in the village. People would avoid their company as they were seen to oppose lucrative development.

Villagers also tended to take sides with the tenant farmer to whom they had rented out their farm ten years earlier. Appalled by his way of treating their house, land, trees, and animals, they felt compelled to send this tenant farmer a termination of his contract in the very same year his tenancy started. They did so in full awareness that according to Swiss law the minimal period of a tenancy of any farm was ten years. After having to watch how their farm was being "run into the ground", year after year throughout a decade, they wrung themselves through to selling it. They sold it not to one of the contending villagers, but to the second son of a farmer from the catholic part of the canton. In their once distinctively reformist municipality, the selling of their farm to a catholic would make anyone to an outcast, and it no doubt consolidated their outcast position in the village. To be sure, "it was a social thing," Rebecca said, "not that religion really mattered that much".

Interestingly, the study of Christian religion featured more importantly in this study than anyone living in these regions would admit, and yet its historically given incursion into these remote regions had important socio-ecological implications. In the Ticino village the church was situated centrally, and the sociality fuelled by the wine and cheese from the *grotto* took place on the outskirts of the village in a joyous liminality before the exodus to America and the land flight of modernity depopulated the place (Wolf, in Hut and Burla 1995: 5). In the Petit-Val, the church featured through its absence. Here, where no forebears had built a church, an ethos of autonomy, if not rebelliousness was cultivated. And even in the Unterengadin, where alongside the catholic, the reformist church was also present, locals maintained an observable and explicit resistance, as they enacted practices that interlaced heathen with Catholic ones. Figurations of fermentation which kept these localities recognisably autonomous persisted in these areas not merely for gustatory and nutritional reasons, but also for body political ones, and for how they shaped the 'affective household' of the villagers. Interestingly, it was primarily for affective reasons that the social practices so central to the body ecological feasting on fermented foods were discontinued in the Petit-Val and this secluded household.

In this context it occurred to me that it was a special treat to be offered a cake, instead of, for instance, a slice of *Zopf* (braided white bread) to a cup of coffee. Naturally, making bread requires time, the time to ferment (*zum gaa la;* lit. to let it go) takes half an hour at least, and baking a cake takes about the same time. Yet cakes are culturally highly valued, presumably because they contain comparatively expensive ingredients. Bread is made of water and flour, white bread additionally of milk and an egg or two, while cake is made of sugar, butter, eggs, and flour (in the case of a *Gleichschwer* cake, all to equal amounts). A loaf of home-baked bread tends to be offered fresh to large groups of family and friends, but Rebecca and her husband lived a very quiet life; they had for instance no plans to celebrate National Day. The cake was thus not only a special treat for an honoured guest, with whom one wished to speak in quiet conversation, a cake could be preserved for weeks in that characteristic metal storage box for sweets, inaccessible to mice and other pests. Due to its precious ingredients, a cake would not become stale and dry instantly, as does white bread, but could be eaten slowly, day after day, or it could be served to a future guest, particularly if injected with a refreshing zest of lemon.

## Discussion

By viewing fermentation as a culinary art that involves an enskilment into the environment, human beings become part of the rhythms of the landscape and its taskscapes, and the resonances and concurrent cycles that constitute the generative field of any ecologically vibrant locality. Through engaging in the production and consumption of fermented food, people cultivate their connectedness to the locality, socio-politically and ecologically, meaning-wise and substance-wise, epistemologically and ontologically. Social and medical anthropologists speak of "emplacement" or "empotment" and consider such identity-forging processes to enhance people's sense of self in a way that has the potential to be health-enhancing.

Fermentation as a culinary art is not merely a metaphor but also a process that ontologically transforms place. Fermentation involves mutually attuned and regulated "doings" to ensure the delicate and easily disturbed connectedness between the organisms in a specific locality. There is a vulnerability to their associations, and also an uncertainty about whether they will flourish. While living organisms are to a certain extent self-contained and self-interested actors, the "figurations of fermentation" discussed above highlighted the interdependency of human and non-human "associations" in any locality. As food "stuff" fermented products that are digested shape and maintain social relatedness in material ways. Sometimes, forms of social relatedness can be smelled from the characteristic odours that bodies perspire. The local strains of bacteria, in combination with the local qualities of the soils, waters and airs, as well as the organic produce they sustain, assist human beings enthralled by their scent, taste and psycho-tropic effects which work towards modulating their affective household, to further enskil themselves into the locality and develop locality-specific ways of regulating their growth. Yet however locality-specific the fermented produce may be, its taste often appeals also to the foreign guest, rendering the social configurations fermentation gives rise to, to open systems interfacing with trends beyond the locality.

So, while *The Pasteurization of France* relied on a standard scientific eradication method of specific microbes to stop acute infectious disease from spreading in the 19th century, the figurations of fermentation that we discussed above were associations of indivudual distinctiveness orchestrated into a mutually attuned diversity.

The body ecological ethos of autonomy and egalitarianism that their cultivation enabled seemed to be endangered by the all-pervasive commercialisation of the body politic intrinsic to 21st century, in the Engadin, while, on the other hand, in the Petit-Val, precisely the prospects of commerce seemed to secure its future.

Finally, let us relate to fermentation as a culinary art that ensures the continued cultivation of certain microbial species specific to a certain place. Those species benefit from the locality-specific human art of the hearth. So, through such locality-specific human endeavour to achieve health, fermentation cultivates the proliferation of microbes specific to a specific environment. Fermentation as a socio-ecological figuration thus "makes place" by enhancing "interspecies dependence" (Tsing 2012) and "multi-species entanglement" (Kirksey and Helmreich 2010) and "becoming with" (Haraway 2008: 44), which dissolves the boundaries between "making and growing" (Hallam and Ingold 2014). "Living with microbes" and cultivating their habitat through "the art of the hearth", promises, in enabling ways, through caring for each other, to affectively modulate the living with chronic conditions in the 21st century.

## Acknowledgements

First, I would like to thank Bernhard Hadolt and Andrea Stöckl for their colleagiality and perceptive editing. Special thanks go furthermore to my family and lifelong friends for their hospitality between 2010–2012, a period when I was in the "holistic" care that is offered at the Paracelsus source. The article was initially commissioned by Elizabeth Hallam and Tim Ingold (2014) but not ready for publication then. It elaborates on my paper *Encounters with old friends and microbes* presented at the joint international conference on *Encounters and Engagements* organised by the SMA and the EASA medical anthropology network in Tarragona, Spain, 12-14 June 2013.

## References

Bourdieu, Pierre. 1984. Distinction: A Social Critique of the Judgement of Taste. London: Routledge & Kegan Paul.

Chau, Adam. 2021. Ritual Terroir: The Generation of Site-specific Vitality. Archives des Sciences Sociales de Religion 193: 25–54.

Csordas, Thomas J. 1993. Somatic Modes of Attention. Cultural Anthropology 8(2): 135–156.

Devish, René. 1993. Weaving the Threads of Life: The Khita Gyn-Eco-Logical Healing Cult among the Yaka. Chicago: University of Chicago Press.

Durkheim, Émile. 1915 [1912]. The Elementary Forms of the Religious Life: A Study in Religious Sociology. Transl. J. W. Swain. London: Allen and Unwin.

Elias, Norbert. 1937. Ueber den Prozess der Zivilisation. 2 vols. Frankfurt a.M.: Suhrkamp.

Fainzang, Sylvie. 2017. Self-medication and Society: Mirages of Autonomy. Abingdon: Routledge.

Fainzang, Sylvie, and Claudine Haxaire, eds. 2011. Of Bodies and Symptoms: Anthropological Perspectives on Their Social and Medical Treatment (Antropologia Mèdica). Tarragona: Publicacions Universitat Rovira i Virgili.

Feld, Steven, and KeithBasso, eds. 1996. Senses of Place. Santa Fe: School of American Research Press.

Good, Mary-Jo Delvecchio., Paul E. Brodwin, Byron J. Good, and Arthur Kleinman, eds. 1992. Pain as Human Experience: An Anthropological Perspective. Berkeley: University of California Press.

Hallam, Elizabeth, and Tim Ingold, eds. 2014. Making and Growing: Anthropological Studies of Organisms and Artefacts. London: Routledge.

Haraway, Donna. 2008. When Species Meet. Minneapolis: University of Minnesota Press.

Henare, Amiria, Martin Holbraad, and Sari Wastell, eds. 2007. Thinking Through Things: Theorising Artefacts Ethnographically. London: Routledge.

Hendy, Jessica, Matthäus Rest, Mark Aldenderfer, and Christina Warinner. 2021. Cultures of Fermentation: Living with Microbes. An Introduction to Supplement 24. Current Anthropology 62(Supplement 24): 197–206.

Holbraad, Martin, and Morten Pedersen. 2017. The Ontological Turn: An Anthropological Exposition. Cambridge: Cambridge University Press.

Honkasalo, Marja-Liisa. 2001. Vicissitudes of Pain and Suffering: Chronic Pain and Liminality. Medical Anthropology 19(4): 319–53.

Howes, David. 2005. Introduction. *In* Empire of the Senses: the Sensual Culture Reader. D. Howes, ed. Pp. 1–17. Oxford: Berg.

Hsu, Elisabeth. 1999. The Transmission of Chinese Medicine. Cambridge: Cambridge University Press.

Hsu, Elisabeth. 2002. Die drei Koerper – oder sind es vier? Curare 24(1/2): 57–64.

Hsu, Elisabeth. 2012. "Feeling Lighter": Why the Patient's Treatment Evaluation Matters to the Health Scientist. Integrative Medicine Research 1(1): 5–12.

Hsu, Elisabeth. 2019. Durkheim's Effervescence and Its Maussian Afterlife in Medical Anthropology. Durkheimian Studies 23: 76–105.

Hsu, Elisabeth. 2022. Chinese Medicine in East Africa: An Intimacy with Strangers. Oxford: Berghahn.

Ingold, Tim. 2000. The Perception of the Environment: Essays on Livelihood, Dwelling and Skill. London: Routledge.

Kirksey, Eben, and Stefan Helmreich. 2010. The Emergence of Multispecies Ethnography. Cultural Anthropology 25 (4): 545–576.

Langer, Susanne K. 1953: Feeling and Form: A Theory of Art. New York: Charles Scribner's Sons.

Laplante, Julie. 2016. Becoming-Plant: Jamu in Java, Indonesia. *In* Plants and Health: New Perspectives on the Health-Environment-Plant Nexus (Ethnobiology). Elizabeth Anne Olson and John Richard Stepp, eds, Pp. 17–65. Oxford: Berghahn.

Laplante, Julie, Ari Gandsman, and Willow Scobie, eds. 2020. Search after Method: Sensing, Moving, and Imagining in Anthropological Fieldwork. Oxford: Berghahn.

Latour, Bruno. 1988 [1984]. The Pasteurization of France. Transl. A. Sheridan and J. Law. Cambridge, Mass.: Harvard University Press.

Manderson, Leonore, and Carolyn Smith-Morris, eds. 2010. Chronic Conditions, Fluid States: Chronicity and the Anthropology of Illness. New Brunswick: Rutgers University Press.

Mattes, Dominik, Bernhard Hadolt, and Brigit Obrist. 2020. Introduction: Rethinking Sociality and Health through Transfiguration. MAT-Medical Anthropology Theory 7(1): 66–86.

Mattingly, Cheryl. 1998. Healing Dramas and Clinical Plots: The Narrative Structure of Experience. Cambridge: Cambridge University Press.

Mattingly, Cheryl. 2010. The Paradox of Hope: Journeys through a Clinical Borderland. Berkeley: University of California Press.

Mol, Annemarie. 2008. The Logic of Care: Health and the Problem of Patient Choice. London: Routledge.

Nissen, Nina, and Mette B. Risør, eds. 2018. Diagnostic Fluidity: Working with Uncertainty and Mutability. Tarragona: Publicacions Universitat Rovira i Virgili.

Paxson, Heather. 2013. The Life of Cheese: Crafting Food and Value in America. Berkeley: University of California Press.

Pols, Jeanette. 2014. Care at a Distance: On the Closeness of Technology. Amsterdam: Amsterdam University Press.

Tsing, Anna. 2012. Unruly Edges: Mushrooms as Companion Species. Environmental Humanities 1: 141–54.

Whyte, Susan. R. 2012. Chronicity and Control: Framing 'Noncommunicable Diseases' in Africa. *In* Medical Anthropology in Europe: Shaping the Field. Elisabeth Hsu and Caroline Potter, eds., Special Issue,Anthropology and Medicine 19(1): 63–74.

Whyte, Susan. R., ed. 2014. Second Chances: Surviving AIDS in Uganda. Durham, NC: Duke University Press.

## Local histories

Brahier, Jean-Luc. 1988. Société de Laiterie de Souboz 1938–1988. 68 pp. Self-published.

Claglüna, Jon. 2001 [1985]. Ardez: Gemeindechronik. 64 pp. Self-published by Chesa Solena, Pontresina.

Hut, Ralph, and Thomas Burla (photos). 1995. Grotti, Splüi, Cantine: Anonyme Felsarchitektur im Macciatal, Architectura rupestre anonyma nella Valmaggia, Architecture rupestre anonyme dans le val Maggia. With text by Conradin Wolf, pp. 5–10 (in German), 11–15 (in Italian), 17–22 (in French). Transl. Eliana Perotti and Katia Frey. Zürich: Howeg.

# Appendix

# Contributors

**Rikke Sand Andersen** is professor of medical anthropology at Department of Anthropology, University of Aarhus and Research Unit for General Practice, University of Southern Denmark. Andersen is former editor-in-chief of the medical anthropology journal *Tidsskrift for Forskning i Sygdom og Samfund*, she has written extensively on cancer, family medicine, and care seeking. She recently co-edited *Cancer Entangled, Acceleration, Anticipation and the Danish State*. Currently, her main interest is to further our understanding of "solo living" as an integrated part of human experimentation with being in the world, and its implications for care politics, inter-generational relations and welfare.

**Thierry Buclin** is a physician and an honorary professor in Pharmacology at Lausanne University, Faculty of Biology and Medicine. He served as the chief of the Division of Clinical Pharmacology at University Hospital (CHUV) for over twelve years. With a specialization in clinical pharmacology and toxicology, he has a hospital-academic background. Committed to creative, independent, and critical research, he focuses on effective, rational, appropriate, safe, monitored, and cost-effective drug prescribing. He has collaborated with social anthropologists for several years.

**Sangeeta Chattoo** is a medical anthropologist and a Senior Research Fellow, department of Sociology, at the University of York (UK). Her research and scholarship focus on medical knowledge and practice; inequalities and health, race, ethnicity and citizenship; genetic disorders, gender and caring. She has worked extensively on health and citizenship issues of minoritised ethnic communities in the UK and India. She is an editor for *Frontiers* (Medical Sociology) and is currently co-editing *Handbook on Racism, Ethnicity and Health* (with Hannah Bradby, Edward Elgar Press). Two of her recent articles are in *Anthropology & Medicine* and *Politics & Policy*.

**Rachel Démolis** is a medical anthropologist, research fellow and principal investigator at HESAV (University of Applied Sciences of Western Switzerland, HES-SO). She began her career in the field of religious anthropology and later developed research in medical anthropology. Her PhD focused on the dynamics of medication observance and resistance among polymedicated patients over 65 in the Vaud canton, Switzerland, and she conducted ethnographic fieldwork in a pain clinic. She currently leads a study that explores nurses' COVID-19 vaccine hesitancy and resistance logics in Western Switzerland and co-leads a study on existential and spiritual care among elderly individuals receiving home care.

**Rose-Anna Foley** is a medical anthropologist and associate professor at HESAV (University of Applied Sciences of Western Switzerland, HES-SO). Her research focuses on cancer, comorbidities, and drugs such as chemotherapy and morphine, in a "social lives of medicine" perspective. She collaborates with researchers from diverse domains, including physiotherapists, pharmacists, and doctors. She is the supervising researcher of the project discussed in this book, examining aging individuals living with polymedication and their relationships with their pharmacists. Additionally, she currently leads a study that focusses on the experiential knowledge and long-term trajectories of people aged 70+ living with cancer.

**Sylvie Fortin** is Professor at the Department of Anthropology (and Pediatrics) at the Université de Montréal. Her work centers on the challenges of clinical practice today, namely diversity, religious pluralism, and gender issues in hospital and community health settings as well as the moral and normative concerns entailed by decision-making and the withdrawal of active treatment at various life stages (from newborns to the elderly) for healthcare providers, patients, and their families. More recently, she explores how diversity issues intersect with death and dying experiences. She has edited several anthropological and social sciences journal issues on these themes as well as an upcoming book (Université de Montréal Press).

**Bernhard Hadolt**, a social anthropologist of medicine, is a Senior Lecturer and Director of Studies at the Department of Social and Cultural Anthropology at the University of Vienna. He carried out research in Austria, Japan, and the Philippines on various topics revolving around social practices, social transformation, and policy making in the fields of assisted reproductive technology, genetic testing, vaccination and blood donation. His recent research focussed on the marketing and implementation of HPV-vaccines in health care systems and tissue economies in relation to blood donation.

**Anna Heitger** is a social anthropologist and currently a doctoral candidate at Humboldt University Berlin at the Institute of European Ethnology and IRI THESys. She is part of the research group *Laboratory: Anthropology of Environment|Human Relations* since 2019. After a two-year research on self-tracking technologies and emerging practices in usage and design (Vienna and Berlin), for her PhD she has conducted an ethnographic study of (future) eating practices as critical human-environment relation in different urban field sites across Berlin. Ongoing research interests include ontological uncertainties, entanglements of geo- and biopolitics, as well as reconfigurations of more-than-human agency in the Anthropocene.

**Elisabeth Hsu** is Professor of Anthropology at the School of Anthropology and Museum Ethnography of the University of Oxford. Hsu's research interests lie within the fields of medical anthropology and ethnobotany, language and text critical studies. They concern Chinese medicine in cross-cultural perspective; the body and body techniques, movements and skills; pulse diagnosis, culinary technology and, specifically, *qinghao* recipes; touch, pain, affect and atmosphere; feelings, emotions, and sensory experience.

**Sabrina Lessard** is an institutional researcher at the Centre for research and expertise in social gerontology (CREGES) and an adjunct professor at Department of Anthropology, Université de Montréal, Canada. Her work focuses on death and dying in geriatric institutions by exploring how "life worth living" is socially constructed and the consequences of this construction on people's experiences of life and death in institutions. Her interests also focus on the diversity of aging experiences and how institutions (hospital, long-term care homes, collective housing) shape them.

**Lina Masana** is a medical anthropologist and senior independent researcher. She is a member of the Medical Anthropology Research Centre (MARC) at the University Rovira i Virgili (URV) and teaches at the University of Barcelona (UB) and ISGlobal (Institute for Global Health Barcelona). Masana has worked extensively on the experience and management of chronic illnesses (chronicity) and related topics such as disability, dependency, public policies, and global health. She specializes in ethnographic methods, qualitative applied health research and analysis of illness narratives. Her last co-edited volume was *Subjectivities and Afflictions in Medical Anthropology*.

**Antonia Modelhart**, a medical anthropologist, currently is a PhD student at the Faculty of Social Sciences and a researcher at the Department of Political Science at the University of Vienna. She works as a researcher in various research projects on health systems, politics and policies, focusing on topics such as antimicrobial resistance, rare diseases and genetic testing. Since her work on oocytes and egg freezing as part of her master's thesis, she has been interested in the sociomateriality of biological substances and entities. Currently, she explores microbes beyond their pathogenic potential and engages in debates on the gut (microbiome) in conversation with affective structures and gut feelings.

**Nina Nissen** is an independent medical anthropologist; she holds a visiting researcher position at the Centre for General Practice, University of Copenhagen, and was previously an associate professor of medical anthropology at the Department of Public Health, University of Southern Denmark. She is interested in how people negotiate the often competing demands of everyday life and the challenges of living with the uncertainties of diagnosis, fluctuating health condition(s) and wellbeing, as well as in how people assemble and mobilise care practices for themselves and for human and non-human others. She is currently exploring the materiality of feminist archives in Berlin, Germany, as sites of care, memory work and creativity.

**Stefan Reinsch** is a medical doctor and anthropologist working as postdoctoral researcher at Brandenburg Medical School – Theodor Fontane, Neuruppin, Germany, while at the same time completing his residency in paediatrics. Reinsch is a board member of the German *Working Group Anthropology and Medicine* (AGEM). He conducts ethnographic research along the life-course of people with cystic fibrosis and has written on decision-making about prenatal genetic diagnosis and waiting for organ transplantation in advanced illness. He recently started two projects about the experiences of overweight people and their physicians in remote rural areas, and the professional identity formation of tomorrow's doctors.

**Mette Bech Risør** is professor of medical anthropology, Center for General Practice, University of Copenhagen and the General Practice Research Unit, UiT The Arctic University of Norway. Risør has done research primarily within the field of care-seeking and clinical encounters with a special interest in sensorial anthropology and the configuration of symptoms and diagnoses, often with a focus on contested disorders. She is a member of the editorial board of the medical anthropology journal *Tidsskrift for Forskning i Sygdom og Samfund*, also former editor-in-chief. Currently, she is engaged with exploring fatigue as an existential phenomenon across life and illness courses.

**Andrea Stöckl** is a medical anthropologist, who, after working for 20 years in academia, is now a practicing psychotherapist (Existential Analysis) in Innsbruck, Austria. She earned a PhD at the University of Cambridge in 2001 and has been a lecturer at the Norwich Medical School at the University of East Anglia until 2021. She has done research on the role of diagnosis in current medical practice, on the conceptualisation of mind-body in autoimmune disorders, and on the relationship between professional carers and disabled people. Her current area of interest remains the relationship between culture and mental health.

**Sjaak van der Geest** is emeritus professor of Medical Anthropology at the University of Amsterdam, The Netherlands. He has done fieldwork in Ghana, Cameroon and at home on a variety of subjects including kinship, sexual relationships and birth control, the use and distribution of medicines, dying, death and funeral, popular song texts, meanings of growing old, sleeping, concepts of dirt and defecation, and cultural variety in privacy experience. See further: www.sjaakvandergeest.nl.